ESSA's Student Manual
for Exercise Prescription,
Delivery and Adherence

ESSA's Student Manual for Exercise Prescription, Delivery and Adherence

Jeff S. Coombes
BEd(Hons), BAppSc, MEd, PhD, ESSAM, AES, AEP, FACSM, FESSA
Professor of Exercise Science, School of Human Movement and Nutrition Sciences
The University of Queensland, Brisbane, Queensland, Australia

Nicola W. Burton
BSc(Hons), MPsych(Clinical), GCert Higher Ed, PhD, FAPS
Fellow, APS College Health Psychologists, Fellow, APS College of Clinical Psychologists
Associate Professor, School of Applied Psychology
Griffith University, Brisbane, Queensland, Australia

Emma M. Beckman
BAppSci (HMSExSci) (Hons), PhD, ESSAM, AES, AEP
Senior Lecturer in Exercise Physiology, School of Human Movement and Nutrition Sciences
The University of Queensland, Brisbane, Queensland, Australia

ELSEVIER

ELSEVIER

Elsevier Australia. ACN 001 002 357
(a division of Reed International Books Australia Pty Ltd)
Tower 1, 475 Victoria Avenue, Chatswood, NSW 2067

ISBN: 978-0-7295-4270-8

National Library of Australia Cataloguing-in-Publication Data

 A catalogue record for this book is available from the National Library of Australia

Senior Content Strategist: Melinda McEvoy
Content Project Manager: Kritika Kaushik
Copy edited by Leanne Peters
Proofread by Tim Learner
Cover and internal design by Georgette Hall
Index by SPi Global
Typeset by GW Tech
Printed in Singapore by KHL Printing Co Pte Ltd

Last digit is the print number: 9   8   7   6   5   4   3   2   1

FOREWORD

Exercise science is a rapidly growing field in Australia. Qualified exercise scientists are professionals equipped with the knowledge and skills to apply the science of exercise when developing interventions that improve health, fitness, wellbeing and performance, and that assist in the prevention of injury and chronic conditions.

Accredited exercise scientists teach, coach and motivate clients to facilitate self-management of physical activity, exercise and healthy lifestyles. They use models of behaviour change, scientific evidence and critical thinking, while accounting for individual factors and social determinants of health. An accredited exercise scientist practises in a culturally safe and inclusive manner and according to the principles of client-centred care. Therefore, prescription, delivery and adherence are important aspects of exercise and sports science.

This text is a unique book in the Australian setting, providing the theoretical understanding and procedures to allow Australian and New Zealand exercise science graduates to work competently within the health, exercise and sport industries. It is also the second text available in Australia that has considered Exercise & Sports Science Australia's exercise science accreditation framework.

ESSA's Student Manual for Prescription, Delivery and Adherence is a beneficial text for any student undertaking an exercise and sports science degree, providing content related to the knowledge and skills required to undertake the development and delivery of an individualised program, no matter the setting.

The editors of this text are expert educators and researchers who have created and structured this text based on years of experience teaching this content, ensuring they cover important competencies of prescription, delivery and adherence.

Exercise & Sports Science Australia (ESSA) is the peak organisation in Australia committed to establishing, promoting and defending the career paths of tertiary-trained exercise and sports science practitioners. As the peak professional body representing exercise and sports science in Australia, ESSA provides national and international leadership and advocacy on key issues and supports its members and the community by fostering excellence in professional practice, education and training and research.

One of the organisation's key roles as a recognised self-regulating body is to promote professional standards by providing high-quality education, accreditation and management of standards. For this reason, ESSA is pleased to support this text as one way we look to ensure consistent and high standards within our professions.

Anita Hobson-Powell
Chief Executive Officer
Exercise & Sports Science Australia

CONTENTS

PREFACE

Students graduating from an exercise science program require knowledge and skills to design, deliver and manage exercise programs that improve performance, fitness, health and wellbeing. These programs may also assist in the prevention and management of injury and chronic conditions.

To enable the development of knowledge, skill and practice, this manual is divided into three sections: Exercise Programming, Exercise Delivery and Exercise Adherence. Each section contains pragmatic information and practicals with activities designed to integrate knowledge and apply decision-making and problem-solving skills relevant to a range of practice situations.

The Exercise Programming section covers the science of exercise program design with contemporary concepts such as targeting sedentary behaviour and the use of autoregulation and repetitions-in-reserve for resistance training prescription and delivery. In this section, general principles of exercise prescription are detailed along with those principles specific to different training modalities. Practical 3 covers special considerations such as exercise for weight loss, exercise programming for before and after pregnancy and exercise programming for special populations (older individuals, children and adolescents).

The section on Exercise Delivery contains a range of practical sessions that cover different aspects of program delivery. This begins with aerobic exercise in Practical 4 and then moves to resistance-based exercise in Practicals 5 to 9, which cover key regions of the body. The remaining practicals in this section cover the delivery of power, speed, agility, flexibility, neuromotor and functional exercise, as well as program delivery in different contexts such as the group environment and exercise in water.

The Exercise Adherence section first looks at the components and assessment of non-adherence, and presents a framework for appraising contributing factors including motivation, attitudes, knowledge, experiences, social influences and setting. Practical 16 presents a framework for how to promote exercise adherence, with components related to action planning, social support, exercise readiness and relevance, context, coping, efficacy, self-regulation and client satisfaction. Practical 17 discusses client-centred communication and using behavioural counselling as an adjunct to exercise programming and delivery in order to understand and promote exercise adherence.

Jeff S. Coombes, Emma M. Beckman and Nicola W. Burton

ABOUT THE EDITORS

Jeff S. Coombes

Jeff is a professor of exercise science in the School of Human Movement and Nutrition Sciences at the University of Queensland. He obtained an undergraduate education degree and a research masters degree in education from the University of Tasmania before completing a PhD at the University of Florida in 1998. Since then he has been teaching exercise science courses that have informed the activities and pedagogical approaches used in this book. He was national president of Exercise and Sports Science Australia (ESSA) from 2006 to 2011 and is currently national chair of the Exercise is Medicine Australia initiative. He was on the committee that designed ESSA's Exercise Science Elements with responsibility for the study area 'Health, Exercise and Sport Assessment'. His practical experience from over 25 years includes working in health and fitness centres and conducting exercise and sports science research. He has been an accredited exercise physiologist since 2006.

Nicola W. Burton

Nicola is an associate professor at Griffith University, a registered psychologist with endorsements in both clinical and health psychology and has worked in government, private practice, hospital and university settings. She obtained a science honours degree and a Master of Clinical Psychology from the University of Queensland before completing a PhD (Public Health) at QUT in 2007. Nicola has over 25 years' experience in physical activity and health, and has been a consultant to the Queensland Curriculum and Assessment Authority for the endorsed Senior Health syllabus, as well as to local, state and federal government including for the *2014 Physical Activity and Sedentary Behaviour Guidelines for Adults (18–64 years)*. She has provided lectures and courses for a range of university undergraduate and postgraduate programs, as well as presentations and workshops for medical, sport and allied health professionals including ESSA members. At Griffith University she designed and leads a cross-disciplinary course on behaviour change skills. She was the chair of the Australian Psychological Society (APS) State Committee (Queensland) and has been awarded as an APS Fellow in recognition of her significant and innovative contributions to health psychology.

Emma M. Beckman

Emma is a senior lecturer in clinical exercise physiology in the School of Human Movement and Nutrition Sciences at the University of Queensland (UQ). After completing her undergraduate degree in human movement sciences at UQ, she worked as an exercise scientist and clinical exercise physiologist before going overseas to complete her master degree in adapted physical activity and returning to UQ to complete her PhD in 2011. She has been tutoring and lecturing in exercise prescription and programming since 2007. She has volunteered for the ESSA Queensland State Chapter for over 10 years and was elected as a director on the ESSA board in 2020.

ACKNOWLEDGEMENTS

A textbook like this is only possible with the labour, love and commitment of numerous people.

An exceptional group of co-authors ensured that this textbook is based on contemporary evidence and years of industry and teaching experience to provide meaningful and practical guidance for exercise scientists. The patience and support of every single co-author was a testament to their exceptional professional and personal qualities, and we are very grateful.

The textbook was inspired from a lab manual that supported the teaching of many current and previous colleagues within and beyond the University of Queensland's School of Human Movement Studies for many years. It went through iterations, updates and improvements and we are grateful to Matthew Hordern, Angus Ross, Andrew Lonergan, Leisbeth Weisfelt, Denise Kaesler, Melanie Sharman, Tania Brancato, Samantha Fisher and Justin Holland for your contributions over the years. To all the 'Prescription and Programming' practical coordinators, tutors and students, both past and present, we thank you for actively engaging with the thousands of hours of practicals, open labs and exams which have formed the foundations of this textbook.

To Exercise and Sports Science Australia (ESSA): thank you for your support and endorsement of this textbook. Special thanks to the President, Kirsty Rawlings, Executive Officer, Anita Hobson-Powell and the board for their contributions, reviews and feedback.

This textbook was reviewed at length and in detail by many different people, all experts in their field, and your comments and feedback were detailed, constructive and fair. We thank you for your time and expertise; we know that the role of the reviewer is often a hidden and thankless task.

Thank you to all the companies and their representatives who assisted with approval of the numerous protocols, tables and figures used throughout this textbook.

To bring this vision to print, we thank the team at Elsevier, including past and current employees involved both directly and indirectly.

Each of us is grateful for the rest of the team; it truly was the bringing together of decades of expertise in prescription, programming and behaviour change. To see those three topics come together in what we believe is a valuable training and professional resource makes us very proud. Thank you to everyone who helped make this possible.

To our families and friends who have supported us through this process. Thank you for your unwavering support. We dedicate this textbook to the vision of optimising health and wellbeing for everyone.

CONTRIBUTORS

Rosalind Beavers BHumMovSc(Hons), PhD, ESSAM, AES, AEP
Lecturer in Exercise Physiology
Faculty of Health
Southern Cross University
Lismore, New South Wales, Australia

Emma M. Beckman BAppSci (HMS- ExSci) (Hons), PhD, ESSAM, AES, AEP
Senior Lecturer in Exercise Physiology
School of Human Movement and Nutrition Sciences
The University of Queensland
Brisbane, Queensland, Australia

Nicola W. Burton BSc(Hons), MPsych(Clinical), GCert Higher Ed, PhD, FAPS
Fellow, APS College Health Psychologists
Fellow, APS College of Clinical Psychologists
Associate Professor
School of Applied Psychology
Griffith University
Brisbane, Queensland, Australia

Kelly M. Clanchy BAppSci(HMS), GradCert Higher Ed, PhD, ESSAM, AES, AEP
Lecturer in Exercise Science
School of Health Sciences and Social Work
Griffith University
Gold Coast, Queensland, Australia

Jeff S. Coombes BEd (Hons), BAppSc, MEd, PhD, ESSAM, AES, AEP, FACSM, FESSA
Professor of Exercise Science
School of Human Movement and Nutrition Sciences
The University of Queensland
Brisbane, Queensland, Australia

Stephen D. Cousins PGCert(Ed), BSc(Hons), MSc, PhD, ESSAM
Lecturer in Exercise Science
College of Science, Health and Engineering
La Trobe Rural Health School
La Trobe University
Bendigo, Victoria, Australia

Michael J. Dale BAppSci(Hons), PhD, ESSAM
Research Fellow
Health Research Institute
Faculty of Health
University of Canberra
Canberra, Australian Capital Territory, Australia

G. Gregory Haff FNSCA, C.S.C.S.*D, PhD
Professor of Exercise Science and Strength and Conditioning
School of Medical and Health Sciences
Edith Cowan University
Perth, Western Australia, Australia

Justin J. Holland BExSci(Hons – Clin Ex Phys), ESSAM, AES, AEP, PhD
Lecturer in Clinical Exercise Physiology
School of Exercise and Nutrition Sciences
Faculty of Health
Queensland University of Technology
Brisbane, Queensland, Australia

Lachlan P. James BSocSci, MSportCoach, MExSci(S&C), ESSAM, ASpS2, PhD
Lecturer in Strength and Conditioning, and Sport and Exercise Science
School of Allied Health, Human Services and Sport
La Trobe University
Melbourne, Victoria, Australia

Nathan Johnson BMedSc, MHlthSc(Hons), Grad.Cert.(Uni.Teaching & Learning), PhD, ESSAM, AES, AEP
Associate Professor in Exercise Physiology
Faculty of Medicine and Health
The University of Sydney
Sydney, New South Wales, Australia

Shelley Keating BExSciRehab, MExSpSci, PhD, ESSAM, AES, AEP
National Health and Medical Research Council (NHMRC) Research Fellow
School of Human Movement and Nutrition Sciences
The University of Queensland
Brisbane, Queensland, Australia

Justin W.L. Keogh BHSc, BHMS(Hons), PhD, ESSAM, ASpS2
Associate Professor
Exercise and Sport Science
Faculty of Health Sciences and Medicine
Bond University
Gold Coast, Queensland, Australia

Dawson J. Kidgell BAppSci, GradDipExSpSci, MAppSci, PhD
Advanced Research Coordinator
Department of Physiotherapy
Monash University
Melbourne, Victoria, Australia

Paul Marshall PhD, ESSAM, AES, AEP
Research Fellow
University of Auckland
Auckland, New Zealand
Adjunct Associate Professor
School of Health Science
Western Sydney University
Sydney, New South Wales, Australia

Mike R. McGuigan PhD
Professor in Strength and Conditioning
School of Sport and Recreation
Auckland University of Technology
Auckland, New Zealand

Jemima G. Spathis BAppSc(Ex Sci) (Hons), PhD, ESSAM, AES, AEP, ASpS2
Lecturer in Exercise Science
School of Behavioural and Health Sciences
Australian Catholic University
Brisbane, Queensland, Australia

REVIEWERS

Stephen Cousins BSc(Hons), MSc, PhD
Lecturer in Exercise Science
La Trobe Rural Health School
La Trobe University
Bendigo, Victoria, Australia

Paul Nolan
University of Auckland
Auckland, New Zealand

Brad Wall PhD, ESSAM, AES, AEP
Senior Lecturer, Exercise Science
Murdoch University
Perth, Western Australia, Australia

Lennon Wicks BSc(ExSc), BSc(AthTraining), MHPEd, ESSAM, AES, AEP
Clinical Assistant Professor (Exercise Physiology)
Discipline of Sport and Exercise Science
Faculty of Health
University of Canberra
Canberra, Australian Capital Territory, Australia

SECTION 1
EXERCISE PROGRAMMING

Jeff S. Coombes and Shelley E. Keating

PROFESSIONAL STANDARDS AND LEARNING OBJECTIVES

The three practicals in this section aim to address professional standards related to the following:

- identify and describe the principles of current best practice for designing exercise programs, and explaining why various exercise types confer health, fitness or performance benefits (as relevant) for the apparently healthy population
- explain in simple, comprehensible language the risks of performing exercise and describing appropriate strategies to address these risks
- design exercise programs that meet the needs of clients, in consideration of:
  - current, best-practice guidelines for performing exercise
  - the exercise tolerance, physical function and capacity, and motivation level of the client
- integrate knowledge of and skills in exercise prescription with other study areas of exercise science.

By the end of this section, it is anticipated that students will be able to:

- understand the scope of practice of accredited exercise scientists in Australia
- explain how the terms 'exercise' and 'physical activity' are currently used
- describe in simple, comprehensible language the benefits and risks of exercise
- understand how the Adult Pre-exercise Screening System (APSS) is used to evaluate the risk of exercise and in the prescription of exercise at an appropriate intensity
- develop and apply appropriate strategies to address the risks of exercise
- identify, describe and apply the general principles of exercise prescription
- identify, describe and apply the principles of aerobic, resistance and flexibility exercise prescription
- understand, describe and apply advice to reduce sedentary behaviour
- understand and classify different types of exercise
- use different approaches to calculate aerobic exercise intensity
- describe the different phases of an exercise session
- design evidence-based individualised exercise programs for apparently healthy adults
- design evidence-based individualised exercise programs for the four following populations:
  - individuals with a weight loss goal
  - during and after pregnancy
  - older individuals
  - children and adolescents.

DEFINITIONS

Adverse event: An unexpected event resulting in ill health, physical harm or death to an individual.

Aerobic exercise: Physical exercise that depends primarily on an aerobic energy-generating process. Also known as 'cardio'.

Body composition: Relative amounts of muscle, bone and fat in a person's body.

Bone loading exercises: High-impact, weight-bearing exercises that aim to improve bone health.

Cardiorespiratory fitness: The ability of the circulatory and respiratory systems to supply oxygen and support the energy demands during sustained physical activity. Also known as aerobic fitness or aerobic endurance.

Exercise: Planned, structured and repetitive physical activity that will improve or maintain one or more components of fitness.

Exercise prescription: A detailed plan of individualised exercises designed for a specific purpose.

Exercise program: The combination of an exercise prescription and advice on sedentary behaviour.

Fitness: A broad term that is generally used to describe a state of being physically fit and healthy. May be divided into health-related physical fitness, skill-related physical fitness and emotional and mental health.

Flexibility: The range of motion available at a joint.

Functional training: Includes exercises that replicate the demands of activities required for an individual's occupation, sport or leisure activities.

Health-related physical fitness: Consists of cardiorespiratory fitness, neuromuscular fitness, body composition and flexibility.

Muscular failure: Completing a repetition with poor technique.

Muscular fatigue: Unable to do another repetition with correct technique.

Neuromotor exercise: An umbrella term that includes exercises aimed to improve balance, coordination, agility and gait. May also refer to proprioceptive exercises (e.g. exercises with eyes closed) and multimodal activities (e.g. tai chi, yoga).

Neuromuscular fitness: The ability of the nervous and muscular systems to combine to produce muscular strength, endurance and power.

Physical activity: Any bodily movement produced by skeletal muscles that requires energy expenditure.

Range of motion: The capability of a joint to go through its complete spectrum of movements.

Repetition (rep): The number of times you perform a specific exercise.

Repetitions in reserve (RiR): The estimated number of additional repetitions you believe you could have completed with correct technique.

Set: A cycle of repetitions (e.g. 10 repetitions may be 1 set).

Skill-related physical fitness: Consists of components such as power, speed, balance, agility and coordination.

Valsalva manoeuvre: Attempting to breathe out against a closed airway. It often occurs while lifting heavy weights and generally should be avoided as it increases blood pressure.

PRACTICAL 1
INTRODUCTION TO EXERCISE PROGRAMMING

Jeff S. Coombes and Shelley E. Keating

Introduction

This practical has a number of activities designed to provide the exercise science student with the foundation knowledge needed to develop the skills to design an individualised exercise program. This manual uses the following model to define the content of the exercise program.

exercise program = exercise prescription + advice on sedentary behaviour

The model is used to remind students that the exercise program should be more than just the exercise prescription. It is important to think about both exercise behaviour and sedentary behaviour.

The goal of an exercise program could be to improve health, fitness, wellbeing and performance and/or to prevent chronic medical conditions. Broadly speaking, exercise programs can focus on health-related physical fitness and/or skill-related physical fitness. Health-related physical fitness may be divided into four components: 1. cardiorespiratory fitness; 2. neuromuscular fitness; 3. body composition; and 4. flexibility. Aerobic exercise training improves cardiorespiratory fitness, whereas resistance training increases neuromuscular fitness. Both aerobic exercise and resistance training improve body composition.

Skill-related physical fitness generally contains components such as power, speed, balance, agility and coordination.[1] However, a component such as balance can also be an aspect of health-related fitness in certain populations (e.g. older individuals). In this manual, power and speed will be covered in more detail in Practical 10 while balance, agility and coordination will be covered in Practical 14.

1. Role of Accredited Exercise Scientists (AESs)

AESs specialise in the design and delivery of exercise programs for apparently healthy individuals. They also deliver and supervise exercise programs for individuals with pathology or injury that have been designed by an appropriately qualified health professional (e.g. accredited exercise physiologist [AEP]). In Australia, an AEP also holds accreditation as an exercise scientist.

ESSA has developed the Exercise Science Standards to define the minimum professional requirements of graduates working in all areas of exercise science.[2] The standards define the professional attributes of an AES (Box 1.1). These have been translated into the scope of practice of an AES that lists possible roles and settings where an AES may work (Figure 1.1) and guidance regarding regulations, boundaries and adhering to a code of professional conduct and ethical practice.[3]

An AES is trained to integrate relevant information (e.g. assessment data, client goals/preferences/concerns/ training experience, research and professional judgment) into the design of the exercise program.

Box 1.1   Exercise and Sport Science Australia's (ESSA's) Professional Attributes of an Accredited Exercise Scientist*

1. Integrate knowledge and skills from the core subdisciplines of exercise science to deliver a broad range of services.
2. Critically analyse and apply decision-making and problem-solving skills across exercise science practice.
3. Design, deliver and manage physical activity and exercise-based interventions including assessments and programming for the purpose of improving health and fitness, wellbeing or performance.

Box 1.1 Exercise and Sport Science Australia's (ESSA's) Professional Attributes of an Accredited Exercise Scientist*—cont'd

4. Deliver exercise-based interventions for clients with medical conditions, injuries or disabilities that have been prescribed by a health professional qualified in clinical exercise prescription.

5. Apply behavioural change principles to support adherence to physical activity and exercise-based interventions.

6. Use a range of modalities to communicate effectively with clients and relevant stakeholders including families, carers and other health and exercise professionals, and maintain appropriate documentation and records of services.

7. Practice ethically, collaboratively and innovatively within the scope of exercise science training including referrals to relevant medical and health professionals and/or services as appropriate.

8. Display professional conduct, decision-making, communication, and client-centred care that is consistent with the ESSA Code of Professional Conduct and Ethical Practice.

9. Apply evidence-based practice and compile, critically evaluate and communicate the scientific rationale for professional decision-making and service delivery, including evaluation of outcomes.

10. Commit to professional self-development in the field of exercise science through educational engagement and ongoing learning, self-evaluation of practice, inter-professional working relationships, innovative practice, and support of new graduates.

11. Practice in a safe, respectful and inclusive way that is responsive to the diverse needs of people, including Aboriginal and Torres Strait Islander peoples, gender and sexually diverse persons, persons of culturally and linguistically diverse backgrounds, and persons living with a disability.

12. Critically analyse technology and apply appropriate digital practices.

13. Demonstrate professional leadership and advocate for client access to services and the exercise science profession.

* To come into effect in 2022.

Source: Exercise and Sport Science Australia, 2021. Accredited Exercise Scientist Professional Standards. https://www.essa.org.au/Public/Professional_Standards/The_professional_standards.aspx (accessed 9 June 2021)

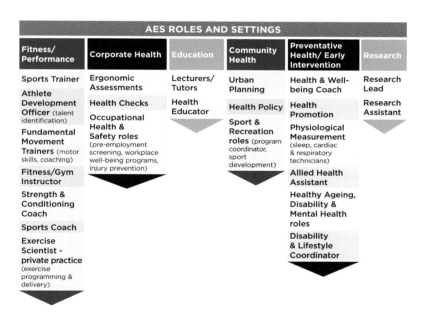

Figure 1.1 Scope of Practice for an Accredited Exercise Scientist
Source: Exercise and Sport Science Australia. 2021. Accredited Exercise Scientist Scope of Practice. https://www.essa.org.au/Public/Professional_Standards/ESSA_Scope_of_Practice_documents.aspx? (accessed 9 June 2021).

Activity 1.1 Accredited exercise scientist scope of practice

AIM:
- To understand the scope of practice of an AES

TASK:
- Complete Worksheet 1.1 by writing Yes/No/Possibly for whether the various scenarios are within the scope of practice of an AES. Add detail to explain your response.

Worksheet 1.1 Accredited Exercise Scientist Scope of Practice	
Scenario	Yes/No/Possibly
An AEP has designed an exercise program for a person with type 2 diabetes and has asked an AES to deliver it.	_____ Explain your response: _____ _____ _____ _____ _____
A woman with hypertension has asked an AES to design and deliver an exercise program for her.	_____ Explain your response: _____ _____ _____ _____ _____
An AES is working in a hospital as a health promotion officer and has been asked to produce a brochure providing physical activity and exercise advice for staff.	_____ Explain your response: _____ _____ _____ _____ _____

2. Exercise, Physical Activity and Sedentary Behaviour

There is often confusion around the terms 'exercise' and 'physical activity'. In the way they are generally used, the terms are not synonymous. The term exercise is used when the activity is carried out to improve or maintain a component of fitness, whereas physical activity refers to any bodily movement.

'Sedentary behaviour' is another term that needs to be considered when designing an exercise program. It refers to any waking behaviour characterised by a low energy expenditure ≤ 1.5 metabolic equivalents (METs) while in a sitting, reclining or lying posture. If a person is not being physically active, they are likely to be sedentary (or inactive). The exception to this is when a person may be required to stand for long periods of time (e.g. in a retail occupation). In this situation they are inactive but not sedentary. There is good evidence that sedentary behaviour is associated with poor health outcomes.[4,5]

An exercise scientist should have the knowledge and skills to provide an individual with both an exercise prescription and physical activity advice to reduce sedentary behaviour. The next activity asks students to recognise the differences between exercise prescription and providing general physical activity advice.

Activity 1.2 Exercise prescription and physical activity advice

AIM:
- To understand differences between 'exercise prescription' and 'physical activity advice' as used in different national guidelines for adults

TASK:
- Complete Worksheet 1.2 by marking the statements as either exercise prescription (EP) or physical activity advice (PAA) based on the following guidance.
  - **Exercise prescription:** When the statement contains specific information (e.g. duration, intensity, frequency) or specific exercises (e.g. resistance, muscle strengthening, balance) are mentioned.
  - **Physical activity advice:** When the statement contains general advice to be physically active or to reduce sedentary behaviour.

Worksheet 1.2 Exercise and Physical Activity	
Australia's Physical Activity and Sedentary Behaviour Guidelines for Adults (18–64 years)[6]	**EP or PAA**
<ul><li>Doing any physical activity is better than doing none. If you currently do no physical activity, start by doing some and gradually build up to the recommended amount.</li><li>Be active on most, preferably all, days every week.</li><li>Accumulate 150 to 300 minutes (2½ to 5 hours) of moderate intensity physical activity or 75 to 150 minutes (1¼ to 2½ hours) of vigorous-intensity physical activity, or an equivalent combination of both moderate and vigorous activities, each week.</li><li>Do muscle strengthening activities on at least 2 days each week.</li><li>Minimise the amount of time spent in prolonged sitting.</li><li>Break up long periods of sitting as often as possible.</li></ul>	_____ _____ _____ _____ _____ _____
American College of Sports Medicine and American Heart Association's Primary Physical Activity Recommendations[7]	
<ul><li>All healthy adults aged 18 to 65 years need moderate-intensity aerobic (endurance) physical activity for a minimum of 30 min on 5 days each week or vigorous-intensity aerobic physical activity for a minimum of 20 min on three days each week.</li><li>Combinations of moderate- and vigorous-intensity activity can be performed to meet this recommendation.</li><li>Moderate-intensity aerobic activity can be accumulated towards the 30-min minimum by performing bouts each lasting 10 or more minutes.</li><li>Every adult should perform activities that maintain or increase muscular strength and endurance a minimum of 2 days each week.</li><li>Because of the dose–response relationship between physical activity and health, persons who wish to further improve their personal fitness, reduce their risk for chronic diseases and disabilities or prevent unhealthy weight gain may benefit by exceeding the minimum recommended amounts of physical activity.</li></ul>	_____ _____ _____ _____ _____
Canadian Physical Activity Guidelines[8]	
<ul><li>To achieve health benefits, adults aged 18–64 years should accumulate at least 150 minutes of moderate- to vigorous-intensity aerobic physical activity per week, in bouts of 10 minutes or more.</li><li>It is also beneficial to add muscle and bone strengthening activities using major muscle groups, at least 2 days per week.</li><li>More physical activity provides greater health benefits.</li></ul>	_____ _____ _____
UK Physical Activity Guidelines[9]	
<ul><li>Adults should aim to be active daily. Over a week, activity should add up to at least 150 minutes (2½ hours) of moderate-intensity activity in bouts of 10 minutes or more— one way to approach this is to do 30 minutes on at least 5 days a week.</li><li>Alternatively, comparable benefits can be achieved through 75 minutes of vigorous-intensity activity spread across the week or combinations of moderate- and vigorous-intensity activity.</li><li>Adults should also undertake physical activity to improve muscle strength on at least 2 days a week.</li><li>All adults should minimise the amount of time spent being sedentary (sitting) for extended periods.</li></ul>	_____ _____ _____ _____

3. Exercise Benefits

The scientific evidence demonstrating the health benefits of exercise is indisputable, and the benefits of exercise far outweigh the risks in most adults.[10] The benefits of exercise can be divided into physical and/or psychological and the following activity provides a list of specific benefits that fall into these categories. The most cited physical benefit is the ability of exercise to decrease all-cause mortality (premature death). Indeed, a person that exercises is likely to live for an additional 4 years.[2] However, what is recognised as more important is the improved quality of life over a lifetime in people that exercise.[3]

One of the most often cited reasons why people exercise is for weight management.[11] However, there is good evidence that exercise without dietary adjustments will have little impact on weight loss.[12] Indeed, when weight loss doesn't happen quickly after starting an exercise program, it is common for people to stop exercising.[13] To 'sell' exercise, we need to promote the numerous other benefits of exercise (listed in the activity below) rather than focusing on weight loss.[14]

In the last decade, the impact that exercise has had on psychological health has become much more apparent. Exercise is associated with decreased anxiety and depression and improved cognitive function.[4] Furthermore, people who exercise are less likely to develop dementia.[5]

Activity 1.3 Personal beliefs on exercise benefits

AIMS:
- To understand your personal beliefs on the benefits of exercise and how the perceived benefits may differ between individuals

TASKS:
- Complete Worksheet 1.3 by ranking the importance of the benefits of exercise to you *personally* as: A = very important; B = slightly important; or C = not important/not applicable.
- Add some additional benefits and rank them.
- Answer the additional questions.

Worksheet 1.3 Personal Beliefs on Exercise Benefits	
Benefit	**Rank** A = very important, B = slightly important or C = not important/not applicable
Improve cardiorespiratory fitness	
Be a good role model for my children	
Manage weight	
Improve strength	
Manage pain	
Look good and improve self-image	
Lose fat	
Help digestion and bowel function	
Increase muscle size	
Improve balance	
Enjoyment	
Boost fertility	
Prevent a chronic health condition	
Manage a chronic health condition	
Improve quality of life	
Manage stress	
Preserve cognitive function	
Improve bone health	

Worksheet 1.3 Personal Beliefs on Exercise Benefits (continued)	
Benefit	Rank A = very important, B = slightly important or C = not important/not applicable
Reduce risk of falling	
Improve mood	
Improve sporting performance	
Allow me to play with children/grandchildren	
Boost energy	
Improve sleep quality	
Improve academic skills/performance	
Maintain independence	
Others:	
_____	_____
_____	_____
_____	_____

Question 1: What determined your choices?

_____

_____

_____

_____

_____

Question 2: How might someone different to you (e.g. different age, gender, health status, occupation, culture) respond?

Demographic you chose (e.g. different age): _____

_____

_____

_____

_____

_____

4. Exercise Risks

There is a very small risk that an adverse event will occur during or after exercise. However, the physical and psychological benefits far outweigh the increased risk.[15] The screening process is where a participant's potential risk factors are determined to minimise the occurrence of an adverse event. A useful screening tool for exercise scientists is the Adult Pre-exercise Screening System (APSS) shown in Figure 1.2.[16] The Worked case study for exercise risks illustrates the APSS. In addition to using a screening tool such as the APSS, it may also be necessary to obtain more detail regarding the participant's medical history.

Most adverse events that are caused by exercise are musculoskeletal injuries. The most common sites for musculoskeletal injuries are knees, feet and ankles, and their likelihood increases with higher intensity

ADULT PRE-EXERCISE SCREENING SYSTEM (APSS)

This screening tool is part of the Adult Pre-Exercise Screening System (APSS) that also includes guidelines (see User Guide) on how to use the information collected and to address the aims of each stage. No warranty of safety should result from its use. The screening system in no way guarantees against injury or death. No responsibility or liability whatsoever can be accepted by Exercise & Sport Science Australia, Fitness Australia, Sports Medicine Australia or Exercise is Medicine for any loss, damage, or injury that may arise from any person acting on any statement or information contained in this system.

Full Name: _____

Date of Birth: _____   Male: ☐   Female: ☐   Other: ☐

STAGE 1 (COMPULSORY)

AIM: To identify individuals with known disease, and/or signs or symptoms of disease, who may be at a higher risk of an adverse event due to exercise. An adverse event refers to an unexpected event that occurs as a consequence of an exercise session, resulting in ill health, physical harm or death to an individual.

This stage may be self-administered and self-evaluated by the client. Please complete the questions below and refer to the figures on page 2. Should you have any questions about the screening form please contact your exercise professional for clarification.

	Please tick your response	YES	NO
1. Has your medical practitioner ever told you that you have a heart condition or have you ever suffered a stroke?			
2. Do you ever experience unexplained pains or discomfort in your chest at rest or during physical activity/exercise?			
3. Do you ever feel faint, dizzy or lose balance during physical activity/exercise?			
4. Have you had an asthma attack requiring immediate medical attention at any time over the last 12 months?			
5. If you have diabetes (type 1 or 2) have you had trouble controlling your blood sugar (glucose) in the last 3 months?			
6. Do you have any other conditions that may require special consideration for you to exercise?			

IF YOU ANSWERED 'YES' to any of the 6 questions, please seek guidance from an appropriate allied health professional or medical practitioner prior to undertaking exercise.

IF YOU ANSWERED 'NO' to all of the 6 questions, please proceed to question 7 and calculate your typical weighted physical activity/exercise per week.

7. Describe your current physical activity/exercise levels in a typical week by stating the frequency and duration at the different intensities. For intensity guidelines consult figure 2.

Intensity	Light	Moderate	Vigorous/High
Frequency (number of sessions per week)	_____	_____	_____
Duration (total minutes per week)	_____	_____	_____

Weighted physical activity/exercise per week

Total minutes = (minutes of light + moderate) + (2 x minutes of vigorous/high)

TOTAL = _____ **minutes per week**

- If your total is less than 150 minutes per week then light to moderate intensity exercise is recommended. Increase your volume and intensity slowly.
- If your total is more than or equal to 150 minutes per week then continue with your current physical activity/exercise intensity levels.
- It is advised that you discuss any progression (volume, intensity, duration, modality) with an exercise professional to optimise your results.

I believe that to the best of my knowledge, all of the information I have supplied within this screening tool is correct.

Client signature: _____   Date: _____

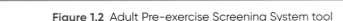

Exe℞cisE is Medicine Australia   Fitness Australia   SPORTS MEDICINE AUSTRALIA   ESSA EXERCISE & SPORTS SCIENCE AUSTRALIA

Figure 1.2 Adult Pre-exercise Screening System tool

FIGURE 1: Stage 1 Screening Steps

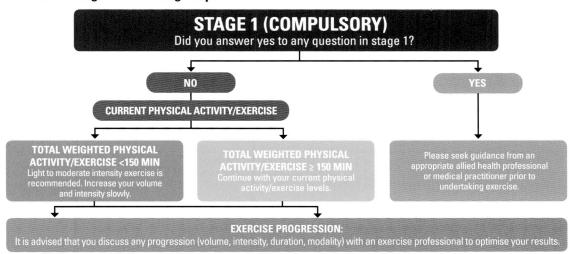

STAGE 1 (COMPULSORY)
Did you answer yes to any question in stage 1?

NO

CURRENT PHYSICAL ACTIVITY/EXERCISE

TOTAL WEIGHTED PHYSICAL ACTIVITY/EXERCISE <150 MIN
Light to moderate intensity exercise is recommended. Increase your volume and intensity slowly.

TOTAL WEIGHTED PHYSICAL ACTIVITY/EXERCISE ≥ 150 MIN
Continue with your current physical activity/exercise levels.

YES

Please seek guidance from an appropriate allied health professional or medical practitioner prior to undertaking exercise.

EXERCISE PROGRESSION:
It is advised that you discuss any progression (volume, intensity, duration, modality) with an exercise professional to optimise your results.

FIGURE 2: Exercise Intensity Guidelines

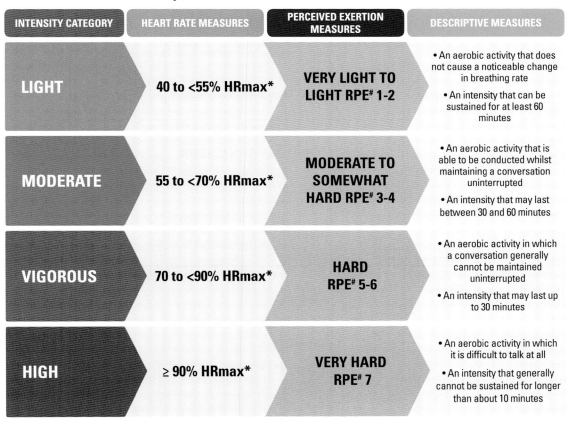

INTENSITY CATEGORY	HEART RATE MEASURES	PERCEIVED EXERTION MEASURES	DESCRIPTIVE MEASURES
LIGHT	40 to <55% HRmax*	**VERY LIGHT TO LIGHT RPE# 1-2**	• An aerobic activity that does not cause a noticeable change in breathing rate • An intensity that can be sustained for at least 60 minutes
MODERATE	55 to <70% HRmax*	**MODERATE TO SOMEWHAT HARD RPE# 3-4**	• An aerobic activity that is able to be conducted whilst maintaining a conversation uninterrupted • An intensity that may last between 30 and 60 minutes
VIGOROUS	70 to <90% HRmax*	**HARD RPE# 5-6**	• An aerobic activity in which a conversation generally cannot be maintained uninterrupted • An intensity that may last up to 30 minutes
HIGH	≥ 90% HRmax*	**VERY HARD RPE# 7**	• An aerobic activity in which it is difficult to talk at all • An intensity that generally cannot be sustained for longer than about 10 minutes

* HRmax = estimated heart rate maximum. Calculated by subtracting age in years from 220 (e.g. for a 50 year old person = 220 - 50 = 170 beats per minute).

= Borg's Rating of Perceived Exertion (RPE) scale, category scale 0-10.

Modified from Norton K, L. Norton & D. Sadgrove. (2010). Position statement on physical activity and exercise intensity terminology. J Sci Med Sport 13, 496-502.

ADULT PRE-EXERCISE
SCREENING SYSTEM (APSS) V2 (2018)

Exe**R**cise is Medicine® Australia   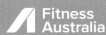 Fitness Australia   SPORTS MEDICINE AUSTRALIA   ESSA·

Figure 1.2, cont'd

STAGE 2 (RECOMMENDED)

 AIM: This stage is to be completed with an exercise professional to determine appropriate exercise prescription based on established risk factors.

CLIENT DETAILS	GUIDELINES FOR ASSESSING RISK
8. Demographics Age: _____ Male ☐ Female ☐ Other ☐	Risk of an adverse event increases with age, particularly males ≥ 45 yr and females ≥ 55 yr.
9. Family history of heart disease (e.g. stroke, heart attack)? Relationship (e.g. father) Age at heart disease event _____ _____ _____ _____ _____ _____	A family history of heart disease refers to an event that occurs in relatives including parents, grandparents, uncles and/or aunts before the age of 55 years.
10. Do you smoke cigarettes on a daily or weekly basis or have you quit smoking in the last 6 months? Yes ☐ No ☐ If currently smoking, how many per day or week? _____	Smoking, even on a weekly basis, substantially increases risk for premature death and disability. The negative effects are still present up to at least 6 months post quitting.
11. Body composition Weight (kg) _____ Height (cm) _____ Body Mass Index (kg/m²) _____ Waist circumference (cm) _____	Any of the below increases the risk of chronic diseases: BMI ≥ 30 kg/m² Waist > 94 cm male or > 80 cm female
12. Have you been told that you have high blood pressure? Yes ☐ No ☐ If known, systolic/diastolic (mmHg) _____ Are you taking any medication for this condition? Yes ☐ No ☐ If yes, provide details _____	Either of the below increases the risk of heart disease: Systolic blood pressure ≥ 140 mmHg Diastolic blood pressure ≥ 90 mmHg
13. Have you been told that you have high cholesterol/ blood lipids? Yes ☐ No ☐ If known: Total cholesterol (mmol/L) _____ HDL (mmol/L) _____ LDL (mmol/L) _____ Triglycerides (mmol/L) _____ Are you taking any medication for this condition? Yes ☐ No ☐ If yes, provide details _____	Any of the below increases the risk of heart disease: Total cholesterol ≥ 5.2 mmol/L HDL < 1.0 mmol/L LDL ≥ 3.4 mmol/L Triglycerides ≥ 1.7 mmol/L

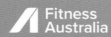   ESSA·

Figure 1.2, cont'd

CLIENT DETAILS	GUIDELINES FOR ASSESSING RISK
14. Have you been told that you have high blood sugar (glucose)? Yes ☐ No ☐ If known: Fasting blood glucose (mmol/L) _____ Are you taking any medication for this condition? Yes ☐ No ☐ If yes, provide details _____	Fasting blood sugar (glucose) ≥ 5.5 mmol/L increases the risk of diabetes.
15. Are you currently taking prescribed medication(s) for any condition(s)? These are additional to those already provided. Yes ☐ No ☐ If yes, what are the medical conditions? _____	Taking medication indicates a medically diagnosed problem. Judgment is required when taking medication information into account for determining appropriate exercise prescription because it is common for clients to list 'medications' that include contraceptive pills, vitamin supplements and other non-pharmaceutical tablets. Exercise professionals are not expected to have an exhaustive understanding of medications. Therefore, it may be important to use common language to describe what medical conditions the drugs are prescribed for.
16. Have you spent time in hospital (including day admission) for any condition/illness/injury during the last 12 months? Yes ☐ No ☐ If yes, provide details _____	There are positive relationships between illness rates and death versus the number and length of hospital admissions in the previous 12 months. This includes admissions for heart disease, lung disease (e.g., Chronic Obstructive Pulmonary Disease (COPD) and asthma), dementia, hip fractures, infectious episodes and inflammatory bowel disease. Admissions are also correlated to 'poor health' status and negative health behaviours such as smoking, alcohol consumption and poor diet patterns.
17. Are you pregnant or have you given birth within the last 12 months? Yes ☐ No ☐ If yes, provide details _____ _____ _____	During pregnancy and after recent childbirth are times to be more cautious with exercise. Appropriate exercise prescription results in improved health to mother and baby. However, joints gradually loosen to prepare for birth and may lead to an increased risk of injury especially in the pelvic joints. Activities involving jumping, frequent changes of direction and excessive stretching should be avoided, as should jerky ballistic movements. Guidelines/fact sheets can be found here: 1) www.exerciseismedicine.com.au 2) www.fitness.org.au/Pre-and-Post-Natal-Exercise-Guidelines
18. Do you have any diagnosed muscle, bone, tendon, ligament or joint problems that you have been told could be made worse by participating in exercise? Yes ☐ No ☐ If yes, provide details _____ _____ _____	Almost everyone has experienced some level of soreness following unaccustomed exercise or activity but this is not really what this question is designed to identify. Soreness due to unaccustomed activity is not the same as pain in the joint, muscle or bone. Pain is more extreme and may represent an injury, serious inflammatory episode or infection. If it is an acute injury then it is possible that further medical guidance may be required.

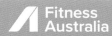

Figure 1.2, cont'd

weight-bearing activities (e.g. running).[6] Methods often used to decrease the risk of a musculoskeletal injury include a warm-up, stretching, a cool-down and progressive overload, even though there is only minimal evidence on the effectiveness of some of these approaches.[1]

A cardiovascular complication is the most concerning exercise risk. In younger individuals the cause of an exercise-related cardiac event is likely to be due to a congenital defect (e.g. hypertrophic cardiomyopathy) whereas in adults it is more likely to be caused by underlying coronary artery disease.[17] The risks of a cardiovascular complication are higher during vigorous intensity exercise[18] and this should be taken into account during screening and exercise prescription. One of the most publicised exercise-related cardiovascular complications is sudden cardiac death. However, it is important for exercise scientists to know and to educate their participants, if questioned, that the absolute risk of an exercise-related sudden cardiac death is very low (1 in 1.5 million episodes of vigorous exercise in men and 1 in 36.5 million with moderate to vigorous exercise in women).[8]

Activity 1.4 Common exercise risks

AIMS:
- To understand how the risks of exercise may differ between individuals, and develop and apply appropriate strategies to address these risks

TASK:
- Complete Worksheet 1.4 by filling in the common exercise risks you would speculate for the different individuals, and strategies you may use to minimise the risks.

Worksheet 1.4 Exercise Risks		
Individual	Exercise Risks	Strategies to Minimise Risk
10-year-old child		
16-year-old youth		
32-year-old adult		
70-year-old older adult		
55-year-old person with diabetes		

Worked Case Study for Exercise Risks

Ralph Macdonald is a 28-year-old male who has come to see you regarding initiating a fitness program for the purposes of 'getting fit and losing some weight'. While Ralph has no signs or symptoms of cardiovascular disease, he explains to you that his motivation to commence regular exercise is based on his father who recently had bypass surgery for ischaemic heart disease at the age of 52, and has commenced a cardiac rehabilitation program that emphasises regular exercise. Ralph wants to reduce his risk of cardiovascular disease later in life.

At your initial appointment, you measure Ralph's height as 179 cm, body mass as 94 kg (body mass index [BMI] = 29 kg/m^2), waist circumference as 96 cm and his blood pressure as 128/78 mmHg. He has brought a recent report from a fasting blood test with the following measures reported: total cholesterol = 4.8 mmol/L, HDL cholesterol = 1.02 mmol/L, triglycerides = 1.6 mmol/L, LDL cholesterol = 2.8 mmol/L and glucose = 5.2 mmol/L. Ralph is a non-smoker who currently does not do any planned, structured exercise. He played soccer in high school but has not participated in sport since. He just enjoys watching it on TV. Ralph is not married nor has any children, and works as an administrative assistant at an accounting firm, which often sees him sitting at the computer for long periods of time over an 8-hour day. On workdays (Monday–Friday) he walks 10 minutes to and from the bus stop each morning and afternoon.

Ralph completes Stage 1 of the APSS tool and, based on the information above, you complete Stage 2 (Figure 1.3).

ADULT PRE-EXERCISE SCREENING SYSTEM (APSS)

This screening tool is part of the <u>Adult Pre-Exercise Screening System (APSS)</u> that also includes guidelines (<u>see User Guide</u>) on how to use the information collected and to address the aims of each stage. No warranty of safety should result from its use. The screening system in no way guarantees against injury or death. No responsibility or liability whatsoever can be accepted by Exercise & Sport Science Australia, Fitness Australia, Sports Medicine Australia or Exercise is Medicine for any loss, damage, or injury that may arise from any person acting on any statement or information contained in this system.

Full Name: *Ralph Macdonald*

Date of Birth: *23.02.1989*   Male: [X]   Female: [ ]   Other: [ ]

STAGE 1 (COMPULSORY)

AIM: To identify individuals with known disease, and/or signs or symptoms of disease, who may be at a higher risk of an adverse event due to exercise. An adverse event refers to an unexpected event that occurs as a consequence of an exercise session, resulting in ill health, physical harm or death to an individual.

This stage may be self-administered and self-evaluated by the client. Please complete the questions below and refer to the figures on page 2. Should you have any questions about the screening form please contact your exercise professional for clarification.

Please tick your response	YES	NO
1. Has your medical practitioner ever told you that you have a heart condition or have you ever suffered a stroke?		✓
2. Do you ever experience unexplained pains or discomfort in your chest at rest or during physical activity/exercise?		✓
3. Do you ever feel faint, dizzy or lose balance during physical activity/exercise?		✓
4. Have you had an asthma attack requiring immediate medical attention at any time over the last 12 months?		✓
5. If you have diabetes (type 1 or 2) have you had trouble controlling your blood sugar (glucose) in the last 3 months?		✓
6. Do you have any other conditions that may require special consideration for you to exercise?		✓

IF YOU ANSWERED 'YES' to any of the 6 questions, please seek guidance from an appropriate allied health professional or medical practitioner prior to undertaking exercise.

IF YOU ANSWERED 'NO' to all of the 6 questions, please proceed to question 7 and calculate your typical weighted physical activity/exercise per week.

7. Describe your current physical activity/exercise levels in a typical week by stating the frequency and duration at the different intensities. For intensity guidelines consult figure 2.

Intensity	Light	Moderate	Vigorous/High
Frequency (number of sessions per week)	*10*		
Duration (total minutes per week)	*10*		

Weighted physical activity/exercise per week

Total minutes = (minutes of light + moderate) + (2 x minutes of vigorous/high)

TOTAL = *100* **minutes per week**

- If your total is less than 150 minutes per week then light to moderate intensity exercise is recommended. Increase your volume and intensity slowly.
- If your total is more than or equal to 150 minutes per week then continue with your current physical activity/exercise intensity levels.
- It is advised that you discuss any progression (volume, intensity, duration, modality) with an exercise professional to optimise your results.

I believe that to the best of my knowledge, all of the information I have supplied within this screening tool is correct.

Client signature: *R Macdonald*   Date: *14.04.2019*

ADULT PRE-EXERCISE SCREENING SYSTEM (APSS) V2 (2018)

ExeRcise is Medicine Australia   Fitness Australia   SPORTS MEDICINE AUSTRALIA   ESSA EXERCISE & SPORTS SCIENCE AUSTRALIA

Figure 1.3 Completed Adult Pre-exercise Screening System Tool for Worked case study for exercise risks

STAGE 2 (RECOMMENDED)

 AIM: This stage is to be completed with an exercise professional to determine appropriate exercise prescription based on established risk factors.

CLIENT DETAILS	GUIDELINES FOR ASSESSING RISK
8. Demographics Age: _28_ Male [X] Female [ ] Other [ ]	Risk of an adverse event increases with age, particularly males ≥ 45 yr and females ≥ 55 yr.
9. Family history of heart disease (e.g. stroke, heart attack)? Relationship (e.g. father) Age at heart disease event _Father_ _52_ _____ _____ _____ _____	A family history of heart disease refers to an event that occurs in relatives including parents, grandparents, uncles and/or aunts before the age of 55 years.
10. Do you smoke cigarettes on a daily or weekly basis or have you quit smoking in the last 6 months? Yes [ ] No [X] If currently smoking, how many per day or week? _____	Smoking, even on a weekly basis, substantially increases risk for premature death and disability. The negative effects are still present up to at least 6 months post quitting.
11. Body composition Weight (kg) _94_ Height (cm) _179_ Body Mass Index (kg/m²) _29.3_ Waist circumference (cm) _96_	Any of the below increases the risk of chronic diseases: BMI ≥ 30 kg/m² Waist > 94 cm male or > 80 cm female
12. Have you been told that you have high blood pressure? Yes [ ] No [X] If known, systolic/diastolic (mmHg) _____ Are you taking any medication for this condition? Yes [ ] No [ ] If yes, provide details	Either of the below increases the risk of heart disease: Systolic blood pressure ≥ 140 mmHg Diastolic blood pressure ≥ 90 mmHg
13. Have you been told that you have high cholesterol/ blood lipids? Yes [ ] No [X] If known: Total cholesterol (mmol/L) _4.8_ HDL (mmol/L) _1.02_ LDL (mmol/L) _2.8_ Triglycerides (mmol/L) _1.6_ Are you taking any medication for this condition? Yes [ ] No [ ] If yes, provide details _____	Any of the below increases the risk of heart disease: Total cholesterol ≥ 5.2 mmol/L HDL < 1.0 mmol/L LDL ≥ 3.4 mmol/L Triglycerides ≥ 1.7 mmol/L

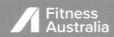
Figure 1.3, cont'd

CLIENT DETAILS	GUIDELINES FOR ASSESSING RISK
14. Have you been told that you have high blood sugar (glucose)? Yes ☐ No ☒ If known: Fasting blood glucose (mmol/L) __5.2__ Are you taking any medication for this condition? Yes ☐ No ☐ If yes, provide details _____	Fasting blood sugar (glucose) ≥ 5.5 mmol/L increases the risk of diabetes.
15. Are you currently taking prescribed medication(s) for any condition(s)? These are additional to those already provided. Yes ☐ No ☒ If yes, what are the medical conditions?	Taking medication indicates a medically diagnosed problem. Judgment is required when taking medication information into account for determining appropriate exercise prescription because it is common for clients to list 'medications' that include contraceptive pills, vitamin supplements and other non-pharmaceutical tablets. Exercise professionals are not expected to have an exhaustive understanding of medications. Therefore, it may be important to use common language to describe what medical conditions the drugs are prescribed for.
16. Have you spent time in hospital (including day admission) for any condition/illness/injury during the last 12 months? Yes ☐ No ☒ If yes, provide details _____	There are positive relationships between illness rates and death versus the number and length of hospital admissions in the previous 12 months. This includes admissions for heart disease, lung disease (e.g., Chronic Obstructive Pulmonary Disease (COPD) and asthma), dementia, hip fractures, infectious episodes and inflammatory bowel disease. Admissions are also correlated to 'poor health' status and negative health behaviours such as smoking, alcohol consumption and poor diet patterns.
17. Are you pregnant or have you given birth within the last 12 months? Yes ☐ No ☒ If yes, provide details _____ _____ _____	During pregnancy and after recent childbirth are times to be more cautious with exercise. Appropriate exercise prescription results in improved health to mother and baby. However, joints gradually loosen to prepare for birth and may lead to an increased risk of injury especially in the pelvic joints. Activities involving jumping, frequent changes of direction and excessive stretching should be avoided, as should jerky ballistic movements. Guidelines/fact sheets can be found here: 1) www.exerciseismedicine.com.au 2) www.fitness.org.au/Pre-and-Post-Natal-Exercise-Guidelines
18. Do you have any diagnosed muscle, bone, tendon, ligament or joint problems that you have been told could be made worse by participating in exercise? Yes ☐ No ☒ If yes, provide details _____ _____	Almost everyone has experienced some level of soreness following unaccustomed exercise or activity but this is not really what this question is designed to identify. Soreness due to unaccustomed activity is not the same as pain in the joint, muscle or bone. Pain is more extreme and may represent an injury, serious inflammatory episode or infection. If it is an acute injury then it is possible that further medical guidance may be required.

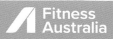

Figure 1.3, cont'd

Stage 1 of the APSS identifies that Ralph has no signs or symptoms of cardiovascular disease and is doing less than 150 minutes per week of physical activity. Based on Figure 1 in the APSS, light to moderate intensity exercise is recommended.

Completing Stage 2 identifies that Ralph has three cardiovascular disease risk factors: family history of heart disease, low physical activity levels and a large waist circumference. While he is not categorised as obese, his BMI is very close at 29.3 kg/m^2, which classifies him as overweight. He also has a sedentary job. Based on this information any progression of exercise intensity and volume should be done slowly. The remaining activities and practicals will provide additional information to develop an individualised exercise prescription.

Activity 1.5 Individual exercise risks

AIMS:
- To assess the risks of exercise for an individual starting an exercise program and apply that information to decisions regarding exercise intensity with an exercise prescription

TASKS:
- Based on the information provided in Case study 1.1 below, complete Stage 2 of the APSS form in Worksheet 1.5.
- Answer the additional questions.

Case study 1.1

You are a self-employed AES. Jill O'Leary is a 54-year-old primary school teacher librarian who works part-time (3 days per week) and has three school-aged children (11, 13 and 16 years old). Jill has come to see you about starting an exercise program to help with weight loss and to improve her energy and sleep. She completes Stage 1 of the APSS indicating that she has no known signs or symptoms of disease (Figure 1.4).

- Her father had a stroke at the age of 68.
- She does not smoke.
- You measure her height as 161 cm, body mass as 74 kg and waist circumference as 79 cm.
- You measure her blood pressure as 124/82 mmHg.
- No one has told her that she has high blood pressure, cholesterol or blood glucose and she has not spent time in hospital in the last 12 months.
- She has no musculoskeletal conditions or injuries.
- She does not take any medication aside from antihistamines when her hay fever flares up (usually with a change of season).

Jill describes her lifestyle as 'hectic' with little time to exercise between work and taking the children to different extracurricular activities after school, with her husband working full-time. Jill used to belong to a gym (she last went about 5 years ago) but says that while she doesn't have time to go to the gym anymore, she would like to start exercising again. She expresses interest in doing exercise that is 'short and sharp'—something more vigorous that would take no more than 30 minutes at home or at the local park on the days that she is not working and the weekends. She has a stationary bike in the garage.

Case study 1.1 (continued)

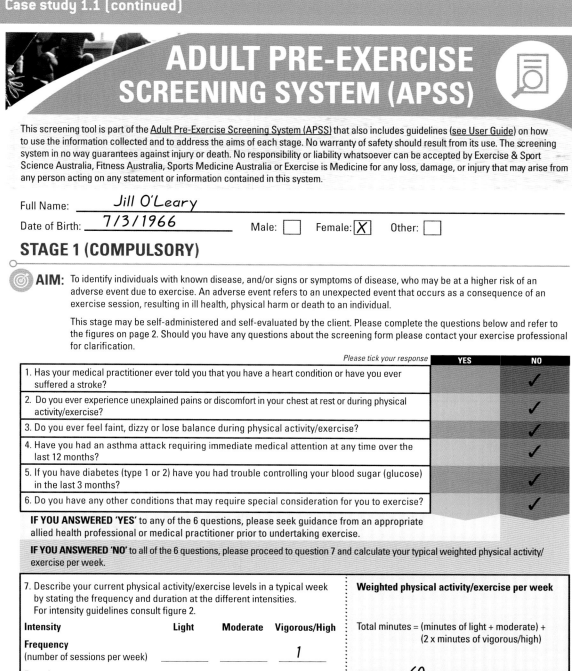

ADULT PRE-EXERCISE SCREENING SYSTEM (APSS)

This screening tool is part of the Adult Pre-Exercise Screening System (APSS) that also includes guidelines (see User Guide) on how to use the information collected and to address the aims of each stage. No warranty of safety should result from its use. The screening system in no way guarantees against injury or death. No responsibility or liability whatsoever can be accepted by Exercise & Sport Science Australia, Fitness Australia, Sports Medicine Australia or Exercise is Medicine for any loss, damage, or injury that may arise from any person acting on any statement or information contained in this system.

Full Name: _Jill O'Leary_

Date of Birth: _7/3/1966_　　　　Male: ☐　Female: ☒　Other: ☐

STAGE 1 (COMPULSORY)

AIM: To identify individuals with known disease, and/or signs or symptoms of disease, who may be at a higher risk of an adverse event due to exercise. An adverse event refers to an unexpected event that occurs as a consequence of an exercise session, resulting in ill health, physical harm or death to an individual.

This stage may be self-administered and self-evaluated by the client. Please complete the questions below and refer to the figures on page 2. Should you have any questions about the screening form please contact your exercise professional for clarification.

Please tick your response	YES	NO
1. Has your medical practitioner ever told you that you have a heart condition or have you ever suffered a stroke?		✓
2. Do you ever experience unexplained pains or discomfort in your chest at rest or during physical activity/exercise?		✓
3. Do you ever feel faint, dizzy or lose balance during physical activity/exercise?		✓
4. Have you had an asthma attack requiring immediate medical attention at any time over the last 12 months?		✓
5. If you have diabetes (type 1 or 2) have you had trouble controlling your blood sugar (glucose) in the last 3 months?		✓
6. Do you have any other conditions that may require special consideration for you to exercise?		✓

IF YOU ANSWERED 'YES' to any of the 6 questions, please seek guidance from an appropriate allied health professional or medical practitioner prior to undertaking exercise.

IF YOU ANSWERED 'NO' to all of the 6 questions, please proceed to question 7 and calculate your typical weighted physical activity/exercise per week.

7. Describe your current physical activity/exercise levels in a typical week by stating the frequency and duration at the different intensities. For intensity guidelines consult figure 2.

Intensity	Light	Moderate	Vigorous/High
Frequency (number of sessions per week)			1
Duration (total minutes per week)			30

Weighted physical activity/exercise per week

Total minutes = (minutes of light + moderate) + (2 x minutes of vigorous/high)

TOTAL = _60_ **minutes per week**

- If your total is less than 150 minutes per week then light to moderate intensity exercise is recommended. Increase your volume and intensity slowly.
- If your total is more than or equal to 150 minutes per week then continue with your current physical activity/exercise intensity levels.
- It is advised that you discuss any progression (volume, intensity, duration, modality) with an exercise professional to optimise your results.

I believe that to the best of my knowledge, all of the information I have supplied within this screening tool is correct.

Client signature: _JOLeary_　　　Date: _18/11/2019_

ADULT PRE-EXERCISE SCREENING SYSTEM (APSS) V2 (2018)

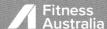 Exe*R*cise is Medicine Australia　 Fitness Australia　 SPORTS MEDICINE AUSTRALIA　ESSA EXERCISE & SPORTS SCIENCE AUSTRALIA

Figure 1.4 Completed stage 1 of Adult Pre-exercise Screening System Tool for Case study 1.1

Worksheet 1.5 Exercise Risks

STAGE 2 (RECOMMENDED)

 AIM: This stage is to be completed with an exercise professional to determine appropriate exercise prescription based on established risk factors.

CLIENT DETAILS	GUIDELINES FOR ASSESSING RISK
8. Demographics Age: _____ Male Female Other	Risk of an adverse event increases with age, particularly males ≥ 45 yr and females ≥ 55 yr.
9. Family history of heart disease (e.g. stroke, heart attack)? Relationship (e.g. father) Age at heart disease event _____ _____ _____ _____ _____ _____	A family history of heart disease refers to an event that occurs in relatives including parents, grandparents, uncles and/or aunts before the age of 55 years.
10. Do you smoke cigarettes on a daily or weekly basis or have you quit smoking in the last 6 months? Yes No If currently smoking, how many per day or week? _____	Smoking, even on a weekly basis, substantially increases risk for premature death and disability. The negative effects are still present up to at least 6 months post quitting.
11. Body composition Weight (kg) _____ Height (cm) _____ Body Mass Index (kg/m²) _____ Waist circumference (cm) _____	Any of the below increases the risk of chronic diseases: BMI ≥ 30 kg/m² Waist > 94 cm male or > 80 cm female
12. Have you been told that you have high blood pressure? Yes No If known, systolic/diastolic (mmHg) _____ Are you taking any medication for this condition? Yes No If yes, provide details _____	Either of the below increases the risk of heart disease: Systolic blood pressure ≥ 140 mmHg Diastolic blood pressure ≥ 90 mmHg
13. Have you been told that you have high cholesterol/blood lipids? Yes No If known: Total cholesterol (mmol/L) _____ HDL (mmol/L) _____ LDL (mmol/L) _____ Triglycerides (mmol/L) _____ Are you taking any medication for this condition? Yes No If yes, provide details _____	Any of the below increases the risk of heart disease: Total cholesterol ≥ 5.2 mmol/L HDL < 1.0 mmol/L LDL ≥ 3.4 mmol/L Triglycerides ≥ 1.7 mmol/L

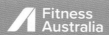

Worksheet 1.5 Exercise Risks (continued)

CLIENT DETAILS	GUIDELINES FOR ASSESSING RISK
14. Have you been told that you have high blood sugar (glucose)? Yes No If known: Fasting blood glucose (mmol/L) _____ Are you taking any medication for this condition? Yes No If yes, provide details _____	Fasting blood sugar (glucose) ≥ 5.5 mmol/L increases the risk of diabetes.
15. Are you currently taking prescribed medication(s) for any condition(s)? These are additional to those already provided. Yes No If yes, what are the medical conditions?	Taking medication indicates a medically diagnosed problem. Judgment is required when taking medication information into account for determining appropriate exercise prescription because it is common for clients to list 'medications' that include contraceptive pills, vitamin supplements and other non-pharmaceutical tablets. Exercise professionals are not expected to have an exhaustive understanding of medications. Therefore, it may be important to use common language to describe what medical conditions the drugs are prescribed for.
16. Have you spent time in hospital (including day admission) for any condition/illness/injury during the last 12 months? Yes No If yes, provide details _____	There are positive relationships between illness rates and death versus the number and length of hospital admissions in the previous 12 months. This includes admissions for heart disease, lung disease (e.g., Chronic Obstructive Pulmonary Disease (COPD) and asthma), dementia, hip fractures, infectious episodes and inflammatory bowel disease. Admissions are also correlated to 'poor health' status and negative health behaviours such as smoking, alcohol consumption and poor diet patterns.
17. Are you pregnant or have you given birth within the last 12 months? Yes No If yes, provide details _____ _____ _____	During pregnancy and after recent childbirth are times to be more cautious with exercise. Appropriate exercise prescription results in improved health to mother and baby. However, joints gradually loosen to prepare for birth and may lead to an increased risk of injury especially in the pelvic joints. Activities involving jumping, frequent changes of direction and excessive stretching should be avoided, as should jerky ballistic movements. Guidelines/fact sheets can be found here: 1) www.exerciseismedicine.com.au 2) www.fitness.org.au/Pre-and-Post-Natal-Exercise-Guidelines
18. Do you have any diagnosed muscle, bone, tendon, ligament or joint problems that you have been told could be made worse by participating in exercise? Yes No If yes, provide details _____ _____	Almost everyone has experienced some level of soreness following unaccustomed exercise or activity but this is not really what this question is designed to identify. Soreness due to unaccustomed activity is not the same as pain in the joint, muscle or bone. Pain is more extreme and may represent an injury, serious inflammatory episode or infection. If it is an acute injury then it is possible that further medical guidance may be required.

ADULT PRE-EXERCISE
SCREENING SYSTEM (APSS) V2 (2018)

Exe℞cise is Medicine® Australia Fitness Australia SPORTS MEDICINE AUSTRALIA ESSA EXERCISE & SPORTS SCIENCE AUSTRALIA

Question 1: Based on Jill's responses, what exercise intensity would be appropriate for Jill to commence, and why? _____ _____

_____

_____

_____

_____

Worksheet 1.5 Exercise Risks (continued)

Question 2: Would you prescribe vigorous-intensity exercise? Justify your answer.

_____

_____

_____

_____

_____

5. General Principles of Exercise Prescription

To design an effective exercise program, it is necessary to know and apply the 10 general principles of exercise prescription provided in Box 1.2. Principles specific to different types of training (i.e. aerobic, resistance, flexibility and neuromotor) will be provided in Practical 2.

Box 1.2   General Principles of Exercise Programming

1. Goal driven

- An exercise scientist should work with a participant to establish his/her goals and then design a program that will achieve them. The SMARTS principle can be used for effective goal setting and tracking.

Specific: target specific areas for improvement

Measurable: quantify progress

Action oriented: indicate what needs to be done

Realistic: achievable

Timely: when the results can be achieved, in both the short and long term

Self-determined: developed in collaboration with the participant and consistent with his/her values and preferences

2. Guidelines based

- An exercise program should be based on current exercise guidelines and contain aerobic and resistance exercises as well as advice to reduce sedentary behaviour. Additional exercises may be indicated for special groups (e.g. balance exercises for older individuals).

3. Specificity

- Responses and adaptations to exercise are specific to the type of exercise and the muscles involved.
  - For example, resistance training is necessary to improve muscular strength.

4. Progressive overload

- A higher load than that which the body is used to is necessary to continue to improve an aspect of fitness.
- Progressive overload should always consider the risk of musculoskeletal injury that is more likely to occur when the load is increased too quickly.
- Stages of progression are: 1. initial; 2. improvement; and 3. maintenance.

Box 1.2   General Principles of Exercise Programming (continued)

- *Initial phase:* usually 4 weeks, depending on the rate of improvement and aims to prepare the individual for a long-term exercise program.
- *Improvement phase:* gradual progression of exercise load by adjusting duration, frequency and intensity until the desired goals (e.g. maintenance) are reached.
  - For example, after training at a moderate intensity for a few months there will be a plateau in the improvement in cardiorespiratory fitness. One option to continue to improve this aspect of fitness would be an increase in intensity (e.g. completing some high-intensity interval training sessions).
- For older and less fit individuals it is recommended to increase the duration rather than the intensity.
- Progressing one element at a time is also advisable.
- *Maintenance phase:* maintaining desired goals

5. Initial levels

- A person with a low level of fitness will have greater relative improvements compared to someone with a high level of fitness.
  - For example, a person with poor muscular strength will have a greater increase in relative strength when doing the same resistance training volume compared to someone with high muscular strength.
- In deconditioned individuals it is important to 'start low and go slow'.

6. Diminishing returns

- Each individual has a maximum genetically determined level to which they can improve their level of fitness.
- Adaptations become less and less as this maximum value gets closer.
  - For example, a person's genetically determined possible maximal cardiorespiratory fitness ($\dot{V}O_2$max) is 65 mL/kg/min. If their initial level is 45 mL/kg/min they will increase this a lot more quickly between 45 and 50 mL/kg/min than between 60 and 65 mL/kg/min, even when doing the same training.

7. Inter-individual variability

- There can be significant variability in the response to exercise training between individuals.
  - For example, two people with the same initial level of flexibility doing the same flexibility exercises can have significantly different improvements in flexibility.

8. Variety

- Continuing with the same exercise program for too long can lead to a plateau in fitness improvements and may decrease motivation to continue.
- Diversifying the exercise prescription with a variety of activities should be considered.
  - For example, have a range of resistance exercises that a participant may choose to complete for each body region.
- For people who are exercising at a high frequency ($>$ 5 days/week), varying the mode is recommended.

9. Reversibility

- When individuals stop exercising they will lose the physical and health benefits gained from the exercise.

10. Something is better than nothing

- If a person cannot meet the recommended exercise prescription targets, performing some exercise will be beneficial (unless there are safety concerns), especially in inactive or deconditioned individuals.

Activity 1.6 General principles of exercise prescription

AIMS:
- To identify and describe the general principles of exercise prescription

TASK:
- Answer the questions in Worksheet 1.6.

Worksheet 1.6 General Principles of Exercise Prescription

Clint is a recreational cyclist who has had a 6-month break from cycling due to knee surgery. His doctor has now given him the 'all clear' to resume his cycling. At his peak level of fitness, just prior to injury, Clint had a $\dot{V}O_2$max of 65 mL/kg/min. Clint wants to know his current fitness level, so you conduct a graded exercise test on a stationary cycle and record his $\dot{V}O_2$max as 44 mL/kg/min.

Question 1: What principle(s) from Box 1.2 best describe what has happened over the last 6 months since his previous $\dot{V}O_2$max test? _____

You re-assess Clint's cardiorespiratory fitness after 8 weeks and then 16 weeks of training and record $\dot{V}O_2$max values of 54 mL/kg/min and 59 mL/kg/min respectively. Clint is disappointed in his improvement from 8 weeks to 16 weeks.

Question 2: Which principle(s) from Box 1.2 is this an example of, and how would you describe this to Clint?

_____

_____

_____

Vera is a 42-year-old business associate who has come to your gym to 'tone up and lose weight'. She tells you that she wants to lose as much weight as possible and feel fit.

Question 3: Which principle(s) from Box 1.2 do you need to use with Vera before you design her exercise

program? _____

Question 4: Give an example of how you could apply the principle(s) in Question 3 to Vera's situation.

_____

_____

_____

Inger is a 33-year-old mother of two who has come to see you to start a new exercise program. She has repeatedly tried to do regular exercise but usually lasts 2–3 weeks before her interest drops off and she stops altogether. You question Inger about her past programs and she tells you that she always aims to jog every day for 20 minutes but gets bored easily.

Question 5: What principle(s) could you use to help Inger maintain her new exercise program?

_____

_____

Question 6: Give an example of the principle(s) you selected in Question 5.

_____

_____

_____

_____

Worksheet 1.6 General Principles of Exercise Prescription (continued)

Jane and her best friend Mariyam start an 8-week fitness bootcamp run by their local gym. They start off with relatively similar levels of cardiorespiratory fitness (which was measured via the group-based field test called the 'beep test'), with both girls achieving the same initial level. Despite doing the same training in terms of type and weekly volume, Mariyam improves her beep test score by four levels after the 8 weeks, while Jane only improves hers by two levels.

Question 7: What principle(s) from Box 1.2 is this an example of?

References

1 American College of Sports Medicine. 2018. *ACSM's Guidelines for Exercise Testing and Prescription,* 10th Edition. Baltimore, MD, USA: Lippincott, Williams and Wilkins.

2 Exercise and Sport Science Australia. 2021. Accredited Exercise Scientist Professional Standards. https://www.essa.org.au/Public/Professional_Standards/The_professional_standards.aspx (accessed 9 June 2021).

3 Exercise and Sport Science Australia. 2021. Accredited Exercise Scientist Scope of Practice. https://www.essa.org.au/Public/Professional_Standards/ESSA_Scope_of_Practice_documents.aspx? (accessed 9 June 2021).

4 Thorp AA, Owen N, Neuhaus M, et al. 2011. Sedentary behaviors and subsequent health outcomes in adults: a systematic review of longitudinal studies, 1996-2011. *Am J Prev Med.* 41:207–215.

5 de Rezende LF, Rodrigues Lopes M, Rey-Lopez JP, et al. 2014. Sedentary behavior and health outcomes: an overview of systematic reviews. *PLoS One.* 9:e105620.

6 Australian Government Department of Health. 2014. Australia's Physical Activity and Sedentary Behaviour Guidelines for Adults (18-64 years). https://www1.health.gov.au/internet/main/publishing.nsf/Content/health-pubhlth-strateg-phys-act-guidelines (accessed 26 March 2021).

7 Haskell WL, Lee IM, Pate RR, et al. 2007. Physical activity and public health: updated recommendation for adults from the American College of Sports Medicine and the American Heart Association. *Circulation.* 116:1081–1093.

8 Tremblay MS, Warburton DE, Janssen I, et al. 2011. New Canadian physical activity guidelines. *Appl Physiol Nutr Metab.* 36:36–46; 47–58.

9 United Kingdom—Department of Health and Social Care. 2011. UK Physical Activity Guidelines. https://www.gov.uk/government/publications/uk-physical-activity-guidelines (accessed 26 March 2021).

10 Melzer K, Kayser B, Pichard C. 2004. Physical activity: the health benefits outweigh the risks. *Curr Opin Clin Nutr Metab Care.* 7:641–647.

11 Allender S, Cowburn G, Foster C. 2006. Understanding participation in sport and physical activity among children and adults: a review of qualitative studies. *Health Educ Res.* 21:826–835.

12 Johansson K, Neovius M, Hemmingsson E. 2014. Effects of anti-obesity drugs, diet, and exercise on weight-loss maintenance after a very-low-calorie diet or low-calorie diet: a systematic review and meta-analysis of randomized controlled trials. *Am J Clin Nutr.* 99:14–23.

13 Lemstra M, Bird Y, Nwankwo C, et al. 2016. Weight loss intervention adherence and factors promoting adherence: a meta-analysis. *Patient Prefer Adherence.* 10:1547–1559.

14 Segar ML, Eccles JS, Richardson CR. 2011. Rebranding exercise: closing the gap between values and behavior. *Int J Behav Nutr Phys Act.* 8:94.

15 Franklin BA, Billecke S. 2012. Putting the benefits and risks of aerobic exercise in perspective. *Curr Sports Med Rep.* 11:201–208.

16 Exercise and Sport Science Australia. 2019. Adult Pre-exercise Screening System (APSS). https://www.essa.org.au/Public/ABOUT_ESSA/Adult_Pre-Screening_Tool.aspx (accessed 26 March 2021).

17 Thompson PD, Franklin BA, Balady GJ, et al. 2007. Exercise and acute cardiovascular events placing the risks into perspective: a scientific statement from the American Heart Association Council on Nutrition, Physical Activity, and Metabolism and the Council on Clinical Cardiology. *Circulation.* 115:2358–2368.

18 Albert CM, Mittleman MA, Chae CU, et al. 2000. Triggering of sudden death from cardiac causes by vigorous exertion. *N Engl J Med.* 343:1355–1361.

PRACTICAL 2
DESIGNING AN EXERCISE PROGRAM

Jeff S. Coombes, Shelley E. Keating and Dawson J. Kidgell

Introduction

Accredited exercise scientists should have the skills to design an individualised exercise program that contains: 1. an exercise prescription; and 2. advice to reduce sedentary behaviour. The success of the exercise program will be determined by the participant's adherence to it. This should result in the program having a positive impact on the participant's health and/or performance. Designing an effective exercise program is often described as being as much an art as it is a science. The art component refers to the successful integration of the principles of exercise programming, both general (Practical 1) and specific to the training type (covered in this practical). Furthermore, integrating these principles with strategies to promote exercise adherence (Section 3) will result in better adoption and maintenance of the program, and the attainment of goals.

Practical 1 covered the 10 general principles of exercise programming. Described below are the principles specific to aerobic, resistance and flexibility exercise prescription that need to be considered during the process of designing an exercise program. These principles are based on the position stand from the American College of Sports Medicine.[1]

1. Principles of Aerobic Exercise Prescription

A. Type
- Uses large muscle groups
- Is rhythmical
- Can be maintained continuously
- Requires little skill to perform
- Includes activities such as brisk walking, jogging, cycling, swimming, rowing, dancing and playing certain sports

B. Intensity
- Moderate to vigorous intensity is recommended for most individuals, although factors such as a person's age and current physical activity level will impact on this (e.g. light to moderate intensity for people who are inactive).

Monitoring
- Various approaches to prescribe and monitor exercise intensity are provided in Box 2.1. Table 2.1 indicates how some are categorised (e.g. moderate, vigorous) and equated to each other.
- The optimal approach to set desired aerobic exercise intensity would be to use the % $\dot{V}O_2max$ (approach 3) and monitor using expired gas analysis while exercising. However, this is not feasible or practical in a non-research setting.
- If data from a maximal exercise test and a resting heart rate are available then the recommended approach is to set intensity as a % of heart rate reserve (HRR) (approach 2).
- If no exercise test data is available, the following are recommended based on the aim:
   - if the aim is to set exercise intensity as moderate or vigorous, use the talk/sing test (approach 7).
   - if the aim is to set exercise intensity in any of the intensity categories use % of HRmax (approach 1) and/or rating of perceived exertion (approach 8).

Box 2.1   Methods to Prescribe and Monitor Aerobic Exercise Intensity

The following methods are the most common approaches to selecting a target aerobic exercise intensity.

1. *% of maximum heart rate (HRmax).* This is the most common approach as it is the easiest to use. It requires the participant's maximal or peak heart rate that is either determined from an exercise test or estimated from an equation (e.g. 208 − [0.7 × age]).[5] The following formula is then used to find the target heart rate, or rates when using a range (e.g. 64−76% HRmax for moderate intensity).

$$\text{target HR} = \text{HRmax} \times \text{\% intensity desired}$$

2. *% of heart rate reserve (HRR).* This approach requires: 1. the participant's maximal or peak heart rate, that is either determined from an exercise test or estimated from an equation (e.g. 208 − [0.7 × age]);[5] and 2. his/her 'resting' heart rate (HRrest). A true resting heart rate is defined as a measure taken on awakening in a neutrally temperate environment and before the person has been subjected to any recent exertion or stimulation, such as stress or surprise. The following formula is then used to find the target heart rate, or rates when using a range (e.g. 40−59% HRR for moderate intensity).

$$\text{target HR} = ([\text{HRmax} - \text{HRrest}] \times \text{\% intensity desired}) + \text{HRrest}$$

Note: For both heart rate based approaches, for longer durations cardiovascular drift will likely increase heart rate when exercising at the same work rate. Therefore, work rate may need to be decreased to keep the heart rate on target, or in the target zone (see Activity 4.3, Task 1).

3. *% of $\dot{V}O_2$max.* This approach is used less as it requires the participant's $\dot{V}O_2$max value. This can be determined using indirect calorimetry from a graded exercise test to volitional exhaustion or estimated from a submaximal test. The following formula is then used to find the target $\dot{V}O_2$, or range (e.g. 46−63% $\dot{V}O_2$max for moderate intensity).

$$\text{target } \dot{V}O_2 = \dot{V}O_2\text{max} \times \text{\% intensity desired}$$

4. *% of $\dot{V}O_2 R$.* This approach requires: 1. the participant's $\dot{V}O_2$max value, that is either determined using indirect calorimetry from a graded exercise test to volitional exhaustion or estimated from a submaximal test; and 2. the participant's 'resting' $\dot{V}O_2$ (usually estimated as 3.5 mL/kg/min). The following formula is then used to find the target $\dot{V}O_2$, or range (e.g. 40−59% $\dot{V}O_2$R for moderate intensity).

$$\text{target } \dot{V}O_2 = ([\dot{V}O_2\text{max} - \dot{V}O_2\text{rest}] \times \text{\% intensity desired}) + \dot{V}O_2 \text{ rest}$$

Note: For both $\dot{V}O_2$-based approaches, once the target(s) have been calculated: 1. the participant has $\dot{V}O_2$ measured during exercise (unusual); or 2. the participant has the work rate set from data from the $\dot{V}O_2$max test (i.e. the work rate that corresponded to this $\dot{V}O_2$ measured during the test); or 3. if a submaximal test was used to estimate $\dot{V}O_2$max then data from this test is used to set the work rate (see Activity 4.3, Task 2). These approaches are more likely to be used in a research setting.

5. *METs.* More common in physical activity and clinical examples (e.g. cardiac rehabilitation). The intensity is set based on the activity. For example, a person may be prescribed to exercise at 5 METs. The work rate required to elicit this intensity for the participant can be calculated using metabolic equations (see Table 2.2). This is an absolute approach that does not take into account the participant's cardiorespiratory fitness (e.g. 5 METs may be high intensity for one person and light intensity for another). If a $\dot{V}O_2$max value is available for a participant then this can be used to determine a relative intensity level (see Table 2.1).

6. *Ventilatory/lactate threshold.* This approach is more likely used in a research setting. It uses either the $\dot{V}O_2$ or the heart rate corresponding to a ventilatory/lactate threshold to monitor the exercise intensity.

7. *Talk/sing test.* This is a more practical and subjective approach arising from knowledge that the ability to hold a conversation during exercise represents an exercise intensity below the ventilatory/lactate threshold (i.e. moderate intensity).[1] The notion is that you can talk, but not sing, during moderate-intensity activity. If you are doing vigorous-intensity activity, you will not be able to say more than a few words without pausing for a breath. During high-intensity exercise, it is very difficult to talk.

8. *Rating of perceived exertion (RPE).* This is generally recommended as an adjunct method for monitoring aerobic exercise intensity (i.e. used in addition to an objective measure). However, it may also be

---

Box 2.1   Methods to Prescribe and Monitor Aerobic Exercise Intensity (continued)

used independently (e.g. in people taking medication such as beta blockers that limit the heart rate response to exercise). It is best used if it can be first compared with an objective measure (e.g. used concurrently) to show the association. There are two commonly used RPE scales for aerobic exercise: the Borg 6–20 scale (Appendix A) and the Borg category ratio scale (CR10). The 6–20 scale was chosen as a simple way to estimate heart rate. Multiplying the Borg score by 10 gives an approximate heart rate for a particular aerobic activity (e.g. resting heart rate of 60 bpm [= 6] and maximal heart rate of 200 bpm [= 20] for a 20 year old). The Borg 6–20 scale is used as the RPE scale of choice for aerobic exercise in this manual. However, to use RPE effectively the participant and exercise scientist should be aware of a number of factors that are detailed in Appendix A.

TABLE 2.1   Thresholds and Ranges for Methods to Prescribe and Monitor Aerobic Exercise Intensity, and Their Relationships to Each Other (Based on Recommendations from the American College of Sports Medicine[6])

Intensity Category	Method to Prescribe and Monitor Intensity						
	% of HRmax	% of $\dot{V}O_2$max	% of HRR or % of $\dot{V}O_2$ R	METs[a]	Ventilatory/ Lactate Threshold	Talk/Sing Test	RPE
Very light	< 57	< 37	< 30	< 2.0	Below	Able to sing	< 9
Light	57–63	37–45	30–39	2.4–4.7		Able to sing	9–11
Moderate	64–76	46–63	40–59	4.8–7.1		Able to talk but unable to sing	12–13
Vigorous[b]	77–95	64–90	60–89	7.2–10.1	Above	Not comfortable talking	14–17
High[b]	80–100	70–100	65–100	10.2–11.3		Very difficult to talk	15–18
Supra-maximal[c]	N/A	≥ 100	N/A	> 11.3		Unable to talk	≥ 18

[a]For a person with a $\dot{V}O_2$max of 40 mL/kg/min.
[b]Note: There is overlap between the ranges for vigorous and high intensities. High-intensity ranges are provided due to widespread use of this term (e.g. high-intensity interval training).
[c]Due to the short duration of this exercise, heart rate cannot be used to monitor intensity.

C. Frequency
- Moderate-intensity aerobic exercise should be completed ≥ 5 days/week.
- Vigorous-intensity aerobic exercise should be completed ≥ 3 days/week.
- Separate with a rest day where possible.

D. Duration
- Minimum of 150 min/week of moderate intensity or 75 min/week of vigorous intensity.
- If using a combination of different intensities, multiply the duration of vigorous by 2 to be equivalent to moderate (e.g. 100 min/week of moderate-intensity exercise + 25 min/week of vigorous-intensity exercise is equivalent to 150 min/week of moderate-intensity exercise).

		Most accurate between
TABLE 2.2 Metabolic Equations for the Estimation of $\dot{V}O_2$ (mL/kg/min) During Cycle Ergometry, Treadmill Walking and Running, and Stepping		
Cycle ergometry[2]	$1.74 \times$ (work rate[a] $\times$ 6.12/kg of body weight) + 3.5	150–750 kpm/min
Treadmill walking and running[3]	speed[b] $\times$ (0.17 + [grade[c] $\times$ 0.79]) + 3.5	
Stepping[4]	3.5 + (0.2 $\times$ steps/min) + (1.33 $\times$ [1.8 $\times$ step height[d] $\times$ steps/min])	12–30 steps/min

[a]work rate in watts
[b]speed in m/min where 1 km/h = 16.7 m/min
[c]grade in % expressed as a decimal
[d]step height in m

2. Principles of Resistance Exercise Prescription

A. Type
- Resistance can be provided by the person's body weight, weights, springs, pneumatic/hydraulic machines or other approaches (e.g. resistance bands/tubes, chains).
- Dynamic exercises are preferred to isometric exercises as they generally replicate activities of daily living/sport. An exception are exercises for the trunk such as the prone bridge.
- Train all six major body regions: 1. trunk (see Practical 5); 2. chest (see Practical 6); 3. shoulders (see Practical 7); 4. arms (see Practical 7); 5. back (see Practical 8); and 6. legs (see Practical 9).
- Use both multi-joint and single-joint exercises.
- First complete multi-joint exercises that impact on more than one body region (e.g. chest press = chest and arms) before single-joint exercises (e.g. triceps extension).
- Correct technique (controlled movements through the full range of motion [ROM]) is vital to optimise benefits and minimise the risk of injury (Practicals 5–10 in this manual are devoted to teaching the correct techniques).

B. Frequency
- Each of the six body regions should be resistance trained at least two times/week.
- There is the option to divide the regions across weekly sessions (e.g. upper body on Monday and Thursday and legs on Wednesday and Saturday). If providing this split routine, ensure that each body region is trained at least 2 days/week.
- Separate resistance exercise training for the same body region by 2 days to allow for adequate recovery of the muscle.

C. Volume (sets, intensity, repetitions, rest and duration)*
Due to the interaction between sets, intensity, repetitions, rest and duration with resistance training, these are covered together under the heading Volume.
- Depends on the training state of the individual and the goals of the program. Table 2.3 provides recommendations on resistance training prescriptions.
- Although Table 2.3 provides ranges for all components in the prescription (sets, reps, intensity, rest, frequency), the participant should be provided with a specific prescription for sets, reps and frequency (e.g. 2 sets of 10 reps, 3 sessions/week). This will avoid participant confusion and the possibility they may just choose the lowest number in a range that is provided. It also allows the exercise scientist

TABLE 2.3	Resistance Training Prescriptions Based on Resistance Training Experience and Goals[a]				
	Goals				
	Strength	**Hypertrophy**	**Power**	**Endurance**	**Combination**
Deconditioned/ sedentary	Use another goal approach (e.g. combination) for 2 weeks then prescribe as a Novice if strength or hypertrophy is a goal		• 1–2 sets • 10–15 reps • 4–6 RiR (5–6 RPE) = light intensity or • 20–50% 1RM • Focus on speed • Longer rest (3–4 minutes) between sets • 2–3 sessions/ week	• 1–2 sets • 15–25 reps • 4–6 RiR (5–6 RPE) = light intensity or • 30–50% 1RM • shorter rest (1–2 minutes) between sets • 2–3 sessions/ week	• 1–2 sets • 10–15 reps • 4–6 RiR (5–6 RPE) = light intensity or • 40–50% 1RM • shorter rest (1–2 minutes) between sets • 2–3 sessions/ week
Novice	• 2–3 sets • 3–8 reps • 1–3 RiR (7–9 RPE) = moderate to heavy intensity or • 70–83%% 1RM • longer rest (3–5 minutes) between sets • 2–3 sessions/ week	• 2–3 sets • 8–15 reps • 3–5 RiR (5–7 RPE) = light to moderate intensity or • 67–80% 1RM, shorter rest (1–2 minutes) between sets • 2–3 sessions/ week	• 2–3 sets • 5–8 reps • 4–6 RiR (5–6 RPE) = light intensity or • 30–45% 1RM • focus on speed • longer rest (5–8 minutes) between sets • 2–3 sessions/ week	• 1–3 sets • 15–20 reps • 4–6 RiR (5–6 RPE) = light intensity or • 40–50% 1RM • shorter rest (60–90 seconds) between sets • 2–3 sessions/ week	• 2–3 sets • 8–12 reps • 3–5 RiR (5–7 RPE = light to moderate intensity) or • 67–80% 1RM • shorter rest (90 seconds) between sets • 2–3 sessions/ week

TABLE 2.3	Resistance Training Prescriptions Based on Resistance Training Experience and Goals (continued)				
	Goals				
	Strength	**Hypertrophy**	**Power**	**Endurance**	**Combination**
Intermediate	• 3–4 sets • 3–5 reps • 0–2 RiR (8–10 RPE) = moderate to heavy intensity or • 80–93% 1RM • longer rest (3–5 minutes) between sets • 3 sessions/week	• 3–4 sets • 10–15 reps • 1–3 RiR (7–9 RPE) = moderate to heavy intensity or • 70–80% 1RM, shorter rest (60–90 seconds) between sets • 3–4 sessions/week	• 3–4 sets • 3–5 reps • 4–6 RiR (5–6 RPE) = light to moderate intensity or • 30–60% 1RM • focus on speed • longer rest (5–8 minutes) between sets • 3–4 sessions/week	• 3–4 sets • 15–20 reps • 4–6 RiR (5–6 RPE) = light to moderate intensity or • 40–60% 1RM • shorter rest (30–60 seconds) between sets • 3–4 sessions/week	• 3–4 sets • 8–12 reps • 1–3 RiR (7–9 RPE) = moderate to heavy intensity) or • 67–80% 1RM • shorter rest (60–90 seconds) between sets • 2 sessions/week
Experienced resistance trained	• 3–5 sets • 1–5 reps • RiR (9–10 RPE) = heavy intensity or • ≥ 80% 1RM • longer rest (3–5 minutes) between sets • 4–5 sessions/week	• 4–6 sets • 8–15 reps • 0–2 RiR (8–10 RPE) = moderate to heavy intensity or • 67–85% 1RM • shorter rest (45–60 seconds) between sets • 3–5 sessions/week	• 3–5 sets • 1–5 reps • 3–5 RiR (5–6 RPE) = light to moderate intensity or • 40–70% 1RM • focus on speed • longer rest (5–8 minutes) between sets • 4–6 sessions/week	• 3–5 sets • 15–20 reps • 3–5 RiR (5–6 RPE) = light to moderate intensity or • 50–60% 1RM • shorter rest (30–45 seconds rest) between sets • 3 sessions/week	• 3–4 sets • 8–12 reps • 1–3 RiR (7–10 RPE = moderate to heavy intensity) or • 70–85% 1RM • shorter rest (45–60 seconds) between sets • 3 sessions/week

aRanges for sets and reps are for the exercise scientist to consider when prescribing the exercise program. The exercise prescription for the participant should provide specific numbers for sets and reps (rather than ranges). The recommendations are based on evidence from various sources.[7–14] If using % 1RM to set intensity, there will be large individual differences, thus the prescription may need to be adapted quickly based on individual needs. reps = repetitions; RiR = repetitions in reserve; RPE = rating of perceived exertion; RM = repetition maximum.

to apply effective progression of the sets and reps (see Progression below). The intensity and rest components are usually provided as a range to accommodate autoregulation (see Box 2.2).

- General recommendation to set a specific prescription is for between 2 and 4 sets with 2–3-minute rest intervals between sets; however:
  - ○ a single set may be effective among novices and deconditioned/sedentary individuals
  - ○ ≥ 2 sets is effective in improving muscular endurance
  - ○ for muscular strength and/or power, longer rest periods between sets (2–4 minutes) are recommended
  - ○ for muscular hypertrophy the total volume is important leading to more sets prescribed (up to 6 for experienced resistance-trained individuals)
  - ○ for muscular endurance shorter rest periods between sets (1–2 minutes) is recommended.
- Complete either as a circuit (moving from one exercise to the next) or complete all sets of one exercise before moving to the next exercise.
- Two sets of eight exercises with a 2-minute rest period in between with a 5-minute warm-up and cool-down should take around 45 mins. As this is a common amount of time allocated to exercise, it is usual to have eight resistance exercises in the prescription.
- Volume needs to be continually increased at regular intervals (as strength improves) to obtain continual gains in muscular fitness. For this reason, it is often referred to as progressive resistance training.

Box 2.2   Autoregulation

Autoregulation is the adjustment of a resistance training prescription based on an individual's readiness to train on a daily or weekly basis. This is based on certain 'readiness factors' (e.g. sleep status, level of anxiety) that impact on a participant's perception of the difficulty of the set/session leading to an adjustment of training intensity or volume.[15] In this regard, autoregulation is a method that can be used to implement the principle of individualisation into a resistance training program. A simple approach to individualise resistance training is to autoregulate the training load prescription through the use of the repetitions in reserve (RiR)-based rating of perceived exertion (RPE) scale (Box 2.3). Autoregulation is a subtype of periodisation that enables the adjustment of the acute resistance training variables (sets, repetitions, load, velocity, etc.) that meet the individual rate of adaptation to training stimuli. Because individuals adapt to training stimuli at different rates, autoregulating training (based on participant feedback) may lead to greater strength gains when compared to traditional percentage-based fixed loading programs (e.g. % 1RM loading) because it accounts for fluctuations in strength capabilities across a training period.[21]

Monitoring intensity

- Box 2.3 provides various approaches for prescribing and monitoring resistance exercise intensity. The main consideration should always be correct technique when completing the exercise.

Box 2.3   Methods to Prescribe and Monitor Resistance Exercise Intensity

The most important consideration when prescribing and monitoring intensity is the technique of the participant completing the exercise. A poor technique does not optimise muscle function and increases the risk of injury in deconditioned individuals and novices. For whichever of the following approaches is applied, a repetition should only be counted if the correct technique is used. If the exercise scientist is directly supervising the participant while they are attempting the exercise then using his/her skills of observing correct dynamic postures will allow for a more accurate choice of resistance intensity.

The following methods are the most common approaches to prescribe and monitor resistance training intensity. They can be separated into: 1. perception based; or 2. resistance/load based. Perception-based approaches are recommended to prescribe and monitor resistance exercise intensity for the majority of participants. Perception-based approaches use an RPE scale and have a number of advantages over load-based methods: 1. they avoid maximal tests that are less safe in deconditioned individuals; 2. in the early stages of a resistance training program load-based prescriptions are likely to change more regularly due to

Box 2.3   Methods to Prescribe and Monitor Resistance Exercise Intensity (continued)

neural adaptations; 3. are easier to use; and 4. allows for easier autoregulation. Autoregulation refers to the adjustment of the training load based on an individual's readiness to train. Autoregulation is discussed in more detail in Box 2.2.

Examples of load-based approaches are % of 1RM and repetition maximum (RM) range. When using a load-based approach, the number of repetitions needs to be the first consideration when setting the resistance. The more repetitions prescribed or completed, the greater the intensity of the set. For example, if a participant completes three repetitions with a load of 50 kg this may be a light intensity. However, if the participant is asked to complete 25 repetitions at the same resistance then this could be heavy.

Perception-based approaches

1. *Repetitions in reserve (RiR)-based rating of perceived exertion (RPE) scale:* For the general population, using the RiR-based RPE scale is a practical and preferred approach to setting and monitoring resistance training intensity. RiR refers to the estimated number of additional repetitions a participant believes they could have completed with the correct technique. RiR = 0 means that another repetition could not have been completed (also known as 'going to failure'). The following scale is based on the work of Zourdos et al. (2016)[16] and provides guidance for setting intensity using RiR and RPE together. Using RiR and RPE together increases the accuracy of prescribing training load and autoregulating training; however, RiR can be used by itself for simplicity.

RPE	RiR/Description	Intensity
10	Maximal effort	Heavy
9.5	No RiR, but could increase load	
9	1 RiR	
8.5	Definitely 1, maybe 2 RiR	Moderate
8	2 RiR	
7.5	Definitely 2, maybe 3 RiR	
7	3 RiR	
5–6	4–6 RiR	Light
3–4	Very light effort	
1–2	Little to no effort	

2. *OMNI RPE scale:* The OMNI scale (Appendix B) uses illustrations that attempt to make it easier for individuals to determine the intensity of resistance training. OMNI is a contraction of the word omnibus, meaning having broadly generalisable properties.[17]

3. *Borg RPE scales:* There are two Borg RPE scales: the Borg 6–20 scale (Appendix A) and the Borg category ratio scale (CR10). The Borg scales were developed to prescribe and monitor aerobic exercise intensity and have limitations when used for resistance training.[18] The shorter time spent completing a resistance training set compared to a bout of aerobic exercise means there is usually a faster increase in perceived exertion. For example, if completing a set of 8 repetitions, the perceived load may increase after each repetition, especially towards the end of the set. In addition, there can be confusion on what a participant is supposed to rate (e.g. intensity of the overall set or final repetition).

Load-based approaches

1. *% of 1RM:* This requires conducting RM strength tests on the exercises being prescribed. The most accurate approach to obtain the 1RM value is to complete a 1RM test; however, this is not always

> ### Box 2.3   Methods to Prescribe and Monitor Resistance Exercise Intensity (continued)
>
> suitable for all individuals (e.g. older individuals and deconditioned participants). Other numbers of RM tests can be used (e.g. 3RM, 5RM, 10RM) and converted to a 1RM using the formula:[19]
>
> $$1RM = W \times 36/(37 - R)$$
>
> where W = weight (kg) and R = number of repetitions.
>
> These approaches lead to a choice of starting resistance as a % of the 1RM value. However, RM testing is time consuming if done according to valid methods (e.g. adequate rest periods between attempts).
>
> 2. *Repetition maximum (RM) range:* A range of repetitions is provided (e.g. 3–5RM, 6–8RM or 9–11RM) with the last repetition within this range done to 'failure' (another repetition could not be completed with correct technique). This intensity is not suitable for a large number of participants and training to 'failure' may not be the optimum approach for strength development.[20]

- Using the repetitions in reserve (RiR)-based rating of perceived exertion (RPE) scale is the preferred approach to set and monitor intensity. A range can be used in the exercise prescription for the RiR-based RPE scale (e.g. 3 sets of 10 repetitions at 1–3 RiR).

Progression
- When progressing the volume of resistance training it is important to understand that individuals will progress at different rates. Using the RiR-based RPE scale to prescribe and monitor intensity allows for autoregulation (see Box 2.2) and more accurate load progressions.
- To progress the prescription, first increase the number of reps up to the maximum in the range, then the number of sets up to the maximum in the range then the intensity.

3. Principles of Flexibility Exercise Prescription

A. Type
- Flexibility exercises should target the following seven areas: 1. chest; 2. back; 3. arms (anterior); 4. arms (posterior); 5. legs (anterior); 6. legs (posterior); and 7. legs (medial and lateral). (See Practical 11.)
- The following are the different types of flexibility exercises.
  - Static stretching. Slowly stretching a muscle to a challenging position (to the point of tightness or slight discomfort) and holding for a certain amount of time (e.g. 10–30 seconds).
  - Slow dynamic stretching. Slow and repetitive movements from one body position to another with a progressive increase in ROM (e.g. lateral neck flexions, trunk rotations).
  - Proprioceptive neuromuscular facilitation (PNF). Involves both stretching and contracting of a target muscle group using different approaches (see Box 2.4). It is recognised as the most effective means to increase ROM by way of stretching.[2]
  - Ballistic stretching. A swinging, bouncing or bobbing movement that uses the momentum of the moving body segment to produce the stretch of the muscle. During the stretch, the final position in the movement is not held.

B. Frequency
- The frequency should be ≥ 2 days/week, with daily being most effective for improving ROM.

C. Volume (sets, intensity, repetitions, rest and duration)
Due to the interaction between sets, intensity, repetitions, rest and duration with resistance training, these are covered together under the heading Volume.

- Stretch to the point of tightness or slight discomfort (e.g. telling participants that they should be able to 'feel a pull without pain').

Box 2.4	**Types of Proprioceptive Neuromuscular Facilitation (PNF) Stretches**

1. *Hold-relax.* The target muscle is held in a passive stretch for about 20 seconds. Then, that same muscle is contracted isometrically and held for 10–15 seconds before relaxing the muscle for 3 seconds. The passive stretch is then repeated for around 20 seconds and this second stretch should be deeper than the first. This stretch is often facilitated by a partner. An example would be where a participant is lying supine and flexes their hip (with the assistance of a partner) to raise one leg straight to place the target muscle (hamstrings) on stretch. This is held for about 20 seconds. Following this, the participant is asked to isometrically contract the hamstrings by attempting to move the leg towards the partner. The partner resists the movement for 10–15 seconds. The participant then relaxes for 3 seconds and then the partner moves the leg into another passive stretch a little deeper than the first.

2. *Contract-relax.* This is similar to the hold-relax stretch except the muscle is contracted concentrically after the passive stretch. Using the previous example, following the passive stretch the participant lowers the leg while it is being slightly supported by the partner before the partner then moves the leg into another passive stretch a little deeper than the first.

3. *Hold-relax with antagonist contract:* Similar to the hold-relax stretch except the antagonist muscle is contracted concentrically after the passive stretch. Using the previous example, following the passive stretch the participant contracts the antagonist muscle (quadriceps) by attempting to move the leg away from the partner, while it is being resisted by the partner. The participant then relaxes for 3 seconds and then the partner moves the leg into another passive stretch a little deeper than the first.

- For PNF, the contraction should be less than 50% maximum voluntary contraction and if there is an assisted stretch it is also to a point of tightness or slight discomfort.
- Hold a static stretch for 30 seconds.
- In older individuals, holding for 30–60 seconds may be more beneficial.
- For PNF, use a 3–6-second hold of the light to moderate contraction followed by a 10–30-second assisted stretch.
- Do enough sets so that each muscle group is stretched for $\geq$ 60 seconds.
- Stretching each muscle group for 60 seconds will take around 10 minutes.

4. Other Exercise Types

In addition to aerobic, resistance and flexibility exercises, there are certain populations/individuals who are likely to benefit from other types of exercise such as neuromotor and bone loading exercises. *Neuromotor exercises* aim to improve balance, coordination, agility and gait. These may also refer to proprioceptive exercises (e.g. exercises with eyes closed) and multimodal activities (e.g. tai chi, yoga). *Bone loading exercises* aim to improve bone health. They include high-impact, weight-bearing exercises that provide forces through the bones that exceed those experienced by daily living activities (e.g. vertical and multidirectional jumping, bounding, hopping, skipping rope, drop jumps and bench stepping).

Neuromotor and bone loading exercises may be interspersed between aerobic and resistance training exercises in the same session. An exercise prescription for older individuals should include both neuromotor and bone loading exercises (see Boxes 3.5 and 3.6).

5. Advice to Reduce Sedentary Behaviour

Sedentary behaviour refers to low energy expenditure behaviour done sitting or lying down when awake. The exercise program should contain a list of personalised strategies and advice to reduce and break up prolonged sedentary behaviour. The exercise scientist should increase a participant's knowledge and understanding of the importance of all forms of movement, including the view that movement should be seen as an opportunity rather than an inconvenience. When working with a participant, it will be helpful to first assess their usual levels of sedentary behaviour and when this occurs. The advice to reduce sedentary behaviour can then be developed. Table 2.4 provides a number of suggestions. The strategies should be agreed upon and recorded on the exercise program as a reminder to the participant.

TABLE 2.4   Suggested Advice for Reducing Sedentary Behaviour

At Home/Leisure	At work	While Travelling
• Get off the couch and stand/walk around the home during TV commercial breaks. • Do household chores, such as folding clothes, washing dishes or ironing, while watching television. • Stand to read the morning newspaper. • Wash your car by hand rather than using a drive-through carwash. • Stand or move around the house while talking on the phone, checking text messages and/or email on your mobile phone. • Catch up with friends with a walk, even if it is to the local coffee shop.	• Stand and take a break from your computer every 20–30 minutes. • Take breaks in sitting during long meetings. • Take a walk to clear the head when problem-solving. • Stand to greet a visitor to your workspace. • Stand during phone calls. • Walk to your colleague's desk rather than phoning or emailing. • Drink more water—going to the water cooler and toilet more frequently will break up sitting time. • Move your printer/bin away from your desk so you have to get up to put something in it. • Use a height-adjustable desk so you can work standing or sitting. • Have standing or walking meetings. • Use headsets or the speaker phone during teleconferences so you can stand. • Take a short walk during the lunch break • Stand at the back of the room during presentations.	• Leave your car at home and take public transport so you walk to and from stops/stations. • Walk or cycle at least part-way to your destination. • Park your car further away from your destination and walk the rest of the way. • Plan regular breaks during long car trips. • On public transport, stand and offer your seat to a person. • Get on/off public transport one stop/station earlier and walk the rest of the way.

Source: Heart Foundation[22]

There are also phrases to remind people of the benefits of movement that could be used in a written exercise program. Some examples are:

- walk more, sit less and exercise
- make your move, sit less, be active for life.

Activity 2.1 Different types of exercise

AIMS:
- To understand and classify different types of exercise

TASK:
- Complete Worksheet 2.1 to classify the different types of exercise based on the categories below. Choose the one category that best represents the exercise.

A: Low–moderate-intensity aerobic exercise (requires minimal skill or cardiorespiratory fitness)

B: Moderate–vigorous-intensity aerobic exercise (requires minimal skill but higher levels of cardiorespiratory fitness)

C: Recreational sport (requires skill and higher levels of cardiorespiratory fitness)

D: Flexibility exercise

E: Muscular strength exercise

Worksheet 2.1 Different Types of Exercise	
Exercise	Category (A, B, C, D or E)
Machine weights	
Walking	
Yoga	
Jogging	
Basketball	
Cycling (for leisure)	
Rowing	
Tai chi	
Aqua jogging	
Cross-country skiing	
Swimming	
Soccer	
Track sprinting	
Slow dancing	
Rowing	
Zumba	
Free weights	
Static stretching	
Volleyball	

6. Interval Training

Aerobic exercise interval training involves alternating periods of usually higher intensity exercise with light recovery exercise or no exercise between intervals.[3] This will generally result in an increase in the average exercise intensity of the session and greater and faster improvements in cardiorespiratory fitness.[4] The appeal of interval training is based on: 1. being more time efficient (larger increase in cardiorespiratory fitness over the same training period (e.g. 8 weeks) compared to lower intensities of exercise; and 2. more variety compared to exercising continuously at the same intensity. Two of the more common approaches are high-intensity interval training (HIIT) and sprint interval training (SIT). Figure 2.1 shows the differences between HIIT and SIT (i.e. SIT intervals are supramaximal, all-out efforts).[23]

HIIT may be further divided into high- and low-volume HIIT based on the total duration of the high-intensity intervals. Any protocol with a total high-intensity duration < 15 minutes (e.g. 10×1 minute) is low-volume HIIT.[22] A common high-volume HIIT protocol is the 4×4 approach that consists of four 4-minute high-intensity intervals separated by 3 minutes of recovery at a light intensity. This results in 16 minutes of high-intensity exercise and is therefore considered high-volume HIIT (≥ 15 minutes of high-intensity intervals).

Designing an interval training session requires consideration of seven parameters as shown in Figure 2.2. Of these, the intensity and duration of the work and recovery intervals are the most important influencing factors for physiological benefits.[6] Practical 4 provides opportunities for students to experience interval training and develop an understanding of how to set work rates to achieve target intensities.

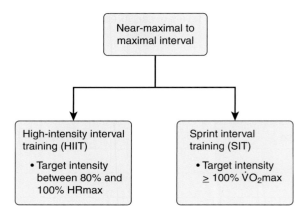

Figure 2.1 Classification scheme for interval training based on exercise intensity
Source: Weston, Wisloff & Coombes[4]

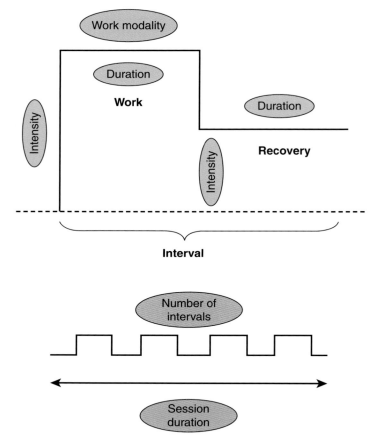

Figure 2.2 Seven components of an interval training session that can be changed
Source: Buchheit & Laursen[23]

Activity 2.2 Calculate aerobic exercise intensity
. . . .

AIM:
- To use different approaches to calculate aerobic exercise intensity

TASKS:
- Complete Worksheet 2.2 by calculating the desired exercise intensity ranges for exercise prescription in each case study by using the information provided in Box 2.1.
- Answer the additional questions.

Worksheet 2.2 Calculate Aerobic Exercise Intensity

1. Percentage of heart rate maximum

Edward is a 20-year-old recreational runner who has come to you for advice on training. He would like to vary his training as he currently undertakes two slow long-distance runs and two tempo runs (currently 8 km at 4 min/km pace). After screening, you determine that high-intensity interval training (HIIT) is appropriate for Edward and you discuss with him the benefits of including one or two sessions of HIIT per week. Edward is enthusiastic about trying something new. The HIIT program you prescribe is the '4 × 4': four minutes at high intensity (85–95% HRmax) interspersed with 3-minutes moving 'rest' periods at 50–60% HRmax, repeated four times.

Question 1: Calculate the target heart rate zone for Edward's 4-minute intervals using the % HRmax method. Show your workings. _____

_____

_____

_____

_____

Question 2: Calculate the target heart rate zone for Edward's 3-minute moving 'rest' periods using the % HRmax method. Show your workings. _____

_____

_____

_____

_____

2. Heart rate reserve (HRR)

Anahera is 29 years old and wishes to start exercising to lose some weight. She prefers walking at a moderate intensity and tells you that her heart rate upon waking is 62 bpm.

Question 3: Calculate the target heart rate zone for Anahera to exercise at a moderate intensity using the HRR method. Show your workings. _____

_____

_____

_____

3. HRR and ratings of perceived exertion (RPE)

Carol is a 53-year-old office worker who wishes to commence an exercise program to improve her fitness and body composition on the recommendation of her general practitioner. Her resting heart rate is 74 bpm. After screening, you decide she should exercise at an intensity of 50–60% HRR. Carol has signed up to a once-weekly work-based lunchtime exercise class in which she can use a heart rate monitor. However, she would like to fit at least two to three additional walks in during the week when she will not have access to a heart rate monitor.

Question 4. Calculate Carol's target heart rate zone based on % HRR. Show your workings.

_____

_____

_____

_____

Worksheet 2.2 Calculate Aerobic Exercise Intensity (continued)

Question 5. How could she monitor her intensity without a heart rate monitor? _____

_____

_____

_____

_____

You reassess Carol after 12 weeks of regular attendance at her work-based class with an average of three additional walking sessions per week. Her resting heart rate is 68 bpm.

Question 6. Recalculate the target heart rate zone based on % HRR. Show your workings.

_____

_____

_____

_____

Activity 2.3 Interval training session

AIM:
- To design a HIIT session

TASK:
- Revisit the story of Jill (Case study 1.1 in Practical 1) who wanted to do a vigorous 'short and sharp' exercise session that would take no longer than 30 minutes. Complete Worksheet 2.3 by designing an interval training session for Jill based on the seven parameters in Figure 2.2.

Worksheet 2.3 Interval Training Session

Principle	Prescription
Work modality	
Interval intensity	
Interval duration	
Recovery intensity	
Recovery duration	
Number of intervals	
Session duration	

Worked Case Study for Exercise Programming

Tariq, aged 45, visits your business for an exercise program he can use at his gym to 'build muscle strength and lose his belly fat'. He has not used a gym before. You undertake an initial assessment that includes a submaximal graded aerobic exercise test and collect relevant information that you enter into your exercise program template (below). You measure his waist circumference at 96 cm and resting blood pressure at 122/82 mmHg. You also assist Tariq to develop some SMARTS goals before designing the exercise program. Tariq is married with two teenage children. He spends a lot of his spare time driving his children to sport and dancing practice and competitions. He works in a pathology laboratory from Monday to Friday, 8.30 am to 5.00 pm, with a 30-minute lunch break. He spends most of his day sitting down and at lunchtime he will usually walk across the road to buy a sandwich and a diet cola. Aside from Thursday nights, in which he plays soccer, Tariq spends most evenings watching television. He takes a bus to work with a bus stop 50 m from his house that takes him right outside his building.

Exercise Program

Participant Details	Participant Goals (Specific, Measurable, Action-orientated, Realistic, Timely, Self-determined)
Name: *Tariq Akhtar* Age: *45*	1. *Undertake four exercise sessions per week for 8 weeks: three gym-based sessions (prescription detailed below) and one soccer game*
Gender: *Male*	2. *Reduce waist circumference from 96 cm to 94 cm after 8 weeks of exercise training*
Body mass: *88 kg*	
Body mass index: *29.1 kg/m^2*	3. *Improve muscular strength and endurance (3RM leg press and 1RM bench press scores increase by 10% after 8 weeks of exercise training)*
Waist circumference: *96 cm*	
Resting heart rate: *68 bpm*	4. *Improve cardiorespiratory fitness into the good category after 8 weeks of exercise training*
Blood pressure: *122/82 mmHg*	
Maximal heart rate: *177 bpm* Age predicted / Measured (circle)	
Initial fitness/activity levels:	
Submaximal bike test (YMCA), estimated $\dot{V}O_2$max = 28 mL/kg/min (good)	
3RM leg press = 210 kg (average)	
1RM bench press = 75 kg (poor)	
Maximal push up test: 4 (poor)	
One 60-minute 'friendly' soccer match per week (two 30-minute halves with a 10-minute half-time break)	
No previous gym experience	

Initial Exercise Prescription (_8_ weeks)

Aerobic exercise

Type	Frequency	Intensity	Duration
Treadmill jogging	*3 times/week*	*112–132 bpm (40–59% HRR, RPE 1–13)*	*30 minutes*
Soccer match	*1 time/week*	*Game dependent, but aim to keep RPE > 12*	*60 minutes*

Resistance exercise

Type/exercise/body region	Frequency	Intensity	Sets/repetitions/rest
Circuit-based program (complete one full set of each exercise before starting next set) 1. *Seated leg press* 2. *Chest press* 3. *Hamstring curl* 4. *Lat pulldown* 5. *Seated leg extension* 6. *Calf raise* 7. *Triceps pulldown* 8. *Biceps curl* 9. *Prone hold (30 seconds)*	*3 times/week*	*3–5 RiR (5–7 RPE)*	*2 sets, 10 repetitions. No rest between sets as moving between exercises as part of circuit. Minimal rest between exercises.*

Flexibility exercise

Type/exercise	Frequency	Intensity	Sets/repetitions/rest
Static stretching: hamstrings, quadriceps, calves, pectorals, shoulders, neck, gluteals	*3 times/week*	*Stretch until feel 'pull without pain'*	*1 set, 1 repetition held for 60 seconds, no rest between stretches*

Exercise Program (continued)
Advice to Reduce Sedentary Behaviour:
• *Instead of watching TV each night, go to the gym or soccer 4 nights per week.* • *At work, set an alarm to stand up and move every 30 minutes. Every hour walk up and down one flight of stairs.* • *On 2 days per week (e.g. non-gym days), pack lunch from home and walk for 15 minutes during the lunch hour.* • *On 2 days per week (e.g. non-gym days), get off the bus one stop earlier and walk the remaining distance to work.*
Progressions for Improvement (with Timelines for Progression):
Aerobic exercise: *From week 8, increase the intensity of the aerobic work to 60–89% HRR and/or add in a 45-minute moderate-intensity jog on the weekends.* Resistance training: *from weeks 8–16, if confident with the exercises and techniques, increase reps to 12, then sets to 3 then intensity to 1–3 RiR (7–9 RPE).*
Target Activity Levels (Maintenance):
Aerobic exercise training: *150–300 minutes per week of moderate-intensity aerobic activity (or 75–150 minutes per week of vigorous-intensity aerobic activity) or an equivalent mix of moderate- and vigorous-intensity activity.* Resistance exercise training: *2–3 sessions per week targeting all major body regions. As strength is a primary goal, one session/week should include lower repetitions (n=3) for 3 sets at an intensity of 0–2 RiR (8–10 RPE).* Flexibility training: *2–3 days per week targeting all major muscle groups.*

7. The Exercise Session

A single exercise session should include four phases: 1. warm-up; 2. conditioning; 3. cool-down; and 4. stretching.

1. Warm-up. This involves 3–10 minutes of light- to moderate-intensity aerobic activity (e.g. walking) and active full range-of-motion exercises (e.g. leg swings, arm swings, calf pumps, walking lunges).

2. Conditioning. This generally consists of aerobic and/or resistance exercise. The exercise program should include aerobic and resistance exercises but they may not necessarily both be completed in the one session (e.g. Monday is aerobic training and Tuesday is resistance training). For this reason the 'and/or' is used here. When aerobic and resistance exercises are in the same session, the order that they are completed will depend on the aims of the program. If there is a greater desire to improve cardiorespiratory fitness then it is recommended to complete the aerobic component first. If muscular fitness is the primary goal then resistance training should come first. In addition to general stretching (see point 4 below) more flexibility exercises may be included in the conditioning phase. However, given the lack of evidence supporting the benefits of stretching, these should not replace other exercises. Neuromotor and/or bone loading exercises may also be added depending on the participant's goals.

3. Cool-down: Following a session that has contained aerobic exercise (perhaps with resistance exercise), 3–10 minutes of light- to moderate-intensity aerobic activity is recommended (e.g. walking).

4. Stretching: This may be performed after the warm-up or cool-down (see Practical 11).

Worked Case Study for the Exercise Session

Miles is 29 years old and has joined your fitness centre. As a member he receives a fitness assessment and you supervise his first session to prescribe weights/resistances and ensure the correct technique is being used. He has previous experience with weight training (he went to the gym 3 times per week for 3 years while at university approximately 10 years ago) but has only continued with infrequent body weight exercises at home since starting work as an electrical engineer. He would like to develop and maintain his muscle strength and endurance.

After conducting the fitness assessment (that does not include RM testing) you prescribe an exercise program with resistance exercises targeting all major body regions at a moderate intensity (see Exercise Log). During the initial exercise session, you set the resistance by observing Miles' technique during the repetitions. At the end of each set, you ask him to estimate how many more repetitions he could have completed with correct technique. You tell him that, as you wish him to exercise at a moderate intensity; when he finishes the set he should be able to complete 2–3 more repetitions with the correct technique. You explain that this is known as repetitions in reserve and noted as RiR on his Exercise Log.

Exercise Log

Name: Miles Stevens

Date

Warm Up

Activity	Time/Distance	Intensity	Completed
Elliptical Trainer	10 min	Moderate	✓

Aerobic

Activity	Time/Distance	Intensity	Completed
-	-	-	✓

Resistance

Exercise	Weight	Sets/Reps	Intensity	
Chest Press	70 kg	2/10	2–3 RiR [7–8 RPE]	Weight / Sets/Reps
Seated Leg Press	220kg	2/10	2–3 RiR [7–8 RPE]	Weight / Sets/Reps
Lat Pulldown	70 kg	2/10	2–3 RiR [7–8 RPE]	Weight / Sets/Reps
Hamstring Curl	30 kg	2/10	2–3 RiR [7–8 RPE]	Weight / Sets/Reps
Dumbbell Shoulder Press	12 kg	2/10	2–3 RiR [7–8 RPE]	Weight / Sets/Reps
Dumbbell Calf Raise	15 kg /hand	2/10	2–3 RiR [7–8 RPE]	Weight / Sets/Reps
Dumbbell Biceps Curl	10 kg	2/10	2–3 RiR [7–8 RPE]	Weight / Sets/Reps
Triceps Pulldown	20 kg	2/10	2–3 RiR [7–8 RPE]	Weight / Sets/Reps
Prone Hold	Hold 30s/rest 30s	2	-	Weight / Sets/Reps
Abdominal Crunches	-	2/10	-	Weight / Sets/Reps

Cool Down

Activity	Time	Sets/Reps	Intensity	Completed
Elliptical Trainer	5 min		Level 2–3	✓
Stretch all major muscle groups	10 min	2/30s	-	✓

Activity 2.4 Exercise risks

AIM:

- Modify an exercise program for an individual currently exercising based on potential risk of a musculoskeletal injury

TASK:

- Complete Worksheet 2.4 by answering the question based on the information provided in the Worked case study for the exercise session (Miles).

Worksheet 2.4 Exercise Risks
Question 1: How would you modify Miles' current training program to minimise the risk of a serious musculoskeletal injury? _____ _____ _____ _____ _____ _____ _____ _____

Activity 2.5 The exercise session

AIM:

- To design an exercise session

TASK:

- Complete Worksheet 2.5 by designing an initial session at the gym for Tariq (Worked case study for exercise programming under Activity 2.3) containing the warm-up, conditioning, cool-down and stretching stages (include the time of each component).

Worksheet 2.5 Exercise Session

Exercise log

Name: _____ Date: _____

Warm-up

Activity	Time/distance	Intensity	Completed
			✓

Aerobic

Activity	Time/distance	Intensity	Completed
			✓

Resistance

Exercise	Weight	Sets/reps	Intensity
	Weight		
	Sets/reps		
	Weight		
	Sets/reps		
	Weight		
	Sets/reps		
	Weight		
	Sets/reps		
	Weight		
	Sets/reps		
	Weight		
	Sets/reps		
	Weight		
	Sets/reps		
	Weight		
	Sets/reps		
	Weight		
	Sets/reps		
	Weight		
	Sets/reps		

Cool-down

Activity	Time	Sets/reps	Intensity	Completed
				✓
				✓

Activity 2.6 Exercise programming for an apparently healthy individual – A

AIM:
- To design an exercise program for an apparently healthy individual that: applies the general principles of exercise prescription; applies the principles of aerobic, resistance and flexibility training; and incorporates advice to reduce sedentary behaviour

Case study 2.1

Fiona is a 36-year-old woman who wants to 'tone up and lose weight', especially for her best friend's wedding in 6 months' time, in which she is a bridesmaid. Fiona works in retail (9.00 am to 5.30 pm, 5 days per week) and is on her feet most of the day. She drives to and from work, although there is a train stop nearby her work with a connecting station 1 km from her home. You measure Fiona's body weight at 73 kg and she is 168 cm tall, with a waist circumference of 82 cm, resting heart rate of 70 bpm and blood pressure of 116/70 mmHg. Fiona currently does no structured exercise during the week. On the weekends she attends a 90-minute yoga class. She would like to exercise before work two mornings each week and could also do more exercise on the weekend.

TASKS:
- Based on the information provided in Case study 2.1, complete Worksheet 2.6 by designing an exercise program for Fiona.
- Answer the additional questions below.

Worksheet 2.6 Designing an Exercise Program

Exercise Program	
Participant Details	**Participant Goals** *(Specific, Measurable, Action-orientated, Realistic, Timely, Self-determined)*
Name:	
Age:	
Gender:	
Body mass:	
Body mass index:	
Waist circumference:	
Resting heart rate:	
Blood pressure:	
Maximal heart rate: Age predicted/Measured (circle)	
Initial fitness/activity levels:	

Worksheet 2.6 Designing an Exercise Program (continued)

Initial Exercise Prescription (___ weeks)			
Aerobic exercise Type	Frequency	Intensity	Duration
Resistance exercise Type/exercise/body region	Frequency	Intensity	Sets/repetitions/rest
Flexibility exercise Type/exercise	Frequency	Intensity	Sets/repetitions/rest

Advice to reduce Sedentary Behaviour:

Progressions for Improvement (with Timelines for Progression):

Target Activity Levels (Maintenance):
Aerobic exercise training: Resistance exercise training: Flexibility training:

Worksheet 2.6 Designing an Exercise Program (continued)
Question 1: Fiona had started a gym program about 5 years ago, but only lasted 3 months before she gave up (stating that she 'got bored'). Which general principle of exercise programming (Box 1.2) might you address to prevent this happening with your program? _____
Question 2: Explain how you would address this principle to ensure that Fiona continues with your prescribed program. _____ _____ _____ _____ _____ _____ _____ _____ _____ _____

Activity 2.7 Exercise programming for an apparently healthy individual – B

AIM:

- To design an exercise program for an apparently healthy individual that: applies the general principles of exercise prescription; applies the principles of aerobic, resistance and flexibility training; and incorporates advice to reduce sedentary behaviour

Case study 2.2
Alberto is a 22-year-old university student who comes to see you to 'tone up his muscles and get stronger'. He studies information technology, is on campus 4 days per week and has just purchased a membership for the university gym. Alberto works Saturday and Sunday at a grocery store so would like to fit his exercise in during the week. He played sport throughout high school (mainly rugby league in the winter and cricket in the summer) but has never been to a gym or lifted weights. Alberto currently cycles 7 km to and from university but drives to work on the weekends. You measure his body weight as 80 kg and height as 181 cm with a waist circumference of 79 cm and blood pressure of 126/82 mmHg.

TASKS:

- Based on the information provided in Case study 2.2, complete Worksheet 2.7 by designing an exercise program for Alberto.
- Answer the additional questions below.

Worksheet 2.7 Designing an Exercise Program			
Exercise Program			
Participant Details		**Participant Goals** *(Specific, Measurable, Action-orientated, Realistic, Timely, Self-determined)*	
Name:			
Age:			
Gender:			
Body mass:			
Body mass index:			
Waist circumference:			
Resting heart rate:			
Blood pressure:			
Maximal heart rate: Age predicted/Measured (circle)			
Initial fitness/activity levels:			
Initial Exercise Prescription (_____ weeks)			
Aerobic exercise **Type**	**Frequency**	**Intensity**	**Duration**
Resistance exercise **Type/exercise/body region**	**Frequency**	**Intensity**	**Sets/repetitions/rest**

Worksheet 2.7 Designing an Exercise Program (continued)

Flexibility exercise Type/exercise	Frequency	Intensity	Sets/repetitions/rest

Advice to Reduce Sedentary Behaviour:

Progressions for Improvement (with Timelines for Progression):

Target Activity Levels (Maintenance):

Aerobic exercise training:

Resistance exercise training:

Flexibility training:

You re-test Alberto's muscular strength (chest press) at 8 weeks and at 16 weeks. At 8 weeks he has improved his 1RM by 20% and is extremely happy with this progress. At 16 weeks, he has improved by a further 10% and Alberto expresses a bit of disappointment, as he has been following your program and working hard.

Question 1: Which general principle of exercise programming (Box 1.2) is this an example of? _____

_____

Question 2: How would you communicate this to Alberto? _____

_____

_____

_____

_____

_____

Alberto takes 3 weeks off his training program during the study break and 2 weeks of exams.

Question 3: What do you think will happen to Alberto's strength and muscle mass in this time? _____

_____

_____

_____

_____

_____

Worksheet 2.7 Designing an Exercise Program (continued)

Question 4: Which general principle of exercise programming (Box 1.2) is this an example of? _____

_____

Question 5: Explain how you would adapt the training program to account for this change. _____

_____

_____

_____

_____

References

1   Garber CE, Blissmer B, Deschenes MR, et al. 2011. American College of Sports Medicine position stand. Quantity and quality of exercise for developing and maintaining cardiorespiratory, musculoskeletal, and neuromotor fitness in apparently healthy adults: guidance for prescribing exercise. *Med Sci Sports Exerc*. 43:1334–1359.

2   Sharman MJ, Cresswell AG, Riek S. 2006. Proprioceptive neuromuscular facilitation stretching: mechanisms and clinical implications. *Sports Med*. 36:929–939.

3   Taylor JL, Holland DJ, Spathis JG, et al. 2019. Guidelines for the delivery and monitoring of high-intensity interval training in clinical populations. *Prog Cardiovasc Dis*. Mar–Apr 62(2):140–146.

4   Weston KS, Wisloff U, Coombes JS. 2014. High-intensity interval training in patients with lifestyle-induced cardiometabolic disease: a systematic review and meta-analysis. *Br J Sports Med*. 48:1227–1234.

5   Tanaka H, Monahan KD, Seals DR. 2001. Age-predicted maximal heart rate revisited. *J Am Coll Cardiol*. 37:153–156.

6   American College of Sports Medicine. 2018. *ACSM's Guidelines for Exercise Testing and Prescription,* 10th Edition. Baltimore, MD, USA: Lippincott, Williams and Wilkins.

7   Zourdos MC, Goldsmith JA, Helms ER, et al. 2019. Proximity to failure and total repetitions performed in a set influences accuracy of intraset repetitions in reserve-based rating of perceived exertion. *J Strength Cond Res*. 7 Feb.

8   Schoenfeld BJ, Ogborn DI, Krieger JW. 2015. Effect of repetition duration during resistance training on muscle hypertrophy: a systematic review and meta-analysis. *Sports Med*. 45:577–585.

9   Schoenfeld BJ, Ratamess NA, Peterson MD, et al. 2014. Effects of different volume-equated resistance training loading strategies on muscular adaptations in well-trained men. *J Strength Cond Res*. 28:2909–2918.

10 Bird SP, Tarpenning KM, Marino FE. 2005. Designing resistance training programmes to enhance muscular fitness: a review of the acute programme variables. *Sports Med*. 35:841–851.

11 Cormie P. 2008. Does an optimal load exist for power training? Point/Counterpoint - Pro. *Strength Con J*. 30:67–68.

12 Flanagan S. 2008. Does an optimal load exist for power training? Point/Counterpoint - Con *Strength Con J*. 30:68–69.

13 Cormie P, McGuigan MR, Newton RU. 2011. Developing maximal neuromuscular power: Part 1—biological basis of maximal power production. *Sports Med*. 41:17–38.

14 Baker D, Newton RU. 2005. Methods to increase the effectiveness of maximal power training for the upper body. *Strength Con J*. 27:24–32.

15 Helms ER, Byrnes RK, Cooke DM, et al. 2018. RPE vs. Percentage 1RM loading in periodized programs matched for sets and repetitions. *Front Physiol*. 9:247.

16 Zourdos MC, Klemp A, Dolan C, et al. 2016. Novel resistance training-specific rating of perceived exertion scale measuring repetitions in reserve. *J Strength Cond Res*. 30:267–275.

17 Robertson RJ, Goss FL, Rutkowski J, et al. 2003. Concurrent validation of the OMNI perceived exertion scale for resistance exercise. *Med Sci Sports Exerc*. 35:333–341.

18 Testa M, Noakes TD, Desgorces FD. 2012. Training state improves the relationship between rating of perceived exertion and relative exercise volume during resistance exercises. *J Strength Cond Res*. 26:2990–2996.

19 Brzycki M. 2012. *A Practical Approach To Strength Training*, 4th Ed. Indianapolis, IN: Blue River Press.

20 Willardson JM, Norton L, Wilson G. 2010. Training to failure and beyond in mainstream resistance exercise programs. *Strength Cond J*. 32:21–29.

21 Balsalobre-Fernandez C, Munoz-Lopez M, Marchante D, et al. 2018. Repetitions in reserve and rate of perceived exertion increase the prediction capabilities of the load-velocity relationship. *J Strength Cond Res*. 10.

22 Williams CJ, Gurd BJ, Bonafiglia JT, et al. 2019. A multi-center comparison of O2peak trainability between interval training and moderate intensity continuous training. *Front Physiol*. 10:19.

23 Buchheit M, Laursen PB. 2013. High-intensity interval training, solutions to the programming puzzle: Part I: cardiopulmonary emphasis. *Sports Med*. 43:313–338.

PRACTICAL 3
EXERCISE PROGRAMMING FOR HEALTHY POPULATIONS WITH SPECIAL CONSIDERATIONS

Jeff S. Coombes and Shelley E. Keating

Introduction

An accredited exercise scientist should have the knowledge and skills to design exercise programs (including exercise prescription and advice to reduce sedentary behaviour) for healthy populations that have special considerations. This includes people with a weight loss goal, women with uncomplicated pregnancies, older individuals, children and adolescents. If an individual from one of these populations has a clinical condition, an accredited exercise physiologist should design the exercise program.

1. Exercise Programming for Weight Loss

Guidelines recommend weight loss for individuals who are overweight with one or more cardiovascular disease (CVD) risk factors (e.g. hypertension) and for those with obesity.[1] The target weight loss for these individuals is at least 5–10% within 6 months. This amount has been shown to be clinically significant due to its impact on CVD risk factors.[2] However, it should be recognised that beneficial improvements in CVD risk factors have been reported with as little as 2–3% of weight loss.[3] Weight maintenance is defined as sustaining a weight change of < 3% of body weight over a long-term period.[4]

Lifestyle interventions for weight loss should include both dietary adjustments to decrease energy intake and sufficient exercise to create a significant negative energy deficit. Aerobic exercise that will provide the greatest energy expenditure over a week should be the focus of the exercise component. The following strategies are taken from the position stand on weight management from the American College of Sports Medicine (ACSM)[5] and should guide the design of the exercise program.

Exercise Prescription

- Aerobic exercise
  - Type = prolonged rhythmic activities (e.g. walking, cycling)
  - Frequency = 5–7 days/week
  - Intensity = moderate to vigorous (refer to Box 2.1 for approaches to monitor intensity)
  - Duration = 300–470 min/week
  - Volume ≥ 8400 kJ/week
- Resistance and flexibility exercises
  - Types, frequencies and volumes of resistance and flexibility training should be the same as for the general population, taking into account the individual's experience, goals and needs.

Additional Considerations

- If previously inactive, start slowly (lower intensity, shorter durations, less exercises).
- The inclusion of resistance and flexibility training should not be at the expense of the aerobic training.

- More exercise (energy expenditure) will result in greater weight loss (when caloric intake is kept constant).
- Additional physical activity via reducing sedentary behaviour should be integrated into the exercise program.
- Exercise should be included into a person's lifestyle for weight loss maintenance.[6,7]
- Use goal setting for short- and long-term weight loss (e.g. lose 5% of body weight over 6 months).

Worked Case Study for Weight Loss

The purpose of this worked case study is to explain weight loss calculations that take into account changes in energy expenditure (from exercise prescription) and energy intake.

Robert is a 47-year-old sales representative who weighs 108 kg with a height of 178 cm (BMI = 34 kg/m^2 [class I obesity]) and waist circumference is 109 cm (abdominally obese). He currently does not exercise and reports some minor knee pain when walking/taking the stairs. His GP has recommended he start an exercise program to lose 10% of his body weight. Robert underwent a medically supervised cardiopulmonary exercise test and his $\dot{V}O_2$max was 32 mL/kg/min with a maximal heart rate of 179 bpm. His resting heart rate was 78 bpm. He had no signs or symptoms of cardiovascular disease during the test.

Based on the recommendations from his GP, Robert needs to lose 11 kg to achieve 10% weight loss. Your target for him is to achieve $\geq$ 8400 kJ/week energy expenditure with moderate-vigorous exercise. Given his current level of activity, you commence a moderate intensity aerobic exercise prescription (46–63% $\dot{V}O_2$max) on 3 days per week for 30 minutes per day. Due to the reported knee pain, you discuss with Robert the types of aerobic exercise which may best suit him. You agree that stationary cycling is the best option to begin.

Estimated fat loss from the initial prescription

It is estimated that you need to have a caloric deficit of 39 000 kJ to lose 1 kg of body fat.[8] Therefore, if Robert wants to lose 11 kg (ideally of body fat) he will need to expend 39 000 kJ $\times$ 11 = 429 000 kJ. We also know that a $\dot{V}O_2$ of 1 L/min expends approximately 21 kJ,[8] and thus we are able to determine approximately how long it will take to expend a set number of kilojoules at a set work rate. For this volume of exercise to result in an 11 kg weight loss, it is assumed there is no change to his caloric intake.

Your initial exercise prescription was stationary cycling for 30 minutes, 3 days per week at an intensity the equivalent of 46–63% $\dot{V}O_2$max. You know that Robert's $\dot{V}O_2$max was estimated at 32 mL/kg/min, so your prescription will aim to have him exercise between 14 and 20 mL/kg/min. In absolute terms (knowing his body weight is 108 kg)* this is equivalent to 1.5–2.2 L/min and thus 31.5–46.2 kJ/min (using 1 L/min = 21 kJ expenditure). Therefore, each week Robert will expend between 2835 kJ (31.5 kJ $\times$ 30 min $\times$ 3 sessions per week) and 4158 kJ (46.2 kJ $\times$ 30 min $\times$ 3 sessions per week). At this exercise prescription it would take Robert approximately 103–151 weeks to expend the 429 000 kJ to lose 11 kg of body fat.

Dietary component

As weight loss is Robert's primary goal, he has also been referred to a dietitian who has placed him on a dietary program that results in a 2100 kJ/day (14 700 kJ/week) caloric restriction. This means that Robert's weekly energy deficit is now between 17 535 kJ (14 700 kJ [diet] + 2835 kJ [exercise]) and 18 858 kJ (14 700 kJ [diet] + 4158 kJ [exercise]). Thus, it would now take Robert an estimated 23–24 weeks to lose 11 kg of body fat.

Activity 3.1 Exercise programming for weight loss

. . . .

AIM:
- To apply principles of weight loss to make relevant calculations regarding energy balance

TASK:
- Based on the information provided in Case study 3.1, complete Worksheet 3.1 by answering the questions.

(*To make the calculation easier, Robert's weight will stay the same. This would overestimate the amount of energy needed to be expended by a slight amount. This would be potentially balanced against a slight decrease in resting metabolic rate with weight loss.)

Case study 3.1

Robert (from the previous worked case study) revisits you after 4 weeks of his lifestyle program. He reports that he has adhered well to both the dietary recommendations from the dietitian and his exercise program. Robert has lost 3 kg (body weight is now 105 kg and he is 'feeling fitter'). He would like to increase the intensity of his sessions and to add in an additional day per week, but currently doesn't have time to do more than 30 minutes per session. You re-measure his $\dot{V}O_2$max as 35 mL/kg/min and progress his exercise prescription accordingly to stationary cycling for 30 minutes, 4 days per week at an intensity the equivalent of 70–90% $\dot{V}O_2$max (moderate to vigorous intensity). The dietitian has kept their caloric restriction recommendations the same (2100 kJ deficit per day).

Worksheet 3.1 Exercise Programming for Weight Loss

Question 1: How many kilojoules per week will Robert be expending with this new exercise prescription? Show your workings. _____

_____

_____

_____

_____

_____

_____

Question 2: How many kilojoules per week is Robert expending now by exercise and caloric restriction combined? Show your workings. _____

_____

_____

_____

_____

_____

Question 3: How long would it take to lose an additional 8 kg based on exercise alone at the new prescription? Show your workings. _____

_____

_____

_____

_____

_____

_____

Worksheet 3.1 Exercise Programming for Weight Loss (continued)

Question 4: How long would it take to lose an additional 8 kg based on the combination of diet and exercise at the new prescription? Show your workings. _____

_____

_____

_____

_____

_____

_____

Activity 3.2 Exercise programming for weight loss

AIM:

- To design an exercise program for weight loss that: applies the general principles of exercise prescription; applies the principles of aerobic, resistance and flexibility training; advises to reduce sedentary behaviour; and takes into account special considerations

TASKS:

- Based on the information provided in Case study 3.2, complete Worksheet 3.2 by designing an exercise program for Sumaira.
- Answer the additional questions.

Case study 3.2

Sumaira is a 57-year-old female who is classified as obese, with a BMI of 34 kg/m². She is a high school English teacher and recently visited her doctor as she has been feeling more tired than usual. Her doctor suggested she start exercising. Sumaira doesn't smoke and enjoys 2 or 3 glasses of wine each week, always with dinner. She often snacks on kilojoule-dense energy drinks and snacks to lift her energy as she works. Sumaira does not do any exercise but is on playground duty 3 days a week in which she walks around the school grounds for 30 minutes at lunch time. She does stand up when she teaches, but generally spends up to 6 hours per day sitting at either her classroom or office desk.

Key assessment results from Sumaira's doctor include the following.

- Blood pressure: 132/86 mmHg
- Total cholesterol: 7.1 mmol/L
- HDL cholesterol: 0.8 mmol/L
- LDL cholesterol: 4.9 mmol/L
- Fasting glucose: 5.5 mmol/L
- Waist circumference: 98 cm
- Weight: 82 kg.
- Resting heart rate: 78 bpm

Sumaira is keen to begin exercise training as she is worried that her current lifestyle could lead to type 2 diabetes (for which Sumaira has a family history) or cardiovascular disease. She reports some osteoarthritis in her knees, which gives her pain when she does activities such as stair climbing. You conduct an initial exercise test using a submaximal treadmill protocol which is well tolerated and estimate her cardiorespiratory fitness at 20 mL/kg/min. Her main goal is to lose weight and she hopes that this will also lead to an increase in her energy levels.

In order to establish an initial exercise program for Sumaira, you ask her further about her weekly schedule. Sumaira has after-school activities on Mondays and Wednesdays and on Saturdays she usually spends the day with her young grandchildren. Together you agree that she will begin exercising 3 days per week (after work on Tuesday and Thursday, and on Sundays).

Worksheet 3.2 Exercise Programming for Weight Loss

Exercise Program

Participant Details	Participant Goals (Specific, Measurable, Action-orientated, Realistic, Timely, Self-determined)
Name:	
Age:	
Gender:	
Body mass:	
Body mass index:	
Waist circumference:	
Resting heart rate:	
Blood pressure:	
Maximal heart rate: Age predicted/Measured (circle)	
Initial fitness/activity levels:	

Initial Exercise Prescription (____ weeks)

Aerobic exercise Type	Frequency	Intensity	Duration

Resistance exercise Type/exercise/body region	Frequency	Intensity	Sets/repetitions/rest

Flexibility exercise Type/exercise	Frequency	Intensity	Sets/repetitions/rest

Worksheet 3.2 Exercise Programming for Weight Loss (continued)
Advice to Reduce Sedentary Behaviour:
Progressions for Improvement (with timelines for progression):
Target Activity Levels (maintenance):
Aerobic exercise training:
Resistance exercise training:
Flexibility training:

Question 1: Based on your initial exercise prescription, calculate how many weeks it would take Sumaira to lose 5 kg of body fat with exercise alone. Show your workings. _____ ____

_____

_____

_____

_____

_____

_____

_____

Question 2: What other allied health professionals could Sumaira consult to assist with her primary goal?

_____

_____

_____

_____

_____

_____

_____

_____

_____

_____

2. Exercise Programming for During and After Pregnancy

Exercise during pregnancy and the postpartum period in women without warning signs or contraindications (see Box 3.1) is safe, has health benefits for the mother and her unborn child, and reduces the risks of pregnancy-related complications. All women with an uncomplicated pregnancy should be encouraged to meet exercise guidelines for the general population before, during and after pregnancy. However, some modifications to an exercise program may be required to accommodate the anatomical and physiological changes which occur as the pregnancy progresses. The following strategies are taken from the American College of Obstetricians and Gynaecologists,[9] the Royal Australian New Zealand College of Obstetricians and Gynaecologists (RANZCOG),[10] the Canadian Guidelines[11] and a position statement from Sports Medicine Australia,[12] and should guide the design of the exercise program.

Box 3.1   Warning Signs and Contraindications for Exercising During Pregnancy[9–12,20]

Warning signs

- Severe chest pain
- Persistent excessive shortness of breath—that does not resolve with rest
- Severe headache
- Persistent dizziness/feeling faint—that does not resolve with rest
- Regular painful uterine contractions
- Vaginal bleeding
- Persistent loss of fluid from the vagina—indicating possible ruptured membranes

Relative contraindications

- History of spontaneous miscarriage, premature labour or fetal growth restriction
- Mild/moderate cardiovascular or chronic respiratory disease
- Pregnancy-induced hypertension
- Poorly controlled seizure disorder
- Type 1 diabetes
- Symptomatic anaemia
- Malnutrition, significantly underweight or eating disorder
- Twin pregnancy after the 28th week
- Other significant medical condition

Absolute contraindications

- Incompetent cervix
- Ruptured membranes, premature labour
- Persistent second- or third-trimester bleeding
- Placenta praevia
- Pre-eclampsia
- Evidence of intrauterine growth restriction
- Multiple gestation (triplets or higher number)
- Poorly controlled Type 1 diabetes, hypertension or thyroid disease
- Other serious cardiovascular, respiratory or systemic disorder

Exercise Prescription

- Aerobic exercise
  - Type = variety of weight bearing (e.g. walking) and non-weight bearing (e.g. swimming)
  - Frequency = 3–5 days/week
  - Intensity = moderate to vigorous (RPE 12–17)
  - Duration = 30–60 min/day
  - Volume = 150–300 min/week
- Resistance exercise
  - Type = machines, free weights, body weight exercises, resistance bands
  - Frequency = 2–3 non-consecutive days/week
  - Volume = 8–10 exercises to train all six major body regions: trunk; chest; shoulders; arms; back; and legs; 1–3 sets of 8–12 repetitions (beginners start at 1 set)—light to moderate intensity (3–5 RiR [5–7 RPE])
  - Additional exercises to strengthen the pelvic floor are recommended (see Box 3.2)
- Flexibility exercise
  - Type = target seven areas: 1. chest; 2. back; 3. arms (anterior); 4. arms (posterior); 5. legs (anterior); 6. legs (posterior); and 7. legs (medial and lateral) (see Practical 11)
  - Frequency = ≥ 2–3 days/week with daily being most effective
  - Volume = stretch to the point of tightness or slight discomfort and hold for 30–60 seconds; stretching each area/muscle for 60 seconds will take around 10 minutes

---

Box 3.2   Exercises to Strengthen the Pelvic Floor During and After Pregnancy*

1. Identify pelvic floor muscles. Let the participant know that the pelvic floor muscles can be identified by attempting to stop urinating in midstream. If they succeed, they have used their pelvic floor muscles. This 'stop test' is not recommended as a regular exercise.

2. Positioning. They can do the exercises in any position.

3. Technique. Contract the pelvic floor muscles and hold for 5 seconds, then relax for 5 seconds. Complete this five times and repeat three times a day. Progress to keeping the muscles contracted for 10 seconds at a time and then relaxing for 10 seconds between contractions. It is important to relax the muscles after each contraction.

4. Maintain focus. Concentrate on gently tightening the pelvic floor muscles, avoiding tension in muscles in the abdomen, thighs or buttocks. Breathe normally during the exercises.

*Due to the difficulty in performing pelvic floor exercises, assistance from an appropriate allied health professional (e.g. women's health physiotherapist) may be needed. Any woman with symptoms of pelvic floor dysfunction (e.g. pain, incontinence) should also seek advice.

Additional Considerations

- A tool should be used for screening (Appendix C).
- If previously inactive, start slowly (lower intensity, shorter durations, fewer exercises).
- Exercise prescription should be modified based on exercise history, discomforts and abilities across the time of pregnancy.
- The 'talk/sing test' or RPE should be used to monitor aerobic exercise intensity.
- Extended warm-ups and cool-downs (both 10–15 minutes) consisting of light intensity physical activity are recommended.
- Pregnant women should be educated on the warning signs to stop exercising (Box 3.3).
- Avoid heat stress/hyperthermia, especially in the first trimester. Adjust physical activity/exercise in excessively hot weather, especially when there is high humidity. Prolonged exercise should preferably be indoors in an air-conditioned environment.

Box 3.3   Warning Signs to Stop Exercising During Pregnancy[8–12]

- Vaginal bleeding or (amniotic) fluid leakage
- Shortness of breath prior to exertion
- Dizziness, feeling faint or severe headache
- Chest pain
- Decreased fetal movement
- Regular painful uterine contractions
- Preterm labour

- Avoid contact sports or activities that may increase risk of trauma to mother or fetus (e.g. football, rugby, soccer, basketball, horseback riding, rock climbing).
- Avoid significant changes in pressure (e.g. skydiving, scuba diving).
- Avoid using the Valsalva manoeuvre during any activity.
- Avoid dehydration and inadequate nutrition. Staying well hydrated and ensuring energy intake is leading to the appropriate gestational weight gain is recommended.
- Avoid long periods of motionless posture (standing still, or lying in a supine position), especially if this causes light headedness or dizziness. After 28 weeks, exercises normally done in the supine position may be modified by tilting the upper body to 45 degrees or completing the exercises while lying on the side. Some yoga poses may also have to be modified later in pregnancy.
- Avoid physical activity/exercise at high altitude (above 2000 m) unless acclimatised and trained to do this prior to pregnancy. Regular high-altitude high-intensity athletes should seek advice/supervision from an appropriately qualified healthcare professional.
- Women who are considering high volumes of exercise training (high intensity, prolonged duration, heavy weights etc.) should seek advice and guidance from a healthcare professional who is knowledgeable about the effects of high-level training on maternal and fetal outcomes.
- After pregnancy, gradually resume light to moderate exercise after 4–6 weeks for vaginal delivery and 8–10 weeks for caesarean (with medical guidance). Women with higher fitness and more vigorous exercise programs prior to, and during, pregnancy may resume exercise sooner.
- Always wear appropriate shoes for the activity, non-restrictive clothing and a supportive bra. When it is hot, wear loose clothing made from 'breathable' fabric.
- Be aware of diastasis recti and how this may impact on exercise prescription (Box 3.4).

Box 3.4   Diastasis Recti

Pregnant or postpartum women may develop diastasis recti, or abdominal separation. It is a gap of around 3 cm between the two sides of the rectus abdominis muscle made up of connective tissue (linea alba). It is caused by stretching of the abdominal muscle during pregnancy or birth and is more common when: 1. the woman is over 35 years of age; 2. the baby has a high birth weight; 3. it is a multiple-birth pregnancy; or 4. the woman has had multiple pregnancies. Excessive abdominal exercises after the first trimester of pregnancy are also a cause.

Typically, the separation of the abdominal muscles will decrease within the first 8 weeks after childbirth. The weakening of the abdominal muscles may make it difficult to lift objects and cause lower back pain. Additional complications include weakened pelvic alignment and altered posture. Consultation with an appropriate allied health professional (e.g. women's health physiotherapist) is recommended for the prescription of correct abdominal exercises for women with diastasis recti.

Worked Case Study for Exercise Programming for During and After Pregnancy

Melissa is a 28-year-old woman who is pregnant with her second child and is in her second trimester (19 weeks' gestation). She is referred to you by her GP with permission to undertake regular exercise within her capabilities, so long as her pregnancy continues without complications. Melissa also has a son who is 2 years old and she works part-time with a desk job (3 days per week—Monday, Wednesday and Friday). She takes care of her 2 year old on her days off. Prior to her first pregnancy, Melissa participated recreationally in triathlons, and when her son was 8 months old she gradually recommenced swimming and cycling, but did not return to jogging due to experiencing some knee pain. Melissa has experienced moderate morning sickness during her first trimester and reports feeling significant fatigue. As a consequence she has not continued to regularly swim and cycle. She undertook a few runs and swims early in her pregnancy, but since 8 weeks' gestation she has only been walking to and from the train station 3 days/week (10 minutes each way at a low intensity).

Melissa has told you that she would like to have a more structured exercise program. During her last pregnancy she was able to continue swimming, stationary cycling and walking until 30 weeks' gestation and gradually modified/reduced her activity according to her energy levels and physical size/comfort. Upon discussion, Melissa agrees with you that the primary goals will be to maintain physical activity at a level likely to maintain health and fitness during pregnancy. Melissa owns an aerobic stepper, a moderate-strength resistance band and a fitball.

You undertake an initial assessment and develop a plan with Melissa (information from the assessment and prescription in Worked example: Exercise programming for pregnancy).

Worked Example: Exercise Programming for Pregnancy

Exercise Program

Participant Details	**Participant Goals** *(Specific, Measurable, Action-orientated, Realistic, Timely, Self-determined)*
Name: *Melissa*	The main goal is to continue to be physically active throughout pregnancy within the limitations of the physical changes that occur, working part-time and caring for a 2 year old.
Age: *28*	Specifically:
Gender: *Female*	1. From weeks 19–30:
Body mass: *62 kg*	• walk 2 × 15 minutes 3 days per week at a moderate intensity (workdays)
Body mass index: *N/A given pregnancy*	• swim once per week for 45 minutes at a moderate intensity (weekend)
Waist circumference: *N/A given pregnancy*	• two home-based resistance sessions per week (while husband looks after their child)
Resting heart rate: *76 bpm, note: resting heart rate increases during pregnancy*	• pelvic floor exercises daily
Blood pressure: *124/84 mmHg*	2. From weeks 31–40:
Maximal heart rate: Age predicted/Measured (circle) *N/A, given maximal heart rate decreases during pregnancy and that maximal testing is not recommended unless medically indicated*	• modify the above depending on physical capabilities (review at 30 weeks)
Initial fitness/activity levels: *Previous exercise history: high activity (triathlon training—running, swimming, cycling and Pilates)* *Current exercise history: 2 × 10-minute walks to and from train station at 'low' intensity, 3 days per week*	

Initial Exercise Prescription (<u>11</u> weeks)

Aerobic exercise **Type**	**Frequency**	**Intensity**	**Duration**
Walk	*3 times/week (Monday, Wednesday and Friday)*	*Moderate: RPE 13–14*	*2 × 15 minutes*
Swim	*1 time/week (Saturday or Sunday)*	*Moderate: RPE 13–14*	*1–1.5 km swim (30–40 minutes)*

Worked Example: Exercise Programming for Pregnancy (continued)

Resistance exercise Type/exercise/body region	Frequency	Intensity	Sets/repetitions/rest
Home-based session: Warm-up (5 minutes, by using aerobic stepper). Body weight wall squats using fitball to guide lower back, wall push-ups, resistance band seated row, resistance band shoulder press, calf raise—single leg off the aerobic stepper— holding on to support for balance, resistance band biceps curl, resistance band triceps extension, resistance band seated leg extension and leg curl	2 times/week (Tuesday, Thursday)	Light to moderate: 3–5 RiR (5–7 RPE)	10 repetitions, 2 sets
Pelvic floor:	Daily	Varied intensity and duration of holds	10 minutes

Flexibility exercise Type/exercise	Frequency	Intensity	Sets/repetitions/rest
Static stretch for chest, back, arms, legs, neck and shoulders	6 times/week	Stretch to the sensation of tightness; important not to overstretch given increased joint laxity during pregnancy	2 sets

Advice to Reduce Sedentary Behaviour:

At work: stand up from desk every 30 minutes and walk to the end of the corridor to get a glass of water. Twice per day, walk up and down the three flights of stairs.

Progressions for Improvement (with timelines for progression):

Aerobic exercise: 'Progression' for walking and swimming will include being able to maintain RPE with increasing body mass and change in physical capabilities. After the first 6 weeks of the initial prescription, you may choose to vary your walking route to include 1–2 hills to maintain a 'moderate' intensity.

Resistance exercise: Progression in reps to 12, then sets to 3, then resistance band strength to increase the intensity to moderate (2–3 RiR). To progress the resistance, increase the tautness of the resistance band and then use the next resistance band strength grade and continue progression to maintain 2–3 RiR by increasing band tautness.

Target Activity Levels (maintenance):

Aerobic exercise training: 150–250 minutes per week of a combination of brisk walking or swimming at a moderate intensity (RPE 12–14)

Resistance exercise training: Two sessions per week of body weight and resistance band exercises at moderate intensity (23–RiR), 8–10 exercises, 12 reps, 3 sets, with daily pelvic floor exercises.

Flexibility training: Stretch major muscle groups at the end of each aerobic and resistance training session.

Activity 3.3 Exercise programming for during and after pregnancy

AIM:

- To design an exercise program for during and after pregnancy that: applies the general principles of exercise prescription; applies the principles of aerobic, resistance and flexibility training; incorporates advice to reduce sedentary behaviour; and takes into account special considerations

TASKS:

- Based on the information provided in Case study 3.3, complete Worksheet 3.3 by designing an exercise program for Li.
- Answer the additional questions.

Case study 3.3
Li is 29 years old and recently learned that she is pregnant with her first child. She is now at 12 weeks' gestation, weighs 58 kg and is 164 cm tall. Prior to this pregnancy, Li was attending two yoga sessions per week and using the gym in her townhouse complex three times per week in which she would do 20 minutes of aerobic work at a 'moderate' intensity and used the weight machines (seated leg press, calf raise, dumbbell lunges with 5 kg in each hand, chest press, lateral pulldown, triceps pulldown and biceps curl). Li is keen to keep fit during her pregnancy but is concerned about continuing her exercise program as she does not know which exercises are safe. Her obstetrician has given her permission to continue the exercises that she is doing, pending no complications arise and that she changes anything that is not comfortable and does not overheat. She also said that she may find it difficult to do regular yoga and suggested to take up an antenatal yoga class instead.

Worksheet 3.3 Exercise Programming for During and After Pregnancy	
Exercise Program	
Participant Details	**Participant goals** *(Specific, Measurable, Action-orientated, Realistic, Timely, Self-determined)*
Name:	
Age:	
Gender:	
Body mass:	
Body mass index:	
Waist circumference:	
Resting heart rate:	
Blood pressure:	
Maximal heart rate: Age predicted/Measured (circle)	
Initial fitness/activity levels:	

Worksheet 3.3 Exercise Programming for During and After Pregnancy (continued)

Initial Exercise Prescription (___ weeks)

Aerobic exercise Type	Frequency	Intensity	Duration

Resistance exercise Type/exercise/body region	Frequency	Intensity	Sets/repetitions/rest

Flexibility exercise Type/exercise	Frequency	Intensity	Sets/repetitions/rest

Advice to Reduce Sedentary Behaviour:

Progressions for Improvement (with timelines for progression):

Target Activity Levels (maintenance):

Aerobic exercise training:
Resistance exercise training:
Flexibility training:

Question 1: What method will you use to prescribe aerobic exercise intensity, and why? _____

_____

_____

_____

Worksheet 3.3 Exercise Programming for During and After Pregnancy (continued)

Question 2: What additional considerations may you need to consider in the second trimester that may lead to modification of your exercise prescription? _____

_____

_____

_____

_____

Question 3: What additional considerations may you need to consider in the third trimester that may lead to modification of your exercise prescription? _____

_____

_____

_____

_____

Question 4: What are possible considerations that will determine when, what type and how much activity she can return to postnatally? _____

_____

_____

_____

_____

_____

Activity 3.4 Exercise programming for after pregnancy

AIM:

- To design an exercise program for after pregnancy that: applies the general principles of exercise prescription; applies the principles of aerobic, resistance and flexibility training; incorporates advice to reduce sedentary behaviour; and takes into account special considerations

TASK:

- Based on the information provided in Case study 3.4, complete Worksheet 3.4 by designing an exercise program for Gillian.

Case study 3.4

Gillian is a 27-year-old woman who gave birth to her second child 12 weeks ago via a caesarean section. She also has a 2-year-old daughter. Gillian's GP has recommended that she resume physical activity and given that she did not deliver her baby vaginally, has not had an internal pelvic floor examination. During her stay in the hospital post-birth she was examined by a physiotherapist who noted a 3 cm abdominal separation, which has now reduced to 2 cm.

Before her first child, Gillian was quite active, attending a local bootcamp three mornings each week and doing a 5-km Park Run every Saturday. She did not do a lot of activity during her first pregnancy and did not resume her activity after the birth of her daughter. Gillian would like to start exercising again so that she has the energy and fitness to keep up with her children and to manage the housework. She would eventually like to start doing Park Run again and even participate in a 10 km run. Gillian currently weighs 72 kg (she was 60 kg at the start of her second pregnancy and increased to 76 kg by the end of the pregnancy). You measure her height at 164 cm, her blood pressure at 118/70 mmHg and her resting heart rate at 72 bpm.

Worksheet 3.4 Exercise After Pregnancy

Exercise Program

Participant Details	Participant Goals (Specific, Measurable, Action-orientated, Realistic, Timely, Self-determined)
Name:	
Age:	
Gender:	
Body mass:	
Body mass index:	
Waist circumference:	
Resting heart rate:	
Blood pressure:	
Maximal heart rate: Age predicted/Measured (circle)	
Initial fitness/activity levels:	

Initial Exercise Prescription (____ weeks)

Aerobic exercise Type	Frequency	Intensity	Duration

Resistance exercise Type/exercise/body region	Frequency	Intensity	Sets/repetitions/rest

Flexibility exercise Type/exercise	Frequency	Intensity	Sets/repetitions/rest

Worksheet 3.4 Exercise After Pregnancy (continued)
Advice to Reduce Sedentary Behaviour:
Progressions for Improvement (with timelines for progression):
Target Activity Levels (maintenance):
Aerobic exercise training: Resistance exercise training: Flexibility training:

3. Exercise Programming for Older Individuals

For the purposes of this manual, older individuals will be defined as $\geq$ 65 years old. Exercise prescription for older individuals is similar to that for the general population except that neuromotor and bone loading exercises should also be added. These may be able to be interspersed between aerobic and resistance training exercises in the same session. The following strategies are taken from position statements from ESSA[13,14] and a position stand from ACSM[15] and should guide the design of the exercise program.

Exercise Prescription
- Aerobic exercise
  - Type = non-weight bearing (e.g. cycling, swimming) to avoid orthopaedic stress (e.g. from jogging)
  - Frequency $\geq$ 5 days/week for moderate intensity, $\geq$ 3 days/week for vigorous intensity
  - Intensity = moderate to vigorous
  - Duration = 30−60 min/day of moderate intensity or 20−30 min/day for vigorous intensity; may be accumulated in 10-minute bouts
- Resistance exercise
  - Type = progressive resistance training programs or weight-bearing calisthenics, stair climbing and other muscle strengthening activities that aim to improve strength, power and endurance
  - Frequency $\geq$ 2 days/week with daily being most effective; 1 session/week should focus on power training

- o Volume = light intensity (4–6 RiR [5–6 RPE]) for beginners; progress to moderate (2–3 RiR [7–8 RPE]) to heavy (0–1 RiR [9–10 RPE]); 8–10 exercises involving the major muscle groups; 1–3 sets of 8–12 repetitions (beginners start at 1 set); for power training, light to moderate intensity for 6–10 repetitions with high-speed movements
- Flexibility exercise
  - o Type = target seven areas: 1. chest; 2. back; 3. arms (anterior); 4. arms (posterior); 5. legs (anterior); 6. legs (posterior); and 7. legs (medial and lateral) (see Practical 11) with slow movements that end in a static stretch—avoid ballistic movements
  - o Frequency ≥ 2 days/week
  - o Volume = stretch to the point of tightness or slight discomfort and hold for 30–60 seconds; stretching each area for 60 seconds will take around 10 minutes
- Neuromotor exercise
  - o Type = motor skills (balance, agility, coordination, gait), proprioceptive training (e.g. exercises with eyes closed), multimodal activities (e.g. tai chi, yoga) (see Box 3.5 for additional details)
  - o Frequency ≥ 2–3 days/week
  - o Volume = 20–30 min/session
- Bone loading exercise
  - o Type = vertical and multidirectional jumping, bounding, hopping, skipping rope, drop jumps and bench stepping (see Box 3.6 for additional details)
  - o Frequency = 4–7 days/week
  - o Volume = 20 min/session

Additional Considerations

- If previously inactive, start slowly (lower intensity, shorter durations, fewer exercises)
- Progression should be guided by tolerance and be slower compared to a younger individual
- Individuals with sarcopenia should focus on increasing muscular strength

---

Box 3.5   Recommendations for Neuromotor Exercises for Older Individuals

Aim:

- Decrease the risk of falling and improve mobility

Approaches:

- Progressively difficult postures that gradually reduce the base of support (e.g. two-legged stand, semi-tandem stand, tandem stand, one-legged stand)
- Dynamic movements that alter the centre of gravity (tandem walk, circle turns)
- Stressing postural muscle groups (e.g. heel, toe stands)
- Reducing sensory input (e.g. standing with eyes closed)

Box 3.6   Recommendations for Bone Loading Exercises for Older Individuals

Aim:

- Increase and/or maintain bone health to prevent osteoporosis

Approaches:

- Intensity moderate to high as tolerated
- Progress volume by:
  - o increasing heights for activities such as bounding and drop jumping, adding weighted vests and changing directions; and/or
  - o increasing the number of impacts (e.g. start with 3 sets of 10 impacts progressing to 5 sets of 20 impacts)
- Allow 1–2 minutes rest between sets

Worked Case Study for Exercise Programming for Older Individuals

Barry is a frail 79-year-old man who is in residential care. He has a history of falls and uses a walking frame around the residential care unit and while out shopping. The manager of the residential care unit has recently established an exercise facility (including two treadmills, three exercise bikes, weight machines and exercise mats) and has employed you to come in twice per week to write exercise programs for the residents, including Barry. The residents can use the gym at any time. There is also a group tai chi class run by an exercise scientist once a week at the facility with classes tailored to improve balance, agility and coordination. You undertake initial screening/assessment of Barry and obtain the following results.

- Blood pressure: 112/72 mmHg
- Waist circumference: 98 cm
- Height: 166 cm
- Weight: 60 kg
- Resting heart rate: 60 bpm
- 6-minute walk test: 407 m (conducted with a walking aid; result is in the 'poor' category) [16]
- Repeated chair stand (number in 30 seconds) score: 9 (result is in the 'below average' category) [17]
- Fast walking speed (fastest time to walk 6 m): 3.48 seconds

Aside from antacids (taken when needed), vitamin D (daily) and some pain medication (taken when his joints are sore), he is on no other medications. Barry's daily schedule is generally as follows: breakfast at 7.30 am, resting/reading/watching TV between 8.30 and 10.30 am, morning tea at 10.30 am, daily outing, lunch at the facility at 1.30 pm, afternoon nap, TV or card games or family visits from 2.30 pm with dinner at 6.00 pm. He often visits family on weekends. You initially decide to start Barry with a combination of aerobic exercise and resistance training exercise, with some simple balance and bone loading exercises on the 2 days per week you are at the facility, with aims to increase the session frequency over the first few months.

Worked Example: Exercise Programming for Older Individuals	
Exercise Program	
Participant Details	**Participant Goals** *(Specific, Measurable, Action-orientated, Realistic, Timely, Self-determined)*
Name: *Barry*	Short-term goals: 3 months
Age: *79*	1. *Increase functional walking capacity: increase distance covered in the 6MWT by 20% (~80 m); this would move Barry into the 'below average' category.*
Gender: *male*	2. *Reduce waist circumference to 94 cm or less; this is associated with a lower health risk for cardiovascular disease for men.*
Body mass: *60 kg*	
Body mass index: *21.8 kg/m²*	3. *Improve fast walking speed by 10% (to ~3.13 seconds); this would move Barry into the 41st–60th percentile ('average').*
Waist circumference: *98 cm*	Long-term goals
Resting heart rate: *60 bpm*	1. *Increase functional walking capacity: increase distance covered in the 6MWT by 30% (from baseline, to ~530 m); this would move Barry into the 'above average' category.*
Blood pressure: *112/72 mmHg*	
Maximal heart rate: ~~Age predicted~~/Measured (circle) *141 bpm*	2. *Reduce waist circumference to < 92 cm; this is associated with the lowest health risk for cardiovascular disease for men.*
	3. *Improve fast walking speed by 20% (from baseline, to ~2.78 seconds); this would move Barry into the 61st–80th percentile ('good').*
Initial fitness/activity levels: *'Poor' functional capacity as determined by 6MWT score of 407 m* *'Below average' leg power as determined by repeated chair stand test score of 9*	4. *Meet and maintain target physical activity goals for older adults.*

Worked Example: Exercise Programming for Older Individuals (continued)

Initial Exercise Prescription (4 weeks)

Aerobic exercise Type	Frequency	Intensity	Duration
Stationary cycling	2 times/week	Moderate	Week 1: 10 minutes Week 2: 15 minutes Week 3–4: 20 minutes

Resistance exercise Type/exercise/body region	Frequency	Intensity	Sets/Repetitions/Rest
Machine based: Seated chest press Seated leg press Seated row Seated leg extension Hamstring curl Shoulder press Biceps curl Triceps extension	2 times/week	Moderate: 2–3 RiR (7–8 RPE)	1 set, 10 reps, 60 seconds rest

Neuromotor training Type/exercise	Frequency	Intensity	Duration
Tai chi	1 time/week	Light	40 minutes

Bone loading Type/exercise	Frequency	Intensity	Sets/repetitions/rest
Double leg jump: holding on to rail for support	2 times/week	Body weight	2 sets of 5 reps with 30 seconds rest

Flexibility exercise Type/exercise	Frequency	Intensity	Sets/repetitions/rest
Static stretch to ankles, quadriceps, hamstrings, lower hips, lower back, trunk, neck, chest and shoulders Holding on to support rail where necessary	6 times/week	Stretch to a point of tightness or slight discomfort	1–3 sets

Advice to Reduce Sedentary Behaviour:

Break up sitting time: Barry is to set an alarm on his phone for every 30 minutes in the mornings and afternoons when he is sitting. Barry is to stand up and walk up and down the corridor at least once. At least once per day Barry can complete his bone loading exercises (in accordance with your exercise progression).

Progressions for Improvement (with timelines for progression):

Aerobic exercise: Add in an additional aerobic exercise session in weeks 5–8 and again in weeks 9–12, then increase the duration of these sessions until meeting the target guidelines. Aerobic exercise progression thereafter will involve increasing the absolute intensity so that relative intensity is maintained.

Neuromotor: Add in additional balance exercises from week 8 onwards. To further progress balance exercises, add in dynamic movements to upset the centre of gravity and/or reduce sensory input.

Resistance exercise: Increase reps to 12, then add in an additional set in weeks 5–8 and again in weeks 9–12, then increase the load according to principles of progressive resistance training.

Bone loading: Increase session frequency to 5 sessions per week over 12 weeks then progress the exercise to single leg hops, multidirectional jumps etc. (if capable).

Worked Example: Exercise Programming for Older Individuals (continued)

Target Activity Levels (maintenance):

Aerobic exercise training: *150–300 minutes of moderate or 75–150 minutes of vigorous (or a combination of both), using the facility's stationary cycle.*

Resistance exercise training: *2 days per week progressive resistance training using the facility's weight machines targeting 8–10 exercises, 3 sets of 12 repetitions at moderate (2–3 RiR [7–8 RPE]) intensity.*

Neuromotor training: *Attend group tai chi class once per week and undertake balance exercises one other session per week (prior to a resistance training session).*

Bone loading: *Daily 20-minute session of bone loading exercises—target time is before morning tea when Barry is usually watching TV.*

Flexibility training: *Following the aerobic sessions 2–3 times per week.*

Activity 3.5 Exercise programming for older individuals

AIM:

- To design an exercise program for an older individual that: applies the general principles of exercise prescription; applies the principles of aerobic, resistance and flexibility training; incorporates advice to reduce sedentary behaviour; and takes into account special considerations

TASKS:

- Based on the information provided in Case study 3.5, complete Worksheet 3.5 by designing an exercise program for Edith.
- Answer the additional question.

Case study 3.5

Edith is a 78-year-old grandmother of four who currently lives independently with her 82-year-old husband. Edith has significant cervical and thoracic kyphosis. Her measured height is 150 cm and she weighs 47 kg. Her posture leads to often falling off balance and she usually uses a cane for assistance when walking, to minimise the risk of falling. This is a concern to her GP as her recent bone mineral density scan showed that she was osteoporotic in her lumbar spine and left hip. Her waist circumference is 75 cm and resting seated blood pressure is 118/78 mmHg. She is currently taking a statin for high cholesterol, and her recent blood test results were: total cholesterol = 3.6 mmol/L, HDL cholesterol = 1.1 mmol/L, triglycerides = 1.0 mmol/L, LDL cholesterol = 2.5 mmol/L and fasting glucose = 4.8 mmol/L. Edith has never smoked. During weekdays, Edith likes to spend 20 minutes in the garden and attends one 40-minute aquarobics class (held at the local senior citizens club). She otherwise spends her time playing bridge and baking for her grandchildren. On the weekends Edith tends to visit family and enjoys taking her grandchildren to the local park, although she finds it difficult to keep up with her grandchildren on the uneven grass and woodchip surfaces at the local park.

Edith's GP has prescribed her some pharmaceutical agents to help manage her osteoporosis and has referred her to you with recommendations to include some resistance training and neuromotor exercises to improve her balance.

You conduct a 6-minute walk test and she completes 470 m, which is in the 'below average' category.

Worksheet 3.5 Exercise Programming for Older Individuals

Exercise Program

Participant Details	Participant Goals (Specific, Measurable, Action-orientated, Realistic, Timely, Self-determined)
Name:	
Age:	
Gender:	
Body mass:	
Body mass index:	
Waist circumference:	
Resting heart rate:	
Blood pressure:	
Maximal heart rate: Age predicted/Measured (circle)	
Initial fitness/activity levels:	

Initial Exercise Prescription (____ weeks)

Aerobic exercise Type	Frequency	Intensity	Duration

Resistance exercise Type/exercise/body region	Frequency	Intensity	Sets/repetitions/rest

Neuromotor exercise Type/exercise	Frequency	Intensity	Sets/repetitions/rest

Worksheet 3.5 Exercise Programming for Older Individuals (continued)			
Bone loading exercise **Type/exercise**	**Frequency**	**Intensity**	**Sets/repetitions/rest**
Flexibility exercise **Type/exercise**	**Frequency**	**Intensity**	**Sets/repetitions/rest**
Advice to Reduce Sedentary Behaviour:			
Progressions for Improvement (with timelines for progression):			
Target Activity Levels (maintenance):			
Aerobic exercise training: Resistance exercise training: Flexibility training:			
Question: What safety measures will you include to ensure that Edith can complete her exercises without falling? _____ _____ _____ _____ _____ _____			

Activity 3.6 Exercise programming for older individuals

AIM:
- To design an exercise program for an older individual that: applies the general principles of exercise prescription; applies the principles of aerobic, resistance and flexibility training; incorporates advice to reduce sedentary behaviour; and takes into account special considerations

TASKS:
- Based on the information provided in Case study 3.6, complete Worksheet 3.6 by designing an exercise program for Andreas.
- Answer the additional question.

Case study 3.6

Andreas is a 62-year-old Masters athlete. He is a runner who has participated in competitive sport since the age of 16. In his youth he specialised in the 800 m and 1500 m events and then in his late 20s and 30s transitioned into the 5 km and 10 km events. He now primarily competes in the 10 km event and his most recent personal best time is 39:42. He enjoys training and competition and has worked with his club trainer over the last 20 years to modify his training and techniques to compensate for age-related declines in physical parameters.

Andreas is married with three adult children and currently works part-time in building management (Monday, Tuesday and Thursday from 8.30 am to 4.30 pm). He has a gym club membership and is part of a running clinic. Andreas has one competitive 10 km run per month and does a 5 km Park Run every Saturday (except on competition weekends). With his running club he does two track sessions per week and he does a further one long run and one tempo 8–10 km run per week.

Andreas and his running coach have noticed that he is experiencing a few more 'aches and pains' than normal and have sought your advice as to some modifications in his current training schedule, and specifically some advice for adding in progressive resistance training to further prevent age-related muscle loss and to maintain his performance.

You undertake initial screening for Andreas with the following measures.

- Blood pressure: 110/72 mmHg
- Waist circumference: 84 cm
- Height: 176 cm
- Weight: 72 kg
- Resting heart rate: 52 bpm
- Chest press 1RM: 70 kg
- Leg press 3RM: 230 kg

Worksheet 3.6 Exercise Programming or Older Individuals

Exercise Program

Participant Details	Participant Goals (Specific, Measurable, Action-orientated, Realistic, Timely, Self-determined)
Name:	
Age:	
Gender:	
Body mass:	
Body mass index:	
Waist circumference:	
Resting heart rate:	
Blood pressure:	
Maximal heart rate: Age predicted/Measured (circle)	
Initial fitness/activity levels:	

Worksheet 3.6 Exercise Programming or Older Individuals (continued)			
Initial Exercise Prescription (____ weeks)			
Aerobic exercise Type	Frequency	Intensity	Duration
Resistance exercise Type/exercise/body region	Frequency	Intensity	Sets/repetitions/rest
Flexibility exercise Type/exercise	Frequency	Intensity	Sets/repetitions/rest
Advice to Reduce Sedentary Behaviour:			
Progressions for Improvement (with timelines for progression):			
Target Activity levels (maintenance):			
Aerobic exercise training: Resistance exercise training: Flexibility training:			
Question: What other healthcare professional(s) may be important to assist with Andreas's concerns of preventing age-related muscle mass loss? _____ _____ _____ _____ _____			

4. Exercise Programming for Children and Adolescents

Adolescence begins with the onset of normal puberty and ends when an adult identity and behaviour are accepted.[18] For the purposes of this manual, children will be defined as preadolescence. For children there is less distinction between physical activity and exercise. To increase physical activity a key focus should be movement that is enjoyable, age appropriate and includes unstructured active play. The following strategies are taken from the *Australian Guidelines for Healthy Growth and Development for Children and Young People*[19] and should guide the design of the program.

Exercise Prescription

- This should consist of aerobic, resistance and bone loading exercises.
- Exercise/physical activity
  - Aerobic exercise
    - Type = enjoyable and developmentally appropriate activities (e.g. running, swimming, dancing, sports)
    - Frequency = daily
    - Intensity = moderate to vigorous, with vigorous on at least 3 days/week
    - Duration = at least 60 min/day; may be accumulated in shorter bouts
  - Resistance exercise
    - Type = may be unstructured (e.g. playing on playground equipment) or structured (machines, free weights, body weight exercises, resistance bands)
    - Frequency ≥ 3 days/week
    - Volume = use body weight as resistance at moderate intensity (2–3 RiR [7–8 RPE]) with 8–10 exercises involving the major muscle groups; 1–3 sets of 8–12 repetitions (beginners start at 1 set); included as part of 60 min/day
  - Bone loading exercise
    - Type = vertical and multidirectional jumping, bounding, hopping, skipping rope, running, drop jumps, bench stepping and sports (football, rugby, soccer, basketball, tennis)
    - Frequency ≥ 3 days/week
    - Volume = as part of 60 min/day

Additional Considerations

- Children should limit entertainment screen time to ≤ 2 hours/day.
- Avoid sustained heavy exercise in exceptionally hot humid environments.

Worked Case Study for Exercise Programming for a Child

Mason is a 10-year-old boy whose concerned parents have been told is 'overweight' for his height. They have seen a dietitian who has provided guidelines for the family and would like you to assist with increasing Mason's physical activity levels. Mason's favourite activity is playing video games which he is allowed to do for 1 hour after school and for a few hours each Saturday and Sunday. At school he has three physical activity lessons each week and Mason generally spends lunchtimes playing games with his friends. Mason has a bicycle and his favourite video game is World Cup Football (soccer).

Worked Example: Exercise for a Child

Question: Outline the exercise recommendations and suggestions that you would make for Mason's parents to assist with his weight management.

The goal is to have Mason meeting the physical activity recommendations and to establish a positive attitude towards physical activity. Given Mason's love of games, this will likely best be facilitated by incorporating games and play into physical activity. While Mason will undertake the three physical education lessons at school each week, it is important that his parents focus on increasing his activity outside of school hours.

For aerobic-based activity the goal is to achieve 60 minutes of moderate-vigorous physical activity per day, with at least 3 days of vigorous-intensity activity. For resistance-based exercise the goal is to undertake three sessions per week. It is also important to include bone loading exercise where possible.

Worked Example: Exercise for a Child (continued)

To achieve this:

Weekday afternoons are currently spent with 60 minutes of video games. Modify this to 3 days per week of 60 minutes of game-based activity. After discussing with both Mason and his parents what is possible to achieve (and that Mason is keen to do) you come up with the following list of activities.

- *Mason will join a local football club that trains 1 weekday evening and has a 40-minute game on Saturdays.*

- *Two days per week: 30 minutes one-on-one soccer with his mum or dad or 30 minutes Frisbee or 30 minutes bike ride followed by 30 minutes of body loading exercise on the play equipment at the local park.*

- *For the other 2 days per week Mason can do 30 minutes of more vigorous activity (e.g. body weight resistance exercises with his Mum and/or Dad), followed by 30 minutes of video games.*

- *On Sundays the family will choose an activity to do together. On days of good weather this can include a bush walk, bike ride, tennis game or a swim. On wet-weather days this can include indoor laser tag, ice skating or indoor rock climbing.*

Activity 3.7 Exercise for a child

AIM:

- To provide exercise recommendations and suggestions to the parents of a child that takes into account special considerations

TASK:

- Based on the information provided in Case study 3.7, complete Worksheet 3.7 by answering the questions.

Case study 3.7

Kirralee is 8 years old and loves dancing. She is currently in the school dance group which practises two lunch times per week, but this is the only physical activity that Kirralee undertakes outside of school physical education lessons. Kirralee's parents have tried to get her doing more activity at home—including some long walks and playing soccer with her older brother—but Kirralee complains that she is 'too tired'. Her older brother is extremely active and very good at sport and Kirralee's parents are concerned that she is not doing enough. They have asked you to develop a framework for an activity program that they can follow that Kirralee will enjoy.

Worksheet 3.7 Exercise for a Child

Question: Outline the exercise recommendations and suggestions that you would make for Kirralee's parents and explain the reasons behind your choice of activities. _____

_____

_____

_____

_____

_____

_____

_____

_____

_____

Activity 3.8 Exercise programming for an adolescent

AIM:
- To design an exercise program for an adolescent that: applies the general principles of exercise prescription; applies the principles of aerobic, resistance and flexibility training; incorporates advice to reduce sedentary behaviour; and takes into account special considerations

TASKS:
- Based on the information provided in Case study 3.8, complete Worksheet 3.8 by designing an exercise program for Jarred.
- Answer the additional question.

Case study 3.8

Jarred is a 16-year-old male who would like to 'bulk up his muscles'. He has started to do push-ups (20–30 repetitions) and sit-ups (up to 50 repetitions) every day and has bought himself some hand weights. His mother is concerned about the safety of what he is doing and has brought him to see you so that you can develop an age-appropriate exercise program. He weighs 64 kg and is 170 cm tall with a resting heart rate of 68 bpm. Jarred plays basketball with his local team (one weeknight training session and one weekend game) and plays basketball with his friends most lunchtimes at school but has never been involved in a structured resistance training program.

Worksheet 3.8 Exercise Programming for an Adolescent

Exercise Program	
Participant Details	**Participant Goals** *(Specific, Measurable, Action-orientated, Realistic, Timely, Self-determined)*
Name:	
Age:	
Gender:	
Body mass:	
Body mass index:	
Waist circumference:	
Resting heart rate:	
Blood pressure:	
Maximal heart rate: Age predicted/Measured (circle)	
Initial fitness/activity levels:	

Initial Exercise Prescription (___ weeks)			
Aerobic exercise **Type**	**Frequency**	**Intensity**	**Duration**

Worksheet 3.8 Exercise Programming for an Adolescent (continued)

Resistance exercise Type/exercise/body region	Frequency	Intensity	Sets/repetitions/rest

Flexibility exercise Type/exercise	Frequency	Intensity	Sets/repetitions/rest

Advice to Reduce Sedentary Behaviour:

Progressions for Improvement (with timelines for progression):

Target Activity Levels (maintenance):

Aerobic exercise training:

Resistance exercise training:

Flexibility training:

Question: What safety measures will you include? _____

_____

_____

_____

_____

_____

_____

References

1   Jensen MD, Ryan DH, Apovian CM, et al. 2014. 2013 AHA/ACC/TOS guideline for the management of overweight and obesity in adults: a report of the American College of Cardiology/American Heart Association Task Force on Practice Guidelines and The Obesity Society. *Circulation*. 129:S102–S138.

2   Swift DL, Johannsen NM, Lavie CJ, et al. 2016. Effects of clinically significant weight loss with exercise training on insulin resistance and cardiometabolic adaptations. *Obesity (Silver Spring)*. 24:812–819.

3   Truesdale KP, Stevens J, Cai J. 2005. The effect of weight history on glucose and lipids: the Atherosclerosis Risk in Communities Study. *Am J Epidemiol*. 161:1133–1143.

4   Stevens J, Truesdale KP, McClain JE, Cai J. 2006. The definition of weight maintenance. *Int J Obes (Lond)*. 30:391–399.

5   Donnelly JE, Blair SN, Jakicic JM, et al. 2009. American College of Sports Medicine Position Stand. Appropriate physical activity intervention strategies for weight loss and prevention of weight regain for adults. *Med Sci Sports Exerc*. 41:459–471.

6   Ostendorf DM, Caldwell AE, Creasy SA, et al. 2019. Physical activity energy expenditure and total daily energy expenditure in successful weight loss maintainers. *Obesity (Silver Spring)*. 27:496–504.

7   Swift DL, McGee JE, Earnest CP, et al. 2018. The effects of exercise and physical activity on weight loss and maintenance. *Prog Cardiovasc Dis*. 61:206–213.

8   American College of Sports Medicine. 2018. *ACSM's Guidelines for Exercise Testing and Prescription,* 10th Edition. Baltimore, MD, USA: Lippincott, Williams and Wilkins.

9   American College of Obstericians and Gynecologists. 2015. ACOG Committee Opinion No. 650: Physical activity and exercise during pregnancy and the postpartum period. *Obstet Gynecol*. 126:e135–142.

10 The Royal Australian New Zealand College of Obstetricians and Gynaecologists (RANZCOG). 2016. Exercise during pregnancy https://ranzcog.edu.au/RANZCOG_SITE/media/RANZCOG-MEDIA/Women%27s Health/Statement and guidelines/Clinical-Obstetrics/Exercise-during-pregnancy-(C-Obs-62)-New-July-2016.pdf?ext=.pdf (accessed 26 March 2021).

11 Mottola MF, Davenport MH, Ruchat SM, et al. 2018. 2019 Canadian guideline for physical activity throughout pregnancy. *Br J Sports Med*. 52:1339–1346.

12 Hayman M, Brown W, Ferrar K, et al. 2016. Exercise in Pregnancy and the Postpartum Period. Sports Medicine Australia position statement. https://sma.org.au/sma-site-content/uploads/2017/08/SMA-Position-Statement-Exercise-Pregnancy.pdf (accessed 26 March 2021).

13 Tiedemann A, Sherrington C, Close JC, et al. 2011. Exercise and Sports Science Australia position statement on exercise and falls prevention in older people. *J Sci Med Sport*. 14:489–495.

14 Beck BR, Daly RM, Singh MA, Taaffe DR. 2017. Exercise and Sports Science Australia (ESSA) position statement on exercise prescription for the prevention and management of osteoporosis. *J Sci Med Sport*. 20:438–445.

15 American College of Sports Medicine, Chodzko-Zajko WJ, Proctor DN, et al. 2009. American College of Sports Medicine position stand. Exercise and physical activity for older adults. *Med Sci Sports Exerc*. 41:1510–1530.

16 Casanova C, Celli BR, Barria P, et al. 2011. The 6-min walk distance in healthy subjects: reference standards from seven countries. *Eur Respir J*. 37:150–156.

17 Rikli RE, Jones CJ. 1999. Functional fitness normative scores for community-residing older adults, ages 60–94. *J Aging Phys Activity*. 7:162–181.

18 Adolescent Health Committee. 2003. Age limits and adolescents. *Paediatr Child Health*. 8:577–578.

19 U.S. Department of Health and Human Services. 2008. Physical Activity Guidelines for Americans https://health.gov/paguidelines/pdf/paguide.pdf (accessed 26 March 2021).

20 Bo K, Artal R, Barakat R, et al. 2018. Exercise and pregnancy in recreational and elite athletes: 2016/2017 evidence summary from the IOC expert group meeting, Lausanne. Part 5. Recommendations for health professionals and active women. *Br J Sports Med*. 52:1080–1085.

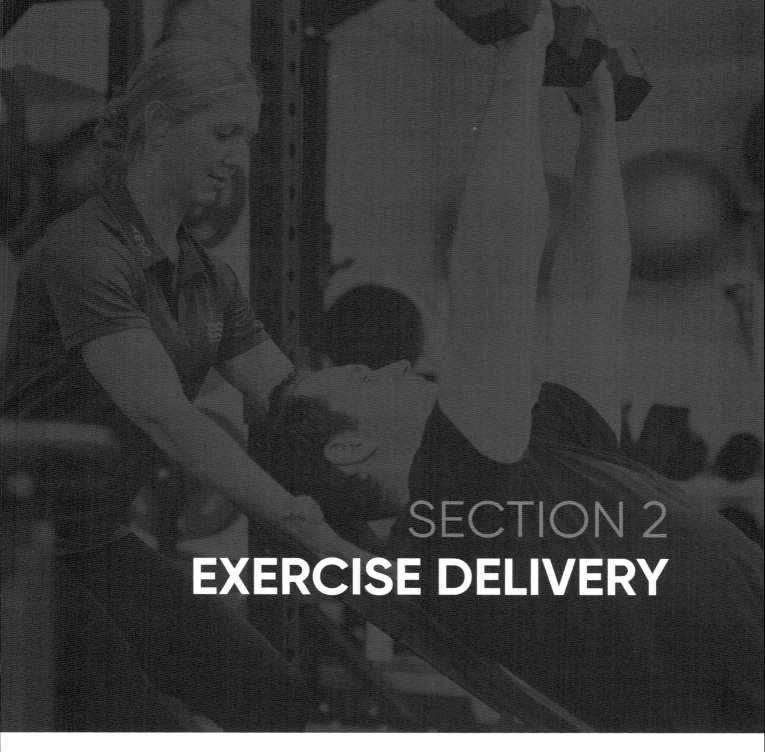

SECTION 2
EXERCISE DELIVERY

Emma M. Beckman

PROFESSIONAL STANDARDS AND LEARNING OBJECTIVES

The 11 practicals in this section aim to address professional standards related to the following:

- identify, describe, analyse and demonstrate a broad range of exercise modalities, and select appropriate exercises and equipment to suit the needs and abilities of clients
- apply the principles of motor control, functional anatomy and biomechanics to assess movement and to recognise the cause of dysfunctional movement patterns and unsafe exercise technique
- apply the principles of motor learning and skill acquisition, including the effective use of learning cues and movement progressions, for teaching and correcting movement and exercise technique
- instruct group-based exercise classes for distinct groups of clients with health, fitness and sports performance goals
- evaluate and adapt the delivery of an exercise prescription to respond to environmental change or change in the needs or capacities of clients
- analyse movement during prescribed exercises, identifying which muscles are active in producing and controlling a movement of a particular joint
- instruct group-based exercise classes for distinct groups of clients with health, fitness and sports performance goals
- modify a group exercise session for individual characteristics
- prescribe and deliver exercise in water environments for a variety of different client goals
- understand the theory that underpins stretching and flexibility and be able to appropriately prescribe flexibility exercises
- effectively prescribe power activities
- understand the development of speed and change of direction and effectively prescribe activities to improve these qualities.

By the end of this section, it is anticipated that students will be able to:

- understand the advantages and disadvantages of different aerobic exercise modes
- deliver an exercise bout for a participant using walking, with consideration of individual differences in the walk-to-run speed transition
- experience different intensities of aerobic exercise and use physiological responses to obtain specific intensities of exercise
- understand how both physiological responses and work rate may be used to achieve and maintain a specific aerobic exercise intensity
- calculate the energy expenditure of an aerobic exercise session
- experience implementing aerobic exercise, including high-intensity interval training, for a home-based setting
- describe the anatomical considerations of key exercises for major muscle groups of the body
- identify musculoskeletal structures from surface anatomy
- demonstrate excellent technique of key exercises for major muscle groups of the body
- describe how variations of exercises change the anatomical consideration and how variations may be used for specific goals
- demonstrate excellent communication of feedback during and after the execution of an exercise to effectively modify technique.

DEFINITIONS

Concentric muscle action: Shortening of a muscle fibre.

Eccentric muscle action: Active lengthening of a muscle fibre.

Isokinetic muscle action: Action in which the rate of movement is constantly maintained through a specific range of motion even though maximal force is exerted.

Isometric muscle action: When a muscle is activated and develops force but no movement at a joint occurs.

Isotonic muscle action: Muscle shortens against a constant load or tension, resulting in movement.

Power: Rate of performing work. When rearranged this represents the product of force and velocity.

Range of motion: The capability of a joint to go through its complete spectrum of movements.

Repetition: One complete movement of an exercise normally consisting of concentric (lifting) and eccentric (lowering) components.

Repetition maximum: Maximum number of repetitions that can be performed at a given resistance. By definition, this means to failure.

Set: A group of repetitions performed continuously without stopping.

Strength: The ability of the neuromuscular system to produce force against an external resistance.

SUGGESTED LEARNING APPROACH

Most practicals in this section contain a large number of exercises and associated variations. For each exercise it is suggested that students work in pairs and are allocated the exercise prior to the practical session. It is then the student's responsibility to prepare their allocated exercise so that they are familiar with how it is performed, the key anatomy of the exercises and how variations might influence the exercise. During the practical session, each pair is then required to demonstrate and instruct the exercise for the class and give some examples of how and why they would use this exercise in a program. This ensures a time-efficient way of utilising peer-based learning within the practical sessions. The use of this approach will depend on class sizes, teaching staff experience in facilitation and the student's confidence. It is recommended that instructors ensure they create a safe environment where feedback is valued and provided in a way that improves confidence and skills.

Below is an example of an activity that could be used throughout the resistance training practicals to facilitate peer-based learning and the feedback process.

Example Activity: Teaching Exercises

Each exercise will be taught to the whole class by a student pair. One student will act as the exercise scientist and one will be the client. The student who acts as the client should also give the class a run-down of the important anatomy and some potential variations of this exercise after the demonstration and instruction.

During the instruction and demonstration of each exercise, an additional student (or a number of students) will act as a peer reviewer. The peer reviewer should watch the exercise closely and give some feedback to the students by answering the following questions.

Question 1: How effective was the demonstration? Include a review of their technique and whether the communication during the initial instruction was effective.

_____

_____

_____

_____

Question 2: During the exercise, was the student giving good cues that effectively improved the technique of the other student?

_____

_____

_____

_____

Question 3: Was the knowledge of the anatomy and variations for this exercise communicated effectively to the class?

_____

_____

_____

_____

PRACTICAL 4
AEROBIC EXERCISE

Nathan A.Johnson, Shelley E. Keating and Jeff S. Coombes

Introduction

Aerobic exercise (also referred to as 'cardio') depends primarily on aerobic energy-generating processes. Common modes of aerobic exercise include walking, jogging, cycling, swimming, dancing and rowing. Usually aerobic exercise is undertaken at a moderate intensity and therefore refers to exercise that can generally be maintained for prolonged periods of time (e.g. 30–45 minutes).

Aerobic exercise can be contrasted with anaerobic exercise of which resistance training and supra-maximal 'all-out' sprinting (e.g. running or cycling) are the most common. 'All-out' sprinting requires the participant to give a maximal effort and depending on the person's fitness and motivation may only last for 5 to 30 seconds. Although not technically aerobic exercise, activities using sprint exercise will be included in this chapter as they are often used in aerobic training programs.

With the increase in popularity of interval training (e.g. high-intensity interval training or HIIT), it is important to delineate between this type of aerobic exercise that is completed at a submaximal intensity and the aforementioned 'all-out' anaerobic sprinting. Indeed, HIIT is often referred to as aerobic interval training or AIT, reflecting its significant contribution from aerobic metabolism. Table 4.1 provides thresholds for exercise intensities that separate high-intensity exercise from supra-maximal 'all-out' sprinting.

The use of the terms 'high intensity' and 'vigorous intensity' can be confusing as they are often used interchangeably. For the purposes of this manual we have used thresholds for vigorous (77–95% HRmax or 64–90% $\dot{V}O_2$max) and high intensity (80–100% HRmax or 70–100% $\dot{V}O_2$max) that overlap (see Table 4.1).

This practical will present an opportunity to gain personal experience in performing and delivering aerobic exercises. Students are encouraged to consider the physiological principles underpinning the exercise response and the benefits of aerobic exercise on cardiorespiratory fitness, weight management, mental and physical health and general wellbeing.

The following will be needed for the activities in this practical: Adult Pre-exercise Screening System (APSS) form (Figure 1.2),[1] various pieces of aerobic exercise equipment (e.g. treadmill, cycle ergometer, rower, step), stop watch, heart rate monitor set (e.g. transmitter, receiver, chest strap), masking tape, body mass scales and a computer with Excel and/or a calculator.

Activity 4.1 Modes of aerobic exercise

There is a considerable variety of aerobic exercise modes. A basic separation is to categorise those using equipment and those needing minimal or no equipment. Walking and running are examples of aerobic exercise modes that may not need equipment. Activity 4.6 gives examples of home-based aerobic activities that do not require equipment. Minimal equipment refers to items such as a skipping rope or a box stepper. When it comes to aerobic exercise equipment, there are many machines such as treadmills, cycle and rowing ergometers and cross-trainers that vary considerably in price and quality. The selection of an appropriate aerobic exercise mode is an important consideration for exercise adherence. For the general population, the choice of mode may be based on considerations such as availability, preferences/enjoyment, participant's mobility level, age and experience. For individuals exercising for sport-related goals, the specificity of the mode is important.

TABLE 4.1   Thresholds and Ranges for Methods to Prescribe and Monitor Aerobic Exercise Intensity, and their Relationships to Each Other (Based on Recommendations from the American College of Sports Medicine[2]). Note: this is a Condensed Version of Table 2.1.

Intensity Category	% of HRmax	% of $\dot{V}O_2max$	Talk/Sing Test	RPE
Very light	< 57	< 37	Able to sing	< 9
Light	57–63	37–45	Able to sing	9–11
Moderate	64–76	46–63	Able to talk but unable to sing	12–13
Vigorous[a]	77–95	64–90	Not comfortable talking	14–17
High[a]	80–100	70–100	Difficult to talk	17–18
Supra-maximal	N/A[b]	≥ 100	Unable to talk	≥ 18

[a] Note: There is overlap between the ranges for vigorous and high intensities. High-intensity ranges are provided due to widespread use of this term (e.g. HIIT).
[b] Due to the short duration of this exercise, heart rate cannot be used to monitor intensity.

AIM:
- Consider advantages and disadvantages of different aerobic exercise modes

TASKS:
- From the options below in Worksheet 4.1, choose an aerobic exercise mode and describe some advantages and disadvantages of its use. Examples are provided for the arm ergometer.
- Present advantages and disadvantages to the class so that classmates can complete the worksheet.
- In the final row list another mode of aerobic exercise not mentioned and describe its advantages and disadvantages.

Worksheet 4.1 Aerobic Exercise Equipment/Modes

Equipment/Mode	Advantages	Disadvantages
Arm ergometer	• Only uses upper body • Useful for lower-limb injuries or people who use a wheelchair for mobility • Could be used to modulate load in people with high lower-limb training loads	• Less muscle mass involvement compared with other modes that use upper and lower body, resulting in lower energy expenditure • Lack of specificity for people who primarily use the lower limbs for locomotion

Worksheet 4.1 Aerobic Exercise Equipment/Modes (continued)		
Equipment/Mode	**Advantages**	**Disadvantages**
Treadmill 		
Cycle ergometer 		
Cross-trainer/elliptical 		

Worksheet 4.1 Aerobic Exercise Equipment/Modes (continued)		
Equipment/Mode	**Advantages**	**Disadvantages**
Rowing machine		
Skipping		
Stepper		

Worksheet 4.1 Aerobic Exercise Equipment/Modes (continued)

Equipment/Mode	Advantages	Disadvantages
Walking		
Nordic pole walking		
Walking up stairs		
Boxing with partner		

Worksheet 4.1 Aerobic Exercise Equipment/Modes (continued)

Equipment/Mode	Advantages	Disadvantages
Boxing with bag 		
Kickboxing 		
Cross-country skiing 		
Other: _____		

Activity 4.2 Walking for exercise: including walk-to-run speed

Walking is the most common form of exercise for adults.[3] A recent survey of Australian adults found that 31% reported walking for exercise on 1–2 days/week, with the next most common activities being jogging/running/ swimming and 'going to the gym'.[4] The popularity of walking may be due to numerous factors including that it:

- is a natural human action
- is accessible and suitable for a considerable portion of individuals
- requires limited exercise knowledge
- is low cost
- has a low risk of injury[5]
- can be easily incorporated into activities of daily living and/or undertaken recreationally
- may be attractive to people with obesity, sedentary and at high risk of cardiovascular disease
- is environmentally friendly
- allows people with poor cardiorespiratory fitness to be able to start with a low intensity and short duration and progress both duration and/or intensity
- allows for intensity progression (e.g. by increasing speed, using stairs or walking up hills).

In the general population regular walking may improve cardiorespiratory fitness, exercise capacity and physical functioning and reduce blood pressure.[6] For many adults walking at a self-selected pace equates with a moderate intensity.[7] It has been estimated that walking at 4.8 km/h would be vigorous intensity for approximately 20% of the population.[8] In this activity students will experience the walk-to-run transition on a treadmill to gain a better understanding of walking speeds and energy expenditure during walking.

As many people exercise to manage body weight, it is important to understand how much energy is expended during various exercise tasks, particularly walking, and consider how this might impact on weight/fat loss. Generally, if a person expends more energy than he/she consumes then weight/fat loss will occur, and the more energy expended the greater the potential weight/fat loss. For example, walking may not be as effective as running for losing weight/fat.[9]

AIM:
- Deliver an exercise bout for a participant using walking, with consideration of individual differences in the walk-to-run speed transition

Safety
- Throughout this practical, students will be required to undertake aerobic exercise, with Activity 4.5 requiring supra-maximal intensity exercise. It is therefore important that all students are screened for any medical condition that may be a contraindication to completing the activities. The APSS (Figure 1.2) and the list of contraindications to exercising (Appendix D) should be used to determine whether a student should participate in the activities.
- Treadmill safety precautions should be provided to the participant (see Appendix E). An assessment of their ability to walk/jog safely should be conducted prior to exercising on a treadmill.

TASKS:
- In pairs, one person completes the activity while his/her partner adds the relevant data to Worksheet 4.2. The pair then swap roles.
- Weigh the participant and record the value.
- Calculate the participant's age-predicted HRmax using the equation i.e. $208 - (0.7 \times age)$.[10] (Note: The formula $220 - age$ is often used to estimate maximal heart rate. However, the above formula used throughout this manual has been shown to be more accurate.)
- Fit a heart rate monitor to the participant.
- The participant starts walking on the treadmill (0% gradient) and slowly increases the speed (over 1–3 minutes) and observes and records the speed at which walking is no longer possible/comfortable and the corresponding heart rate. The partner then stops the treadmill and covers the treadmill speed display with tape so the participant cannot view the speed.

- The participant then does five more similar trials to determine the speed at which walking is no longer possible/comfortable. The partner removes the tape after each trial and records this speed (without allowing the participant to view the speed) and the corresponding heart rate, then replaces the tape.
- Swap roles after completing all six attempts. Record your average walk-to-run speed transition in the worksheet below.
- Complete all questions in Worksheet 4.2.

Worksheet 4.2 Walk-to-Run Speed

Your partner (participant): _____

Participant's body mass: _____ kg

Participant's age-predicted HRmax: _____ bpm

With display visible, speed at which participant's walking is no longer possible/comfortable:

_____ km/h   Heart rate: _____ bpm

With display covered, speed at which participant's walking is no longer possible/comfortable:

Attempt 1: _____ km/h   Heart rate: _____ bpm

Attempt 2: _____ km/h   Heart rate: _____ bpm

Attempt 3: _____ km/h   Heart rate: _____ bpm

Attempt 4: _____ km/h   Heart rate: _____ bpm

Attempt 5: _____ km/h   Heart rate: _____ bpm

Average speed from the 6 attempts _____ km/h

Average heart rate from the 6 attempts _____ bpm

Question 1. What % of HRmax is this intensity equivalent to for the participant? _____

Question 2. Using Table 4.1, circle the intensity/intensities to which this is equivalent (you may need to circle more than one).

    low   moderate   vigorous   high   supra-maximal

Question 3. Comment on any difference between speeds when the display was visible compared to covered.

_____

_____

_____

_____

Question 4. Comment on the within-individual difference in your participant's walk-to-run speeds from the five attempts when the display was covered.

_____

_____

_____

_____

Worksheet 4.2 Walk-to-Run Speed (continued)

Question 5. Comment on any between-individual difference between you and your partner's walk-to-run speeds from the six attempts.

_____

_____

_____

_____

Question 6. Discuss what factors may impact on differences in walk-to-run speeds (e.g. leg length, previous experience).

_____

_____

_____

_____

Question 7. Reflect on how this might influence your treadmill prescription with future clients.

_____

_____

_____

_____

Question 8. Using the appropriate formula in Table 4.2, estimate the participant's oxygen consumption at their average walk-to-run speed. _____ mL/kg/min

Question 9. Using the assumption that an oxygen consumption of 1 L/min uses 21 kJ, estimate the energy expenditure if he/she was to walk for 30 minutes at this speed.

Step 1: Convert oxygen consumption in mL/kg/min to L/min by multiplying by body mass and dividing by 1000. _____ L/min

Step 2: Convert oxygen consumption in L/min to kJ by multiplying by 21. _____ kJ

Step 3: Multiply by 30 for 30 minutes of walking at this speed. _____ kJ

Question 10. Use an internet search to find a food that contains approximately this amount of energy (e.g. 1 slice of white bread contains around 335 kJ). _____

Question 11. For this question assume that: 1. the participant maintains an unchanged energy intake based on their body mass (e.g. 9000 kJ/day); 2. to lose 1 kg of weight/fat requires 37,000 kJ to be expended; and 3. all exercise energy expenditure is from oxidation of fat.[*]

If a participant wishes to lose 3 kg of weight/fat, how long would he/she need to walk for at that speed? _____ minutes.

Question 12. Following on from Question 11, if this participant completes 150 minutes per week of walking at this speed (and gradient), and keeps energy intake stable, how many weeks will it take to lose 3 kg weight/fat? _____ weeks.

[*]Although this is incorrect (as glucose and fat both contribute to aerobic exercise metabolism) we will use this assumption for the purpose of the calculation. Knowing and using the correct macronutrient contributions would not significantly change the result.

TABLE 4.2 Metabolic Equations for the Estimation of $\dot{V}O_2$ (mL/kg/min) During Cycle Ergometry, Treadmill Walking and Running, and Stepping	
Cycle ergometry[11]	
Males	$1.76 \times$ (work rate[a] $\times 6.12$/kg of body weight) $+ 3.5$
Females	$1.65 \times$ (work rate[a] $\times 6.12$/kg of body weight) $+ 3.5$
Treadmill walking and running[12]	speed[b] $\times$ (0.17 + [grade[c] $\times 0.79$]) $+ 3.5$
Stepping[2]	$3.5 + (0.2 \times$ steps/min) $+ (1.33 \times [1.8 \times$ step height[d] $\times$ steps/min])

[a]work rate in watts (150 kpm/min = 25 W)
[b]speed in m/min where 1 km/h = 16.7 m/min
[c]grade in % expressed as a decimal
[d]step height in metres

Activity 4.3 Achieving, maintaining and monitoring aerobic exercise intensity

Prescribing and setting an aerobic exercise intensity is an important skill for exercise professionals. Two common approaches are to use % HRmax or % $\dot{V}O_2$max. Table 2.1 in Practical 2 discusses the use of these and other approaches. Table 4.1 provides thresholds and ranges used to categorise different intensities and how they are equated to each other.

In Task 1 the participant will be required to maintain intensity in the appropriate zone, using % of HRmax. Work rate will be adjusted to maintain the heart rate in the correct zone. At the end of each stage students will also compare with the talk/sing test criteria and the rating of perceived exertion (RPE).

In Task 2 the participant will be required to maintain intensity at a work rate associated with a % of the participant's estimated $\dot{V}O_2$max. Analogous to the use of % 1 repetition maximum (RM) to prescribe a resistance training intensity, in a practical setting, using a % of the participant's estimated $\dot{V}O_2$max is limited by the difficulty in obtaining an accurate $\dot{V}O_2$max value/estimate. This is similar to the difficulty in obtaining a 1 RM, resulting in the use of more practical approaches such as the repetitions in reserve (RIR)-based RPE approach to set resistance training intensity. Using % $\dot{V}O_2$max is more common in a research setting and a considerable amount of research evidence in exercise science concerns the effects of exercise training programs that prescribe exercise using this approach (work rate associated with a % $\dot{V}O_2$max). For example, the research may demonstrate improvements in performance outcomes 'after 12 weeks of cycle training performed 3 days/week at 70% $\dot{V}O_2$max'. This is likely to have been set using the work rate associated with 70% $\dot{V}O_2$max, rather than $\dot{V}O_2$ measured in training sessions.

During these tasks the student will also reflect on the limitations of using different approaches to set exercise intensity, estimate the energy expenditure and observe changes in physiological responses over time. This includes appreciating why basing exercise intensity on physiological responses such as heart rate which varies within a bout (e.g. due to cardiovascular drift) will not necessarily ensure that a %$\dot{V}O_2$max target 'zone' is being achieved and maintained.

AIMS:
- Experience different intensities of aerobic exercise
- Understand how both physiological responses and work rate may be used to achieve and maintain a specific aerobic exercise intensity
- Calculate the energy expenditure of an aerobic exercise session

TASK 1: Aerobic exercise intensity using heart rate
- In pairs, one person completes the exercise while his/her partner adjusts the work rate. Then the pair swaps roles.

Worksheet 4.3.1 Aerobic Exercise Intensity Using Heart Rate

Your partner (participant): _____

Participant's age-predicted HRmax: _____ bpm

57% of participant's age-predicted HRmax: _____ bpm

64% of participant's age-predicted HRmax: _____ bpm

77% of participant's age-predicted HRmax: _____ bpm

Mode: _____

Time (mins)	Intensity	Heart Rate (bpm) at End of Interval	Work Rate at End of Interval (e.g. km/h, watts)	Talk/Sing Test[a]	RPE[b]
1–3	Very light				
3–6	Light				
6–9	Moderate				
9–12	Vigorous				

[a]Select: 1. able to sing; 2. able to talk but unable to sing; or 3. not comfortable talking.

[b]See Appendix A.

Question 1: How many work rate adjustments during the stage were needed to maintain the participant's heart rate in the target zone? Suggest reasons why this was needed.

Very light _____   Light _____   Moderate _____   Vigorous _____

_____

_____

_____

_____

_____

_____

Question 2: Did the participant's responses for the talk/sing test and RPE agree with Table 4.1? Add 'yes' or 'no' to the table below.

Intensity	Talk/Sing Test	RPE
Very light		
Light		
Moderate		
Vigorous		

Worksheet 4.3.1 Aerobic Exercise Intensity Using Heart Rate (continued)

Question 3: Using the work rate and heart rate outcomes from the multistage submaximal exercise session (first three stages), calculate the participant's estimated $\dot{V}O_2$max.*

Intensity	Work Rate (e.g. km/h, watts)	Heart Rate (bpm) – at End of Interval	$\dot{V}O_2$ (mL/kg/min)
Very light			
Light			
Moderate			

Step 1: Calculate the oxygen consumption ($\dot{V}O_2$) for the work rates using the metabolic calculation equations in Table 4.2.

Step 2: Use Figure 4.1 to plot the three points at the three intensities (heart rate versus $\dot{V}O_2$).

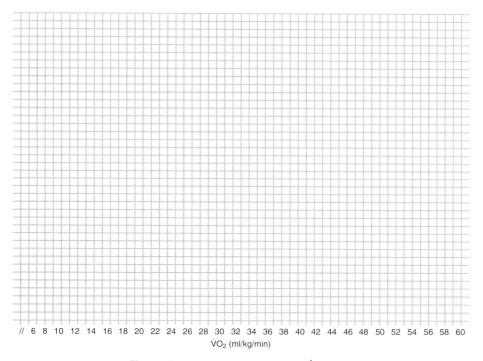

// 6 8 10 12 14 16 18 20 22 24 26 28 30 32 34 36 38 40 42 44 46 48 50 52 54 56 58 60

$\dot{V}O_2$ (ml/kg/min)

Figure 4.1 Graph for calculating $\dot{V}O_2$max

Step 3: Assuming that the HR/$\dot{V}O_2$ relationship is linear, obtain the equation for this line (in the form $y = mx + b$).

Step 4: Solve the equation to predict the $\dot{V}O_2$max (by inserting HRmax value for y into the equation $y = mx + b$ to find x, where $x = \dot{V}O_2$ corresponding with HRmax).

$\dot{V}O_2$max: _____ mL/kg/min

*This approach may not be as accurate in estimating $\dot{V}O_2$max compared to other tests (e.g. YMCA) but should provide a useful value for the next task.

- Calculate the participant's age-predicted HRmax using the equation $208 - (0.7 \times$ age) and the various percentages of this number, as required in Worksheet 4.3.1.[10]
- Fit a heart rate monitor to the participant to monitor intensity.
- Each participant selects a piece of aerobic exercise equipment (treadmill, cycle ergometer or stepper) and completes 3 minutes of exercise at four different intensities: very light, light, moderate and vigorous. The partner adjusts the work rate when necessary to maintain the participant in the intensity

zone or to change to the next intensity. Record how many adjustments in work rate during each stage are required to maintain intensity.

- The partner completes Worksheet 4.3.1. At the end of each interval, the work rate and heart rate are recorded and the talk/sing test details and RPE (use Appendix A) are obtained by asking the participant.
- Complete the additional questions.

TASK 2: Aerobic exercise intensity using work rate

- In pairs, one person completes the exercise while his/her partner sets the work rate and monitors responses.
- Fit a heart rate monitor to the participant.
- Each participant selects a piece of aerobic exercise equipment (e.g. treadmill, cycle ergometer, stepper) and completes 12 minutes of exercise at a vigorous intensity (70% of $\dot{V}O_2$max).
- Work rate at 70% $\dot{V}O_2$max is calculated in Worksheet 4.3.2 and is used to set and maintain the intensity (i.e. work rate is not changed during the activity).
- The partner completes Worksheet 4.3.2. The heart rate is recorded and the RPE (use Appendix A) is obtained by asking the participant every 3 minutes.
- Complete the additional questions.

Worksheet 4.3.2 Aerobic Exercise Intensity Using Work Rate

Your partner (participant): _____

Mode: _____

Participant's $\dot{V}O_2$max: _____ mL/kg/min. If your participant has previously had their $\dot{V}O_2$max measured via a graded exercise test, use this result; otherwise use the estimated $\dot{V}O_2$max from Worksheet 4.3.1.

70% of participant's $\dot{V}O_2$max: _____ mL/kg/min

Calculate the work rate (km/h, watts, steps/min) to elicit 70% $\dot{V}O_2$max using the metabolic equations in Table 4.2 appropriate for the chosen mode of exercise: _____

Time (mins)	Intensity	Heart Rate (bpm)	RPE[b]
0	Rest		
3	70% $\dot{V}O_2$max		
6	70% $\dot{V}O_2$max		
9	70% $\dot{V}O_2$max		
12	70% $\dot{V}O_2$max		

Question 1: Describe the changes to HR and RPE during exercise.

_____

_____

_____

_____

Question 2: Calculate the total energy expenditure of the exercise session (refer to the calculations from Worksheet 4.2): _____ kJ

[b] See Appendix A

Worksheet 4.3.2 Aerobic Exercise Intensity Using Work Rate (continued)

Question 3: Explain why work rate and energy expenditure usually change during exercise sessions that use heart rate, the talk test or RPE to achieve and maintain exercise intensity. Reflect on what this means for determining energy expenditure during exercise if heart rate, the talk test or RPE are used to determine intensity.

_____

_____

_____

_____

Question 4: If you are using heart rate, the talk test or RPE to achieve and maintain intensity of an exercise session, can you be sure that the participant is at a targeted % $\dot{V}O_2$max or receiving the required physiological stimulus?

_____

_____

_____

_____

Activity 4.4 High-intensity interval exercise

High-intensity interval exercise involves alternating periods of high-intensity aerobic exercise with light-to-moderate recovery activity or no activity between intervals.[13] Activity 2.3 required students to design an aerobic high-intensity interval program using seven parameters shown in Figure 2.2.

Completing higher intensity exercise can allow for greater physiological stimulus and adaptation than moderate-intensity continuous exercise.[14] Studies have shown that people undertaking HIIT for as little as 4 weeks have larger improvements in cardiorespiratory fitness than moderate-intensity continuous training (MICT), and can also improve vascular function and skeletal muscle metabolism,[15-17] and prevent primary and secondary cardiometabolic diseases.[18]

Studies using high-intensity exercise have been performed in a variety of settings, with countless variations in duration, intensity and mode. One separation of HIIT protocols is based on volume. High-volume HIIT protocols have been defined as those that accumulate $\geq$ 15 minutes of time spent in the high-intensity intervals in the session, with all other HIIT protocols being defined as low-volume HIIT.[15] The majority of evidence for HIIT improving cardiorespiratory fitness has used the high-volume HIIT approach. Recently, low-volume HIIT protocols (e.g. 1 $\times$ 4 minutes or 10 $\times$ 1 minute) have led to comparable improvements in cardiorespiratory fitness to high-volume HIIT[13,14] and superior to MICT.[13]

AIM:
- Experience a HIIT session and use physiological responses to obtain specific intensities of exercise

TASKS:
- Suggest choosing a different partner to previous activities.
- In pairs, one person completes the exercise while his/her partner adjusts the work rate and provides guidance on when to start/stop the intervals and records data. The pair then swap roles.
- Calculate the participant's age-predicted HRmax using the equation 208 − (0.7 $\times$ age) and 80% of this number, as required in Worksheet 4.4.[10]
- Fit a heart rate monitor to the participant to monitor intensity.
- Each student selects a piece of aerobic exercise equipment (e.g. treadmill, cycle ergometer, rowing ergometer, stepper) and completes 2 $\times$ 4-minute high-intensity intervals (i.e. > 80 HRmax; see Table 4.1), with a 3-minute recovery period in between.
- A 5-minute warm-up should be used.

- The 3-minute recovery period should be completed at an intensity that will result in the heart rate going down to the moderate-intensity zone (64–76% HRmax) by around the first minute of recovery and staying there for the remainder of the recovery period.
- The partner completes Worksheet 4.4. At the end of each minute, the heart rate is recorded and the talk/sing test details and RPE are obtained for the *whole interval* by asking the participant at the end of each of the high-intensity intervals.
- Complete the additional questions.

Worksheet 4.4 High-Intensity Interval Exercise

Your partner (participant): _____

Participant's age-predicted HRmax: _____ bpm

80% of participant's age-predicted HRmax: _____ bpm

Mode: _____

High-intensity exercise interval 1	Heart rate (bpm) – at end of 1 minute	
	Heart rate (bpm) – at end of 2 minutes	
	Heart rate (bpm) – at end of 3 minutes	
	Heart rate (bpm) – at end of 4 minutes	
	Work rate – at end of 4 minutes	
	Talk/sing test[a] – at end of 4 minutes	
	RPE[b] – at end of 4 minutes	
Recovery	Heart rate (bpm) – at end of 5 minutes	
	Heart rate (bpm) – at end of 6 minutes	
	Heart rate (bpm) – at end of 7 minutes	
High-intensity exercise interval 2	Heart rate (bpm) – at end of 8 minutes	
	Heart rate (bpm) – at end of 9 minutes	
	Heart rate (bpm) – at end of 10 minutes	
	Heart rate (bpm) – at end of 11 minutes	
	Work rate – at end of 11 minutes	
	Talk/sing test[a] – at end of 11 minutes	
	RPE[b] – at end of 11 minutes	

[a]Select: 1. able to sing; 2. comfortable talking but unable to sing; or 3. not comfortable talking.

[b]See Appendix A.

Question 1: How many work rate adjustments during the first high-intensity interval were needed to maintain the participant's heart rate in the target zone? _____

Worksheet 4.4 High-Intensity Interval Exercise (continued)

Question 2: How many work rate adjustments during the second high-intensity interval were needed to maintain the participant's heart rate in the target zone? _____ Discuss any differences in work rate adjustments with interval 1. _____

_____

_____

_____

_____

_____

_____

_____

_____

Question 3: Did the participant's responses to the talk/sing test and RPE after the first high-intensity interval agree with Table 4.1? Add 'yes' or 'no' to the table below.

Intensity	Talk/Sing Test	RPE
High		

Question 4: Did the participant's responses to the talk/sing test and RPE after the second high-intensity interval agree with Table 4.1? Add 'yes' or 'no' to the table below. Discuss any differences with interval 1.

Intensity	Talk/Sing Test	RPE
High		

_____

_____

_____

_____

Question 5: If you were using an approach with shorter duration intervals (e.g. 10 × 1 minute), why may heart rate response not be appropriate for achieving exercise intensity? Discuss alternative options for implementing this type of protocol.

_____

_____

_____

_____

Question 6: Critically discuss the suitability of prescribing HIIT for a range of participants.

_____

_____

_____

_____

_____

_____

_____

Activity 4.5 Sprint interval exercise

Although not technically aerobic exercise (there is an aerobic component but also a significant contribution of energy from anaerobic metabolism), activities using sprint exercise are often included in aerobic training. Sprint exercise often requires a person to complete supra-maximal, often 'all-out' efforts, that usually last between 5 and 30 seconds. Figure 2.1 illustrates the differences between high-intensity and sprint exercise. Spin classes and some types of CrossFit training are examples of where you often see sprint interval exercise. Unlike high-intensity intervals that may have interval durations long enough (e.g. $\geq$ 2 minutes) to use the heart rate to monitor intensity, sprint intervals are too short to use this approach. The following activity is designed to demonstrate this.

One of the more common sprint interval protocols uses 30-second 'all-out' efforts on a cycle ergometer. This approach is sometimes called a 'Wingate', based on a 30-second aerobic capacity test developed at the Wingate Institute in Israel.[19] A study showed that 4–6 × 30-second sprints performed 5 times per week for 2 weeks led to comparable benefits to training involving 5 × 90–120-minute sessions/week at moderate-to-vigorous intensity.[20] This contributed to the suggestion that sprint interval exercise can lead to benefits with considerably less time commitment to moderate-to-vigorous intensity continuous exercise. It should be remembered that the actual exercise session time also includes warm-up, cool-down and time for recovery between intervals, and that in the study that used 4–6 × 30-second intervals, the overall exercise session duration was around 30 minutes.[20]

One limitation of sprint interval exercise is that adjusting the work rate for different exercise modes (e.g. cycle ergometers) can be difficult. Electromagnetically braked bikes (e.g. Lode) and rowing ergometers (e.g. Concept) provide resistance proportional to the power output (i.e. the harder a person pedals/rows the greater the resistance), which is ideal for this type of exercise. However, with other ergometers it may be more difficult to set a resistance, which can result in a participant having to overcome a large resistance at the start and/or not having enough resistance at peak power output. On a basic cycle ergometer (e.g. Monark), one approach to overcome this is to have the participant begin pedalling as fast as possible against low resistance (e.g. 2 kg) and after 2 seconds apply a set-load based on body weight (e.g. 0.075 kg/kg body mass). For an 80-kg person this would be equivalent to 6 kg. This approach requires an extra person to adjust the load, which will not always be practical. During the recovery period between sprint intervals the participant can remain on the ergometer and be encouraged to cycle at a low cadence (e.g. 50 rpm) against a light resistance (e.g. 0.5 kg) to reduce venous pooling in the lower extremities and minimise possible feelings of light-headedness and/or nausea.

AIM:
- Experience a sprint interval session and use work rate to achieve specific intensities of exercise

TASKS:
- Suggest choosing a different partner to previous activities.
- In pairs, one person completes the exercise while his/her partner provides guidance on when to start/ stop the intervals and records the heart rate. The pair then swap roles.
- Fit a heart rate monitor to the participant.
- This activity needs to be completed on a suitable cycle ergometer (electromagnetically braked), or one that can be adjusted to provide a work rate that allows the participant to perform 'all-out' cycling.
- The protocol involves 3 × 30-second 'all-out' sprints with 4 minutes recovery (slow pedalling) between each sprint. A 5-minute warm-up should be used if the participant has not completed any exercise in the previous 30 minutes.
- A 5-minute cool-down should be used.
- The partner completes Worksheet 4.5.
- Complete the additional questions.

Worksheet 4.5 Sprint Interval Exercise

Your partner (participant): _____	
Heart rate (bpm) at end of 5-minute warm-up	
Heart rate (bpm) at end of 1st 30-second sprint	
Heart rate (bpm) at end of 1st 4-minute recovery	
Heart rate (bpm) at end of 2nd 30-second sprint	
Heart rate (bpm) at end of 2nd 4-minute recovery	
Heart rate (bpm) at end of 3rd 30-second sprint	

Question 1: Why isn't the heart rate response to exercise used to set or monitor intensity during sprint interval exercise?

_____

_____

_____

_____

_____

Question 2: Critically discuss the suitability of prescribing sprint interval training for a range of participants.

_____

_____

_____

_____

_____

_____

_____

_____

_____

Activity 4.6 Home-based aerobic exercises

For many people, attending a gymnasium to exercise is not an option (e.g. cost) or is undesirable (e.g. not wishing to be seen in that environment). For some people, exercising outside of their home or workplace is not attractive because of environmental constraints (e.g. poor access to paths) or personal safety. In addition, people often state that lack of time is a major barrier to exercise and the time needed to travel to a venue to exercise may waste valuable time that could be spent being active. Therefore, exercising at home needs to be considered for all people, and an exercise professional may consider prescribing home-based programs to overcome these barriers.

Most people will not have access to large pieces of exercise equipment at home, but aerobic training can be performed in this environment with a small amount of, or no, equipment. This activity will look at home-based aerobic exercise modes and the heart rate responses to these activities.

AIM:
- Experience implementing aerobic exercise, including HIIT, for a home-based setting

TASKS:

- Suggest choosing a different partner to previous activities.
- In pairs, one person completes the exercise while his/her partner completes Worksheet 4.6. The pair then swap roles.
- Calculate the participant's age-predicted HRmax using the equation $208 - (0.7 \times age)$ and the various percentages, as required in Worksheet 4.6.[10]
- Fit a heart rate monitor to the participant to monitor intensity.
- Choose one of the home-based aerobic exercise modes from Worksheet 4.6.
- The participant is required to exercise to get his/her heart rate in the moderate-intensity zone (64–76% of age-predicted HRmax) and keep it there for 1 minute.
- Increase the intensity so the heart rate is in the vigorous-intensity zone (77–95% of age-predicted HRmax).
- Present the advantages and disadvantages of each attempt to the class, so that classmates can complete the worksheet.
- In the final row list one other home-based aerobic exercise not mentioned.
- Complete the additional questions.

Worksheet 4.6 Home-Based Aerobic Exercises

Your partner (participant): _____

Participant's age-predicted HRmax: _____ bpm

64% of participant's age-predicted HRmax: _____ bpm

77% of participant's age-predicted HRmax: _____ bpm

Home-Based Exercise	Heart Rate Response
Walking fast on the spot with high knee lifts	Time to achieve moderate-intensity heart rate zone: _____ seconds Heart rate after 1 minute in moderate-intensity heart rate zone: _____ bpm Additional time to get into the vigorous-intensity zone: _____ seconds
Running on the spot	Time to achieve moderate-intensity heart rate zone: _____ seconds Heart rate after 1 minute in moderate-intensity heart rate zone: _____ bpm Additional time to get into the vigorous-intensity zone: _____ seconds
Stepping up and down on a box/step	Time to achieve moderate-intensity heart rate zone: _____ seconds Heart rate after 1 minute in moderate-intensity heart rate zone: _____ bpm Additional time to get into the vigorous-intensity zone: _____ seconds
Shadow boxing	Time to achieve moderate-intensity heart rate zone: _____ seconds Heart rate after 1 minute in moderate-intensity heart rate zone: _____ bpm Additional time to get into the vigorous-intensity zone: _____ seconds

Worksheet 4.6 Home-Based Aerobic Exercises (continued)	
Jumping jacks	Time to achieve moderate-intensity heart rate zone: _____ seconds Heart rate after 1 minute in moderate-intensity heart rate zone: _____ bpm Additional time to get into the vigorous-intensity zone: _____ seconds
Burpees	Time to achieve moderate-intensity heart rate zone: _____ seconds Heart rate after 1 minute in moderate-intensity heart rate zone: _____ bpm Additional time to get into the vigorous-intensity zone: _____ seconds
Walking up and down stairs	Time to achieve moderate-intensity heart rate zone: _____ seconds Heart rate after 1 minute in moderate-intensity heart rate zone: _____ bpm Additional time to get into the vigorous-intensity zone: _____ seconds
Other: _____	Time to achieve moderate-intensity heart rate zone: _____ seconds Heart rate after 1 minute in moderate-intensity heart rate zone: _____ bpm Additional time to get into the vigorous-intensity zone: _____ seconds

Question 1: For the exercise you completed, discuss the heart rate response, including considerations for using this mode for high-intensity exercise.

_____

_____

_____

_____

_____

_____

Question 2: Reflect on whether you would prescribe this type of exercise, and to whom.

_____

_____

_____

_____

_____

_____

_____

References

1   Exercise and Sport Science Australia. 2019. Adult Pre-exercise Screening System (APSS). https://www.essa.org.au/Public/ABOUT_ESSA/Adult_Pre-Screening_Tool.aspx (accessed 26 March 2021).

2   American College of Sports Medicine. 2018. *ACSM's Guidelines for Exercise Testing and Prescription*, 10th Edition. Baltimore, MD, USA: Lippincott, Williams and Wilkins.

3   Ham SA, Kruger J, Tudor-Locke C. 2009. Participation by US adults in sports, exercise, and recreational physical activities. *J Phys Act Health*. 6:6–14.

4   Heart Foundation. 2017. National Physical Activity Plan: 2016 Survey Findings. https://www.heartfoundation.org.au/getmedia/6a32b12f-15b8-4265-ba7e-d1cdfff5bee4/National_Physical_Activity_Plan_Survey_2016_-_Report1.pdf (accessed 26 March 2021).

5   Hootman JM, Macera CA, Ainsworth BE, et al. 2002. Predictors of lower extremity injury among recreationally active adults. *Clin J Sport Med*. 12:99–106.

6   Murtagh EM, Nichols L, Mohammed MA, et al. 2015. The effect of walking on risk factors for cardiovascular disease: an updated systematic review and meta-analysis of randomised control trials. *Prev Med*. 72:34–43.

7   Ainsworth BE, Haskell WL, Herrmann SD, et al. 2011. Compendium of Physical Activities: a second update of codes and MET values. *Med Sci Sports Exerc*. 43:1575–1581.

8   Kelly P, Murphy M, Oja P, et al. 2011. Estimates of the number of people in England who attain or exceed vigorous intensity exercise by walking at 3 mph. *J Sports Sci*. 29:1629–1634.

9   Williams PT. 2013. Greater weight loss from running than walking during a 6.2-yr prospective follow-up. *Med Sci Sports Exerc*. 45:706–713.

10 Tanaka H, Monahan KD, Seals DR. 2001. Age-predicted maximal heart rate revisited. *J Am Coll Cardiol*. 37:153–156.

11 Kokkinos P, Kaminsky LA, Arena R, et al. 2018. A new generalized cycle ergometry equation for predicting maximal oxygen uptake: The Fitness Registry and the Importance of Exercise National Database (FRIEND). *Eur J Prev Cardiol*. 2047487318772667.

12 Kokkinos P, Kaminsky LA, Arena R, et al. 2017. New Generalized Equation for Predicting Maximal Oxygen Uptake (from the Fitness Registry and the Importance of Exercise National Database). *Am J Cardiol*. 120:688–692.

13 Taylor JL, Holland DJ, Spathis JG, et al. 2019. Guidelines for the delivery and monitoring of high-intensity interval training in clinical populations. *Prog Cardiovasc Dis*. 62(2):140–146.

14 Weston KS, Wisloff U, Coombes JS. 2014. High-intensity interval training in patients with lifestyle-induced cardiometabolic disease: a systematic review and meta-analysis. *Br J Sports Med*. 48:1227–1234.

15 Williams CJ, Gurd BJ, Bonafiglia JT, et al. 2019. A Multi-center comparison of $\dot{V}O_{2peak}$ trainability between interval training and moderate intensity continuous training. *Front Physiol*. 10:19.

16 Ramos JS, Dalleck LC, Tjonna AE, et al. 2015. The impact of high-intensity interval training versus moderate-intensity continuous training on vascular function: a systematic review and meta-analysis. *Sports Med*. 45:679–692.

17 Way KL, Sultana RN, Sabag A, et al. 2019. The effect of high-intensity interval training versus moderate intensity continuous training on arterial stiffness and 24h blood pressure responses: A systematic review and meta-analysis. *J Sci Med Sport*. 22:385–391.

18 Hussain SR, Macaluso A, Pearson SJ. 2016. High-Intensity Interval Training Versus Moderate-Intensity Continuous Training in the Prevention/Management of Cardiovascular Disease. *Cardiol Rev*. 24:273–281.

19 Ayalon A, Inbar O, Bar-Or O. 1974. Relationships among measurements of explosive strength and anaerobic power. In: Morehouse N, ed. *International series on sports sciences, Vol. I, Biomechanics IV*. Baltimore: University Park Press; 527–532.

20 Gibala MJ, Little JP, van Essen M, et al. 2006. Short-term sprint interval versus traditional endurance training: similar initial adaptations in human skeletal muscle and exercise performance. *J Physiol*. 575:901–911.

PRACTICAL 5
THE TRUNK

Emma M. Beckman and Paul W. Marshall

Introduction

The region between the rib cage and the pelvis are referred to as the torso, trunk and/or core. We will refer to this area as the trunk. The role of this region can be described and discussed in many ways, and has been debated in the scientific literature over the last decade. The purpose of this chapter is to provide guidance to those wishing to provide exercises for this region.

The role of the trunk in activities of daily living, occupational pursuits, and sports and leisure is often complex. Many activities that individuals will perform in an occupational or sporting context require the generation and transmission of force through the trunk musculature. For example, the maximal throw of a discus requires the generation of trunk rotation from the throwing-arm side, but also the blocking or transferral of forces on the non-throwing side. The same requirements are involved in many rotational activities such as the golf swing, as well as occupational activities that require the swinging of implements or the lifting of loads from one location to another. Not many activities are reliant on forceful movement into flexion and extension. However, tasks often require endurance of trunk flexors and extensors to maintain positions both with and without load. Given the complexities of the trunk in generating and resisting forces, the exercises that are provided in this practical contain a mix of activities to provoke thought as to when the selection of an exercise may be optimal for an individual's training, health and performance goals.

Exercises included in this practical are:

- prone bridge
- side bridge
- bird dog
- Pallof press
- abdominal crunch
- oblique crunch
- back extension.

For each exercise, a primary variation will be presented with actions, starting position, finishing position, equipment set-up and execution of the exercise. This will be followed by a table of technique and cues and a table of variations for the exercise.

Anatomy

The anatomy of the trunk is shown in Figure 5.1 to provide a visual representation of the muscles of interest. The movements and muscles recruited are listed in Table 5.1.

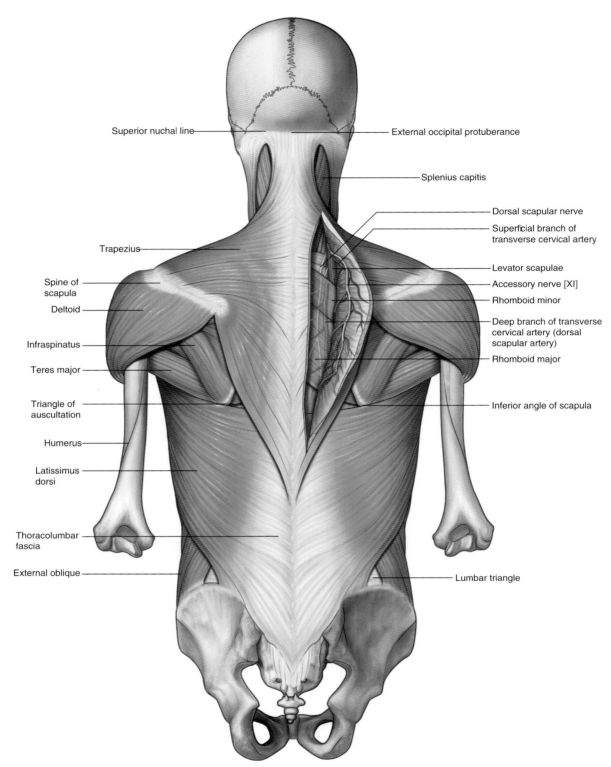

Figure 5.1 Anatomy of the trunk showing the muscles of interest
Source: Drake (2015).[1]

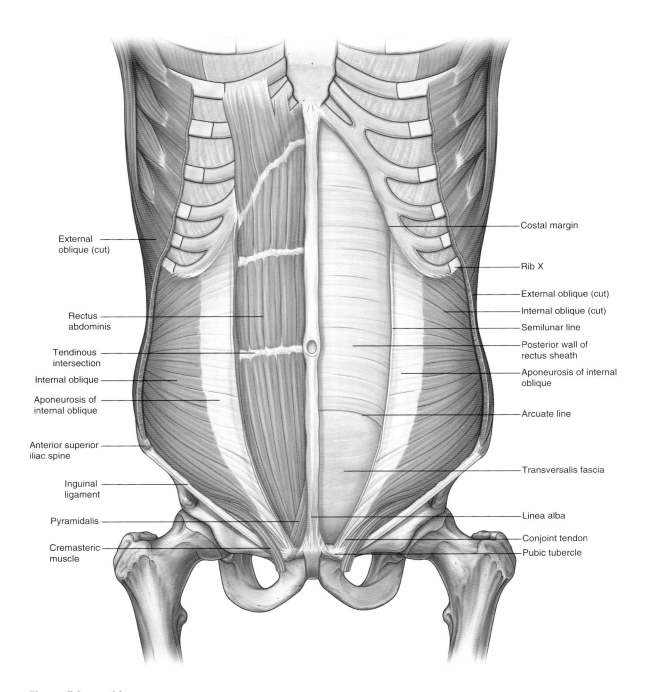

Figure 5.1, cont'd

TABLE 5.1 Anatomy of the Trunk	
Movement	**Muscles Recruited**
Trunk/spine flexion	• Rectus abdominis

Spine extension	• Erector spinae (ES):
	  ○ Iliocostalis (ES)
	  ○ Longissimus (ES)
	  ○ Spinalis (ES)
	• Quadratus lumborum (acting bilaterally)

Trunk lateral flexion	• Iliocostalis (ES) (acting unilaterally) • Longissimus (ES) (acting unilaterally) • Quadratus lumborum (acting unilaterally)
Deep lumbar muscles	• Transverse abdominis • Internal obliques • External obliques • Multifidus • Diaphragm • Pelvic floor
Superficial lumbar muscles	• Iliocostalis (ES) • Longissimus (ES) • Spinalis (ES) • Quadratus lumborum

Exercise 5a: Prone Bridge

Basic Exercise

Primary action:

- Isometric stabilisation of the whole body, predominantly to control trunk flexion and extension

Starting position:

- Lie prone with elbows flexed and positioned underneath shoulders.

Finishing position:

- Knees, hip, head and shoulders are in a straight line, with toes and elbows in contact with the ground and keeping the elbows positioned under shoulders.

Execution of exercise:

- Lift pelvis until finishing position is achieved and hold for the required period of time.
- Suggested ranges are 30 seconds for a novice with 3 sets and a 1-minute rest between efforts.

The primary variation of the prone bridge is shown on elbows and toes (Figure 5.2). This will be followed by technique and cues (Table 5.2) and variations for the exercise (Table 5.3).

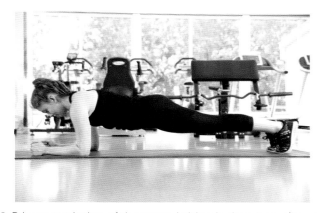

Figure 5.2 Primary variation of the prone bridge is shown on elbows and toes

TABLE 5.2 Cues and Technique for the Prone Bridge	
Poor Technique/Watch for	**Good Cues**
✗ Excessive scapula retraction, elevation or protraction ✗ If pelvis is lowered or level position cannot be maintained ✗ Rotation of pelvis ✗ Raising the pelvis high ✗ Head position and changes in any of the spinal curves in the cervical, thoracic and lumbar regions	✓ 'Keep a straight-line body position' ✓ 'Tuck your tailbone under' ✓ 'Keep your hips level'

TABLE 5.3 Variations for the Prone Bridge			
Variation	**Rationale**		**Considerations**
Position on knees	The prone bridge may be too challenging for some individuals so this regression reduces the resistance to make the exercise easier by reducing the lever length and reducing the load on the muscles.		Issues in technique while attempting the full prone bridge, such as collapsing through the lower back, will be a good indication to try this variation.
Single leg hip extension	This variation reduces the base of support and introduces rotational bias to one side, therefore requiring significantly more control of rotation of the trunk as the leg is lifted.		Initially, consider small repetitions of leg lifts rather than long holds to progress the exercise gradually.

TABLE 5.3	Variations for the Prone Bridge (continued)		
Variation	**Rationale**		**Considerations**
Unstable surface	The elbows or the feet (or knees) may be placed on a surface such as a Bosu ball, swiss ball or wobble board, increasing the need for stabilisation and anti-rotation forces		A strong rationale is required for this variation. Technique of a novice should be carefully observed for safety.

Exercise 5b: Side Bridge

Basic Exercise

Primary actions:

- Isometric resistance of trunk lateral flexion
- Isometric stabilisation through shoulder, elbow, hip, knee and ankle (side closest to the ground working hardest)

Starting position:

- Start by lying on side with the elbow underneath the shoulder; hips, knees and ankles should be in a straight line.

Finishing position:

- Knees, hip, head and shoulders are in a straight line, with only the lateral side of the foot and elbows in contact with the ground.

Execution of exercise:

- Lift the pelvis and trunk until the finishing position is achieved and hold for the required period of time.

The primary variation of the side bridge is shown positioned on elbow and toes (Figure 5.3). This will be followed by technique and cues (Table 5.4) and variations for the exercise (Table 5.5).

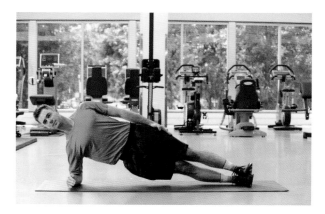

Figure 5.3 Primary variation of the side bridge is shown positioned on elbow and toes

TABLE 5.4	Cues and Technique for the Side Bridge
Poor Technique/Watch for	**Good Cues**
✗ Excessive scapula retraction, elevation or protraction ✗ Raising the pelvis too high ✗ Head position and changes in any of the spinal curves in the cervical, thoracic and lumbar regions ✗ Leaning forwards is encouraged over leaning backwards if it is difficult to remain in a straight line	✓ 'Keep body in a straight line' ✓ 'Tuck your tailbone under' ✓ 'Keep your hips level'

TABLE 5.5	Variations for the Side Bridge			
Variation	**Rationale**			**Considerations**
Position on knees	Reduces the resistance by decreasing the length of the lever. This reduces the load on the muscles to make the exercise easier.			It may be easier to have both knees bent; however, the top knee can be kept straight to provide additional support.
Star side bridge	Raising the top leg will increase the challenge to the hip abductors on the stabilising leg and the lifted top leg.			Individuals should not sacrifice a straight body position in order to lift the top leg. This progression should only be used when the individual is strong enough to maintain a good neutral posture.

Exercise 5c: Bird Dog

Basic Exercise

Primary actions:

- Hip extension
- Shoulder flexion
- Resisting trunk rotation
- Isometric stabilisation through pelvis

Starting position:

- Start in quadruped position with elbows and wrists under shoulders and knees under hips.

Finishing position:

- One arm and the contralateral leg are lifted to be parallel to the floor.

Execution of exercise:

- Static hold exercise or performed with concentric and eccentric repetitions.
- Lift the arm and leg on opposite sides until finishing position is achieved and hold for the required period of time.

The primary variation of the bird dog is shown with alternating arms and legs (Figure 5.4). This will be followed by technique and cues (Table 5.6) and variations for the exercise (Table 5.7).

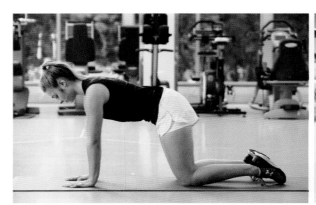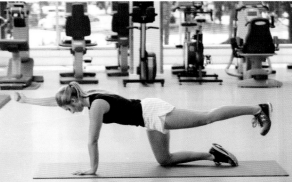

Figure 5.4 Primary variation of the bird dog is shown with alternating arms and legs

TABLE 5.6   Cues and Technique for the Bird Dog

Poor Technique/Watch for	Good Cues
✗ Excessive scapula retraction, elevation or protraction ✗ Excessive lumbar flexion or extension during the limb movements ✗ Head position and changes in any of the spinal curves in the cervical, thoracic and lumbar regions	✓ 'Keep your trunk stable while you move your arms and legs' ✓ 'Keep your hips level' ✓ 'Focus on extending your leg straight before lifting your leg up into line with your body'

TABLE 5.7   Variations for the Bird Dog

Variation	Rationale		Considerations
Around the world	Raise one arm or one leg at a time. Having only one limb in the air at a time will decrease the resistive demands.		To progress this, ask the individual to follow a random pattern by calling out which limb to raise.

TABLE 5.7 Variations for the Bird Dog (continued)			
Variation	**Rationale**		**Considerations**
Resisted bird dog	Adding a TheraBand will increase the resistance to increase the strength of the hip extensors.	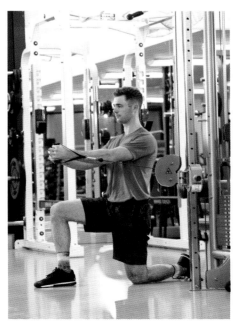	The goal of this exercise is primarily to increase trunk control and resist perturbations; the band should not be so difficult that it adversely affects technique.

Exercise 5d: Pallof Press

Basic Exercise

Primary actions:

- Isometric stabilisation shoulder horizontal flexion and extension
- Resisting trunk rotation

Starting position:

- Start in half-kneeling position, parallel to a cable or TheraBand in the coronal plane; pull the resistance until the trunk is facing forwards, with elbows flexed and held at the level of the sternum.

Finishing position:

- Both arms should be straight and the shoulders and pelvis square.

Execution of exercise:

- The cable or TheraBand tension should not change; it will want to pull the body back to the attachment point, but the body should be held in a forward-facing position.
- Slowly bring the arms out to a straight arm position while keeping the hips and shoulders square, then return to the start position.

The primary variation of the Pallof press is shown in a half-kneeling position (Figure 5.5). This will be followed by technique and cues (Table 5.8) and variations for the exercise (Table 5.9).

Figure 5.5 Primary variation of the Pallof press is shown in a half-kneeling position

TABLE 5.8 Cues and Technique for the Pallof Press	
Poor Technique/Watch for	**Good Cues**
✗ Excessive scapula retraction, elevation or protraction ✗ If the weight is too high, usually there is evidence of using momentum to achieve the exercise	✓ 'Keep your hips square' ✓ 'Keep your hips straight and steady and think of your hip bones as headlights that point forwards at all times' ✓ 'Only continue the exercise while you can maintain the straight body position'

TABLE 5.9 Variations of the Pallof Press			
Variation	**Rationale**		**Considerations**
Standing	This places a lot more resistive demand through the trunk as the base of support has been narrowed.		This should only be performed by an individual with good lumbopelvic control.

Exercise 5e: Abdominal Crunch

Basic Exercise

Primary action:

- Trunk flexion

Starting position:

- Lie supine on the mat, knees and hips flexed, feet flat on mat and arms in desired position.

Finishing position:

- The trunk is flexed maximally without hip flexion.

Execution of exercise:

- Raise the upper body towards the legs, flexing the lower torso.
- Pause slightly to allow elastic energy to dissipate.

The primary variation of crunch is shown in a supine position with the arms across the chest (Figure 5.6). This will be followed by technique and cues (Table 5.10) and variations for the exercise (Table 5.11).

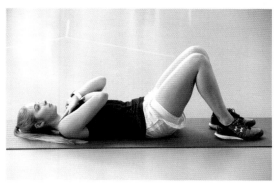 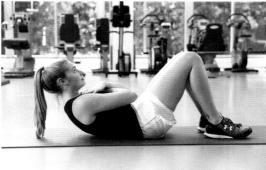

Figure 5.6 Primary variation of crunch is shown in a supine position with the arms across the chest

TABLE 5.10	Cues and Technique for the Abdominal Crunch
Poor Technique/Watch for	**Good Cues**
✗ Feet fixed to allow full 'sit up' range of motion— promotes significant involvement of the hip flexors and the disc pressure involved in this range is significant	✓ 'Roll the vertebrae up and around the movement' ✓ 'Focus on moving your rib cage towards your hips'
✗ Keeping the chin on chest or poking the head out significantly ✗ Using the movement of the neck to contribute to the action	✓ 'Breathe normally—don't hold your breath' ✓ 'Face directly to front not up or down' ✓ 'Try and keep your head in a neutral position'

TABLE 5.11	Variations for the Abdominal Crunch		
Variation	**Rationale**		**Considerations**
Fitball	The use of the fitball allows a greater starting range of trunk extension, increasing the distance of excursion of the exercise.		The lower body should stay relatively stable during this variation; watch for significant movement of the lower limbs.
Reverse crunch	With the legs in the air, the exercise action becomes movement of the pelvis towards the rib cage, rather than the rib cage towards the pelvis.		Legs may swing to use momentum for this exercise; try to minimise the involvement of the legs.
Dead bugs	Starting with the arms and legs in the air, shoulders may remain on the ground and the legs may be lowered towards the ground and back up. Or arms may be flexed while lower body remains still. To challenge obliquely, move opposite arm and leg at once.		

Exercise 5f: Oblique Crunch

Basic Exercise

Primary action:

- Trunk rotation

Starting position:

- Lie supine on the mat, with knees flexed at approximately 80°.

Finishing position:

- The trunk is flexed and rotated maximally without hip flexion.

Execution of exercise:

- Raise the upper body towards the legs, flexing the lower torso and slowly rotating towards one side.
- Pause slightly to allow elastic energy to dissipate.

The primary variation of the oblique crunch is shown in supine with the arms across the chest (Figure 5.7). This will be followed by technique and cues (Table 5.12) and variations for the exercise (Table 5.13).

Figure 5.7 Primary variation of the oblique crunch is shown in supine with the arms across the chest

TABLE 5.12 Cues and Technique for the Oblique Crunch	
Poor Technique/Watch for	**Good Cues**
✘ Often people will try and secure their feet so they can utilise their hip flexors; ensure the feet remain free	✓ 'Keep your heels on the ground' ✓ 'Think about bringing your left side of your rib cage to your right hip bone' (then give the opposite instruction for the other side)

TABLE 5.13 Variations for the Oblique Crunch			
Variation	**Rationale**		**Considerations**
Russian twist	In a sit-up position, this variation emphasises contraction of the hip flexors to maintain the lower body position while the upper body twists. This will allow greater range of rotation to be achieved.	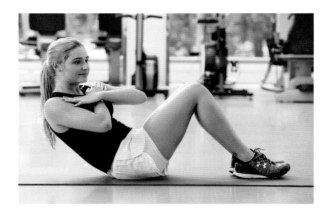	As the trunk is unsupported for this variation, the position of the trunk needs to be adequately maintained.

TABLE 5.13	Variations for the Oblique Crunch (continued)		
Variation	**Rationale**		**Considerations**
Woodchop	This variation can be performed in a lying, kneeling or standing position and requires the rotation of the trunk against resistance. The addition of resistance means this exercise can be used to progress trunk rotation strength.		If performed in a standing position, it is likely that a large element of rotation may occur at the hips rather than the trunk. This might be desirable in sports or activities where combined hip and trunk rotation is required.
Addition of bicycle legs	In a lying position the upper trunk rotates similarly to the original variation; however, the legs are lowered from a tabletop position towards the ground in an alternating fashion. This requires stabilisation of the upper and lower trunk to maintain a neutral spine.		In people who are unable to maintain a neutral spine, the erector spinae muscles are likely to try to contribute to the activity in stabilising the trunk if the abdominals are weak. Watch for changes in the position of the lumbar spine.

Exercise 5g: Back Extension

Basic Exercise

Primary action:

- Trunk extension

Starting position:

- Lie prone on back-extension apparatus with the hips in contact with the apparatus.
- Position the legs so that the knees are level with the hips.
- Place pads in contact with the hips and the back of the ankles.
- Flex hips with the torso hanging towards the ground.
- Place hands on each side of the head or crossed at the chest.

Finishing position:

- Hip extension to achieve a flat body alignment.

Execution of exercise:

- Extend trunk slowly until finishing position is reached.

The primary variation of the back extension is shown in a machine with the hips supported (Figure 5.8). This will be followed by technique and cues (Table 5.14) and variations for the exercise (Table 5.15).

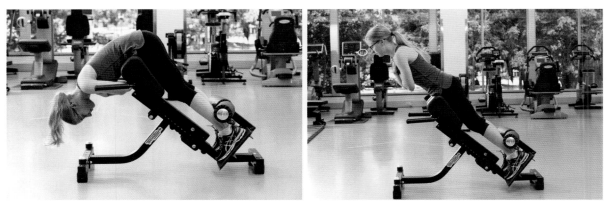

Figure 5.8 Primary variation of the back extension is shown in a machine with the hips supported

TABLE 5.14   Cues and Technique for the Back Extension

Poor Technique/Watch for	Good Cues
✗ Overextension of the trunk ✗ Using momentum to swing up and down	✓ 'Lift upwards in a slow and controlled manner' ✓ 'Don't swing up to the final position—only lift to a straight position'

TABLE 5.15   Variations for the Back Extension

Variation	Rationale		Considerations
Addition of arm movements	With the arms extended, it increases the torque. If this is achievable, the addition of load across the chest can be considered.		In individuals with restricted shoulder flexion range, lifting the arms may change the curve of the lumbar spine. Watch for this throughout the exercise.
Unsupported hips	By performing the same action with the hips positioned above the apparatus, the activity will require extension of the hips and the trunk, including the gluteus muscle and the hamstring group.		This variation is excellent for training the hamstrings.
Cobra	This exercise can be performed without equipment by lying prone on a mat and extending through the trunk.		While this exercise is a regression, the simple act of getting up and down off the floor can be challenging, so check for this ability before prescribing this variation.

Activity 5.1 Progressing trunk exercises

Background

Appropriate training of the trunk muscles should be individualised according to the needs of each client. No single muscle should be targeted or favoured over another for appropriate trunk muscle training. While isolated trunk exercises such as those demonstrated in this chapter have a place for increasing the capacity of the different muscles, trainers should be aware that moderately loaded whole-body exercises such as squats and deadlifts also provide a sufficient training stimulus for the trunk while also having better transfer to activities of daily living. Trunk exercise prescription should be viewed as part of a balanced whole-body prescription and as a means of building a client towards performing large whole-body movements (i.e. squats, deadlifts).

Given the added benefits of engaging in activities that utilise a number of other muscles, especially related to specificity for sport and activities of daily living, it is important that practitioners are skilled in including exercises that help individuals achieve their specific goals.

AIM:
- To develop a spectrum of exercises from simple to advanced that moves a client towards their goals.

TASK:
- Fill in Worksheet 5.1. The first row is done for you using exercises that are not included in this practical but are common progressions or regressions of exercises. Students are encouraged to try out these exercises or use internet resources to find different options.

Worksheet 5.1 Progressing Trunk Exercises

Case study Description	Basic Exercise	Progression 1	Progression 2	Rationale
Swimmer looking to improve their 50 m freestyle time	Dead bug with arm and leg movements	Kneeling TheraBand flutters	Standing, single-arm alternating push down in a straight stance	These progressions move from checking the client can maintain good neutral position, to the addition of distal movements in a supported position, through to the need to resist higher forces in a sport-specific position
A 60-year-old female, avid weekend gardener (**hint:** consider the need to maintain static positions while kneeling and also consider change of positions)				
Golfer looking to improve drive off the tee				
Mother with 2-year-old twins who reports that her back and legs get tired after a long day				

Activity 5.2 Abdominal bracing

Background

Abdominal bracing and hollowing (also known as drawing-in) are specific contraction techniques trainers will encounter in clinical practice. Bracing can be described as a tightening of the abdominal wall and lumbar muscles, without any visible expansion or shortening of the abdominal wall, whereas hollowing is a specific technique advocated as targeting the transverse abdominis and multifidus muscles. The origin of these techniques was based on the thought that stability of the trunk and deep trunk muscle motor control needed to be enhanced during everyday movements and exercise, and might prevent or reduce symptoms of low back pain. Students should be aware that there is no need to apply these techniques for the healthy individuals they will work with as the exercises demonstrated in this chapter are sufficient for appropriately recruiting all the trunk muscles. Indeed, for effective prescription for people with low back pain, students should be encouraged to pursue a balanced whole-body prescription as current evidence suggests there is no need for any specific exercise or contraction technique for the vast majority of clients. While there is some utility for using 'bracing' in high-intensity weightlifting prescription (e.g. powerlifting, Olympic weightlifting), this is typically only used in heavy squat and deadlift movements as an additional cue for maintaining form and should not be advocated in exercise prescription for healthy novice populations.

AIM:

- To obtain, understand and apply information that is applicable to you and how to explain the information to others.

TASKS:

- After reading the background to this activity, you may want to do some further reading.[2] Having thought about the concepts provided, in pairs discuss what this information and evidence means for you and your practice as an exercise scientist.

- With your partner, practise relaying this information in layperson's language to someone who comes to see you and asks to have isolated trunk-specific exercises in their program.

- Complete the questions below.

Worksheet 5.2 Abdominal Bracing

Question 1: What does this information and evidence mean for you and your practice as an exercise scientist?

_____

_____

_____

_____

Question 2: What technical terms would you replace with layperson's language to explain to someone outside of this field?

_____

_____

_____

_____

References

1   Drake R 2015. *Gray's Atlas of Anatomy.* Churchill Livingstone.
2   Marshall PW, Desai I, Robbins DW. 2011. Core stability exercise in individuals with and without chronic nonspecific low back pain. *J Strength Cond Res.* 25(12):3404–3411.

PRACTICAL 6
THE CHEST

Emma M. Beckman and Mike R. McGuigan

Introduction

This practical will cover exercises that use the muscles of the chest (pectoralis) as mobilisers. The group of exercises consist primarily of pushing movements centred about the glenohumeral joint.

Pushing exercises of the chest involve flexion or horizontal flexion of the humerus. The difference between the pulling movements of the upper back and pushing movements of the chest is that the scapula partly contributes to the movement for the pulling movements, whereas in the pushing movements generally it does not. Rather, for several of the pushing movements of the chest the scapula should remain fixated in the set position to allow the humerus to move into flexion. However, as will be discussed in the practical, the technique and specific cues that may be used will depend on different factors such as body position, training age and needs of the client that the student is working with. It should also be noted that while the exercises described in this practical are considered chest exercises, many are multi-joint exercises. Therefore, they will also utilise the deltoids and triceps, in addition to the chest muscles.[1]

This practical and the subsequent practicals on the back and shoulder will all require an understanding and appreciation of the importance of considering the scapula when prescribing exercises for the upper limbs. Therefore, this practical includes a brief introduction on the connections between the upper body and the scapula and the stabilisation that occurs at both the scapula and the humeral head during exercise.

The practical contains activities for students to complete, in addition to case studies on chest exercises that are relevant to a range of populations. The case studies will apply to healthy populations, athletes and populations with special considerations. When analysing the chest exercises, it is important to keep in mind that these exercises need to be considered within the context of the overall training program and the needs of the individual. Chest exercises can be progressed and modified according to these needs and the goals of the training program.

Exercises included in this practical are:

- bench press
- push-up
- fly.

For each exercise, a primary variation will be presented with actions, starting position, finishing position, equipment set-up and execution of the exercise. This will be followed by a table of technique and cues and a table of variations for the exercise.

Anatomy

The chest muscles act predominantly at the shoulder joint. The primary actions that exercises of the chest focus on are shoulder flexion and shoulder horizontal flexion. A primary muscle of interest in this practical is the pectoralis major. This large muscle is divided into two portions: the sternoclavicular head and the sternocostal head. While most of the included exercises consider both of the heads of the pectoralis major to be activated, if there is a specific focus of an individual exercise related to anatomy this will be discussed. It is possible to change the emphasis on particular regions of the muscle, depending on the exercise. The most common combination of actions during chest exercises is shoulder flexion or horizontal flexion in combination with elbow extension. Therefore, the anatomy related to elbow extension is shown in Table 6.1. The anatomy and important role of the shoulder stabilisers is also considered. The anatomy of the chest is shown in Figure 6.1 to provide a visual representation of the muscles of interest. The movements and muscles recruited are listed in Table 6.1.

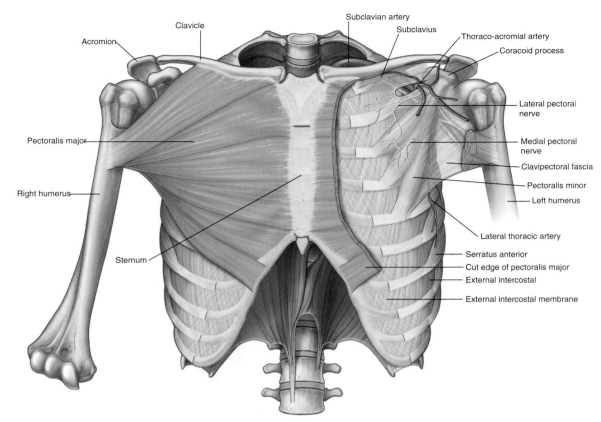

Figure 6.1 Muscles of the chest
Source: Drake (2015).[2]

TABLE 6.1 Anatomy of the Chest	
Movement	**Muscles Recruited**
Glenohumeral horizontal flexion	• Pectoralis major • Deltoid (anterior fibres)
Glenohumeral flexion	• Deltoid (anterior fibres) • Pectoralis major (clavicular fibres) • Coracobrachialis • Biceps brachii
Elbow extension	• Triceps brachii • Anconeus
Scapular stabilisation	• Serratus anterior • Middle/lower fibres of trapezius
Humeral head stabilisation	• Supraspinatus (rotator cuff) • Infraspinatus (rotator cuff) • Teres minor (rotator cuff) • Subscapularis (rotator cuff)

TABLE 6.1 Anatomy of the Chest (continued)	
Movement	**Muscles Recruited**
Lumbar spine stabilisation (deep)	• Transverse abdominis • Internal obliques • External obliques • Multifidus • Diaphragm • Pelvic floor
Lumbar spine stabilisation (superficial)	• Rectus abdominis • Iliocostalis (erector spinae) • Longissimus (erector spinae) • Spinalis (erector spinae) • Quadratus lumborum

Exercise 6a: Bench Press

Basic Exercise

Primary actions:

- Shoulder horizontal flexion
- Elbow extension

Starting position:

- Elbows are fully extended with the glenohumeral joint flexed at 90°.
- Grip will depend on the goal of the exercise; the standard bench press will use an overhand grip slightly wider than shoulder-width apart.

Finishing position:

- The bottom of the pectoral region between the nipples and the xiphoid process.

Equipment set-up:

- Ensure any safety equipment such as stoppers are set up prior to loading the bar.
- One spotter should be positioned immediately behind the bar or, if using two spotters, they can be positioned at either end of the barbell.
- Lie supine on the bench with feet flat on the floor or placed on the end of the bench.
- Line eyes up under the bar before lifting.

Exercise execution:

- Move the bar through a gentle arc towards the chest.
- Contact the bar lightly with the chest.
- Without bouncing, push the bar back towards the starting position.
- Speed of the exercise will depend on the goal of the exercise.

The primary variation of the bench press is shown on a flat bench with a barbell (Figure 6.2). This will be followed by technique and cues (Table 6.2) and variations for the exercise (Table 6.3).

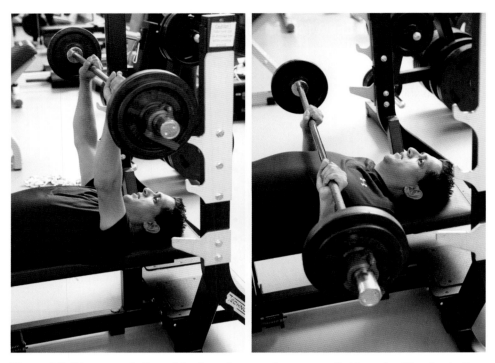

Figure 6.2 Primary variation of the bench press shown on a flat bench with a barbell; starting and finishing position (left) and middle position (right)

TABLE 6.2   Cues and Technique for the Bench Press

Poor Technique/Watch for	Good Cues
✗ Bouncing the bar off the chest, which occurs when lifter allows weight to travel too fast down to chest in the bench press; rib cage bends to absorb the impact and rebounds, and it will also decrease the workload	✓ 'Shoulders set' ✓ 'Control the bar up and down'
✗ Failure to complete range of motion (ROM)	✓ 'Touch the chest' ✓ 'Lockout at the top'
✗ Wrist instability	✓ 'Grip the bar tightly' ✓ 'Line up your wrists under the bar'
✗ Lumbar hyperextension ✗ Abdominal 'curling' ✗ Rounded shoulders/poor control of scapula/poor control of humeral head ✗ Uncontrolled speed of movement ✗ Flexion or extension of cervical spine	✓ 'Keep your bottom on the bench (lying)' ✓ 'Keep a neutral spine' ✓ 'Expand your chest—inhale' ✓ 'Keep your shoulders down—decrease upper trapezius activity' ✓ 'Control the speed' ✓ 'Feet on the bench or firmly on the floor' ✓ 'Keep your head on the bench'
✗ Lack of full extension of the elbows	✓ 'Straighten your elbows at the top of the movement'

TABLE 6.3   Variations for the Bench Press

Variation	Rationale		Considerations
Dumbbell bench press	Greater involvement of humeral head stabilisation muscles. Why? Greater ROM is utilised and there is increased reliance of stabilisation. Each arm is worked equally. Recent research has suggested greater activation in pectoralis major compared to a standard bench press.[3]		Hold dumbbells outside the shoulders.
Incline dumbbell press	Places more emphasis on the sternoclavicular head of the pectoralis major and anterior deltoid than horizontal bench press. The incline press between the angles of 44° and 56° results in significantly greater activation of the sternoclavicular head of pectoralis major than does the horizontal plane.[4] A recent study showed that bench incline angles of 30° and 45° both increased activation of the upper chest.[5]		The amount of incline can be adjusted to suit. Greater incline will also incorporate more anterior deltoid as increased shoulder flexion is performed.
Decline dumbbell press	Places more emphasis on the sternocostal head of the pectoralis major and anterior deltoid than on the horizontal bench press. The decline press at an angle of −15° showed greater activation of the lower chest.[5]		The angle of decline can be adjusted.
Single-arm dumbbell press	Performed with a single dumbbell using one arm. This will allow for complete focus on one side of the body during the exercise.		Hold one dumbbell outside the shoulder and use the other arm to hold the side of the bench to provide stability.

TABLE 6.3   Variations for the Bench Press (continued)

Variation	Rationale		Considerations
Seated chest press	Various machine options are available. There is increased stability provided by the machine, which can be useful for populations with very low levels of upper body strength.		Set up the machine so the handles are in line with the middle of the chest or just above. Maintain feet on the floor and the back against the backrest.
Wide-grip bench press	Wide hand spacing requires more horizontal flexion. Less ROM is required to complete the lift as the path to the chest is shorter, and individuals are generally able to produce more force using a wider grip. The wider grip predominantly emphasises pectoralis major.[6]		Width of the grip. Position the wrists immediately below the bar.
Narrow-grip bench press	Performed with narrow hand spacing. Movement is pure flexion of the shoulders if the elbow is held close to the trunk. This can result in potentially greater activation of the sternoclavicular head of the pectoralis major and triceps.[6]		Width of grip. Position wrists immediately below the bar. Full extension at top of the movement.

TABLE 6.3   Variations for the Bench Press (continued)

Variation	Rationale		Considerations
Smith machine bench press	More stable position. Can be performed as flat, incline or decline bench press variations.		Position of bench and lifter relative to fixed bar. Release bar from safety hooks. Lower bar under control.
Cable chest press	Performed unilaterally or bilaterally in either a seated or a standing position. Allows for increased ROM and to work one side of the body at a time.		Stand facing away from the cable stacks. Use either standing or seated position. Watch for accessory movements of the legs and trunk.
Powerlifters arched back	The vast majority of individuals should attempt to maintain the body position described above with the back in contact with the bench. However, competitive and highly experienced lifters will often extend considerably through the spine.		This variation should only be used with experienced individuals.

TABLE 6.3   Variations for the Bench Press (continued)

Variation	Rationale		Considerations
Bands and chains	Variable resistance such as using elastic bands and chains can alter the length–tension relationship and vary the difficulty of the exercise depending on the set-up.[7]		Position of band or chains on the bar. Method to attach bands using hooks or dumbbells.
High-velocity bench press	Exercises performed with greater velocity will increase power output. Loads between 30% and 70%, 1 repetition maximum (1RM) optimise power output during the bench press.[8]		Bar moved as quickly as possible. Good technique should be maintained during the exercise.
Bench press throw	This exercise overcomes the deceleration that occurs at the end of the standard bench press (even when performed explosively). Loads < 30% 1RM optimise power output during bench press throws.[8]		For safety this should be performed with a spotter, in a Smith machine or using specialised equipment which catches the bar upon release.

Activity 6.1 Questioning bench press prescription

AIM:
- To understand the role of the bench press in an exercise program

TASK:
- Fill in Worksheet 6.1.

Worksheet 6.1 Questioning Bench Press Prescription
Question 1: The bench press is often prescribed (almost automatically) in general fitness training. Justify (using anatomical and physiological principles) why this exercise would be beneficial to a healthy person's strength training program.
_____ _____ _____ _____

Activity 6.2 The sticking point

Background

Bar path kinematics: When performed using heavy resistance (approximately $\geq$ 80% 1RM), the bar path of the bench press can be divided into distinct phases: 1. the acceleration phase (where the highest forces are produced to overcome inertia); 2. the sticking region (an area of decreased velocity, thus negative acceleration); 3. a maximal strength phase (where the primary musculature involved are at the optimal length for force production); and 4, the deceleration phase (where the bar is intentionally decelerated to complete the lift).[9]

AIM:
- To investigate the sticking point in the bench press

EQUIPMENT REQUIRED:
- A linear position transducer or accelerometer is required to optimise the following activity.

TASKS:
- Perform the bench press with three different resistances of light ($>$ 4 RIR), moderate 4–6 RIR) and heavy (1–3 RIR).
- Have two participants (following an adequate warm-up) perform 1–2 repetitions at each load. The participant should be instructed to move the bar as fast as possible.
- The participant should rest for at least 2 minutes between trials.
- Fill in Worksheet 6.2 and record the peak and mean velocity for each of the loads using a linear position transducer (or similar technology).
- Answer additional questions about the activity.

Worksheet 6.2 The Sticking Point		
Measures and Interpretation		
	Mean velocity (m/s)	*Peak velocity (m/s)*
Low load = ___ kg		
Moderate load = ___ kg		
High load = ___ kg		

Worksheet 6.2 The Sticking Point (continued)

Question 1: What happens to velocity as the load gets higher?

_____

_____

_____

Question 2: What is the name of this relationship?

_____

_____

_____

Question 3: For each load, whereabouts during the lift did the participant feel like the lift was slowing down?

_____

_____

_____

Question 4: During the lift, were you able to observe a noticeable decrease in velocity of the bar? Describe your experience.

_____

_____

_____

Question 5: Was the position of the sticking region different for individuals? Describe your experience.

_____

_____

_____

Exercise 6b: Push-up

Basic Exercise

Primary actions:

- Shoulder horizontal flexion
- Elbow extension
- Isometric fixation of trunk and lower body

Starting position:

- Body weight is supported through the heels of the hands and the toes.

Finishing position:

- Chest nearly touching the floor, head in neutral position (nose almost touching the floor), elbows flexed to at least 90°.

Execution of exercise:

- Starting with a straight line between the shoulders, hips and knees, lower the body towards the floor.
- Contact the chest gently to the ground.
- Push back up to the start position.

The primary variation of the push-up is shown on hands and toes (Figure 6.3). This will be followed by technique and cues (Table 6.4) and variations for the exercise (Table 6.5).

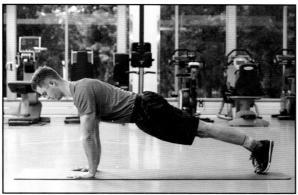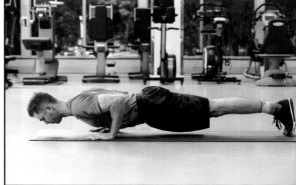

Figure 6.3 Primary variation of the push-up shown on hands and toes

TABLE 6.4 Cues and Technique for the Push-up	
Poor Technique/Watch for	**Good Cues**
✗ Elbows flared out	✓ 'Tuck elbows in'
✗ Scapula not sitting against the rib cage, poor thoracic position	✓ 'Squeeze chest on concentric phase'
✗ Head position dropping down	✓ 'Keep head centred'
✗ Different anthropometry, including high levels of central adiposity, may require modification of the mid position of the exercise	

TABLE 6.5 Variations for the Push-up			
Variation	**Rationale**		**Considerations**
Trunk position: incline, decline, flat	The difficulty of the push-up can be varied by changing the trunk position. Incline is the easiest and decline is the hardest.[10] Load is approximately 40% of bodyweight using an incline position of 61 cm from the ground, 64% for a regular push-up and 74% using a decline position of 61 cm.[10]		Level of incline or decline. Consider varying the amount of incline or decline to vary intensity.

TABLE 6.5   Variations for the Push-up (continued)

Variation	Rationale		Considerations
Width of arm position: wide, narrow	Several hand positions can be used in the push-up. Narrower base of support emphasises the triceps and sternal head of the pectoralis major.[11,12] A wider base of support uses the pectoralis major to a greater extent.[13]		The elbows should be kept tucked in close to the body throughout.
Unstable environment: Swiss ball, medicine balls, foam roller	The difficulty of the push-up can be increased by performing it on an unstable surface such as a Swiss ball. This leads to increased activation of the trunk and triceps muscles.[14]		Make sure the ball or object(s) is held in a stable position during the exercise.
Suspended push-ups using suspension devices (TRX etc.)	Variation that claims to increase activation of chest muscles but little supporting evidence for these claims.		If technique starts to fail the individual should become more upright to reduce the load of the exercise.
Assisted push-up on knees	Useful for clients with insufficient upper body strength to perform a standard push-up. Performing push-ups from a kneeling position requires relative load of approximately 50% bodyweight compared to 64–70% for standard push-ups.[10]		Another way to assist the movement is to use a suspended power band and position the band across the chest so the elasticity in the band makes the movement easier.

TABLE 6.5   Variations for the Push-up (continued)

Variation	Rationale		Considerations
Loaded push-up	Adding load by using weighted vests or putting a weight plate on the back will increase the load during the push-up.		Maintain good technique with additional load. May place a power band around the body to increase the resistance.
Accentuated negative	Due to the increased force production capacity during the eccentric (lowering) portion of the exercise, it is possible to accentuate this. For example, a weight plate could be added and then removed prior to resuming the ascent.		Maintain good technique with additional load.
Power push-up	Power exercise which is performed with high velocity. Various types of plyometric-type push-ups have been compared and have been shown to have greater peak force and rate of force development compared to standard push-ups.[15]		It is important to maintain good technique during high-speed movements and control the landing to reduce the impact on the wrists and hands. Land hands with control to reduce impact forces.
Dips	Performed using bench (dip bars are also an option). Additional load can be added using weights tied around the waist or a weighted vest.		Grip dip bars with arms extended and knees bent with legs crossed. Lower under control until upper arms are parallel with the floor. Press back up to full extension.

Activity 6.3 Progressing the push-up

AIM:

- To work through the various progressions that can be used for the push-up exercise.[16]
- The five levels of progression are:
    1. assisted (e.g. band-assisted push-up)
    2. bodyweight (e.g. standard push-up)
    3. resisted (e.g. weighted push-up [using vest or plate on back])
    4. eccentric (e.g. drop and stick push-up [drop down from boxes either side])
    5. plyometric (e.g. power push-up).

TASKS:

- In small groups, students should attempt each progression and then fill in Worksheet 6.3 with additional examples of progressions.
- Note that the progression is generally based on the movement capability of the individual, so this will provide the opportunity for students of different levels of proficiency to participate.

Worksheet 6.3 Progressing the Push-up	
Can you think of one other example of a push-up variation for each of the progression levels?	
Assisted	
Bodyweight	
Resisted	
Eccentric	
Plyometric	

Exercise 6c: Fly

Basic Exercise

Primary action:

- Shoulder horizontal flexion

Starting position:

- Elbows are slightly flexed with the dumbbells over the shoulders.
- Spotter can stand directly behind.

Finishing position:

- Arms abducted and laterally flexed.

Equipment set-up:

- Lie supine on the bench with feet flat on the floor or placed on the end of bench.

Motion:

- Move the dumbbells through a gentle arch of approximately 90° while maintaining a small (approximately 5°) amount of elbow flexion throughout the motion.
- Return to the starting position focusing on using the chest muscles.

The primary variation of the fly is shown on a flat bench with dumbbells (Figure 6.4). This will be followed by technique and cues (Table 6.6) and variations for the exercise (Table 6.7).

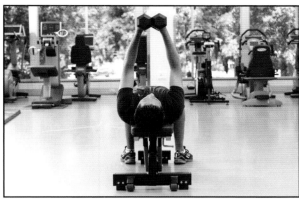 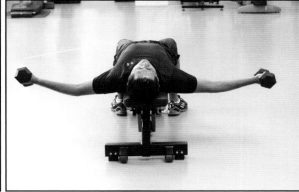

Figure 6.4 Primary variation of the fly is shown on a flat bench with dumbbells; starting and finishing position (left) and middle position (right)

TABLE 6.6 Cues and Technique for the Fly	
Poor Technique/Watch for	**Good Cues**
✗ Keeping elbows locked out	✓ 'Keep a slight bend in your elbows'
✗ Scapula winging, poor thoracic position	✓ 'Keep your chin tucked in and maintain a neutral spine position'
✗ Arching through lumbar spine to increase ROM achievable	

TABLE 6.7 Variations for the Fly			
Variation	**Rationale**		**Considerations**
Trunk position: incline, decline, flat	Dumbbell flys can be performed in various positions, depending on the goal of the movement. There may be less activation in pectoralis major compared to barbell and dumbbell bench press.[17]		Controlled speed of exercise Full ROM should be achieved while keeping a flat back position.
Equipment: Swiss ball, bench	Exercise can be performed on a bench or other surfaces such as a Swiss ball.		The weights may need to be reduced in this variation when compared to a flat surface.

TABLE 6.7	Variations for the Fly (continued)		
Variation	**Rationale**		**Considerations**
Standing cable fly	Cable crossover variations allow the movement to be performed using machines and to isolate the chest muscles. Can also be performed as lying or seated cable fly.		Controlled speed of exercise. Full ROM should be achieved while maintaining limited contributions of the legs and trunk.
Pec deck fly	Machine option that allows for a stable position with back supported to focus completely on chest muscles during the movement.		Set up machine so upper arms are parallel to the floor in the starting position. Full ROM.

Activity 6.4 Case study—chest exercises

AIM:

- To apply what you have learned about chest exercises to real life examples.

TASKS:

- The following case studies provide examples of three different types of clients (older adult, youth athlete and general healthy population).
- These provide examples of how you might make decisions about chest exercise selection and other acute training variables, based on the individual needs of your client.
- For each case study, consider the exercises provided in the table for each scenario and answer the extension questions given.
- If possible, extend your knowledge by considering how you might manipulate other variables that have not been addressed (such as tempo) and the setting of intensity (load).

Worksheet 6.4 Questioning Bench Press Prescription

Scenario 1

Client: Older adult

Goal: Increase upper body strength and power to improve the ability to carry out activities of daily living.

The client is a 70-year-old woman who would like to have increased upper body strength and power to help her cope with everyday activities of daily living such as gardening.

Example training session for older adult

Exercise	Sets	Reps	RIR
Seated chest press or Smith machine bench press	3	10–12	3–5
Incline dumbbell press	2	10–12	3–5
Pec deck fly	3	10–12	3–5

Rest period between sets = 2–3 minutes

Rest period between exercises = 1 minute

Question 1: What is the advantage of using machine-based and seated positions for an older client with limited mobility?

_____

_____

Question 2: What would be the advantages of using free weights with this type of client?

_____

_____

Question 3: What type of considerations would you have to make if she had restricted range of motion at her shoulder?

_____

_____

Scenario 2

Client: Youth athlete

Goal: Increase upper body strength and movement competency

A 15-year-old girl plays a variety of sports, including netball and softball.

Example training session for youth athlete

Exercise	Sets	Reps	RIR
Warm up			
Band-assisted push-ups	3	10–12	2–3
Dumbbell bench press	3	8–10	2–3
Incline dumbbell fly	3	10–12	2–3

Rest period between sets = 2 minutes

Rest period between exercises = 1 minute

Worksheet 6.4 Questioning Bench Press Prescription (continued)

Question 4: What would be a good progression of push-up exercises that you could use with this client?

_____

_____

Scenario 3

Client: 25-year-old man

Goal: Increase muscle hypertrophy

A 25-year-old man is training with the goal of increasing muscle hypertrophy. The chest workout is part of a 4-day split (4 days of training followed by 1 day of rest).

Example training session for client wanting to increase hypertrophy

Exercise	Sets	Reps	RIR
Incline barbell bench press	5	10–12	0
Dumbbell bench press	4	8–10	0
Dumbbell fly	3	10–12	0
Standing cable fly	3	10–12	0
Push-ups	3	To failure	0

Rest period between sets = 1 minute

Rest period between exercises = 1 minute

Question 5: What is the rationale for using shorter rest periods between the sets?

_____

_____

Question 6: Can you think of any advanced training techniques you could introduce into the client's training program for added variety and hypertrophy stimulus?

_____

_____

References

1   Stastny P, Golas A, Blazek D, et al. 2017. A systematic review of surface electromyography analyses of the bench press movement task. *PLoS One.* 12(2):e0171632.

2   Drake R 2015. *Gray's Atlas of Anatomy.* Churchill Livingstone.

3   Farias DA, Willardsen JM, Paz GA, et al. 2016. Maximal strength performance and muscle activation for the bench press and triceps extension exercises adopting dumbbell, barbell and machine modalities over multiple sets. *J Strength Cond Res.* 31(7):1879–1887.

4   Trebs AA, Brandenburg JP, Pitney WA. 2010. An electromyography analysis of 3 muscles surrounding the shoulder joint during the performance of a chest press exercise at several angles. *J Strength Cond Res.* 24(7):1925–1930.

5   Lauver JD, Cayot TE, Scheuermann BW. 2016. Influence of bench angle on upper extremity muscular activation during bench press exercise. *Eur J Sport Sci.* 16(3):309–316.

6   Lehman GJ. 2005. The influence of grip width and forearm pronation/supination on upper-body myoelectric activity during the flat bench press. *J Strength Cond Res.* 19(3):587–591.

7   Kuntz CR, Masi M, Lorenz D. 2014. Augmenting the bench press with elastic resistance: scientific and practical applications. *Strength and Conditioning Journal.* 36(5):96–102.

8   Soriano MA, Suchomel TJ, Marin PJ. 2017. The optimal load for maximal power production during upper-body resistance exercises: a meta-analysis. *Sports Med.* 47(4):757–768.

9   Kompf J, Arandjelović O. 2017. The sticking point in the bench press, the squat, and the deadlift: similarities and differences, and their significance for research and practice. *Sports Med.* 47(4):631–640.

10   Ebben WP, Wurm B, VanderZanden TL, et al. 2011. Kinetic analysis of several variations of push-ups. *J Strength Cond Res.* 25(10):2891–2894.

11   Cogley RM, Archambault TA, Fibeger JF, et al. 2005. Comparison of muscle activation using various hand positions during the push-up exercise. *J Strength Cond Res.* 19(3):628–633.

12   Gouvali MK, Boudolos K. 2005. Dynamic and electromyographical analysis in variants of push-up exercise. *J Strength Cond Res.* 19(1):146–151.

13   Contreras B, Schoenfeld B, Mike J, et al. 2012. The biomechanics of the push-up: implications for resistance training programs. *Strength Cond J.* 34(5):41–46.

14   Marshall P, Murphy B. 2006. Changes in muscle activity and perceived exertion during exercises performed on a swiss ball. *Appl Physiol Nutr Metab.* 31(4):376–383.

15   Dhahbi W, Chaouachi A, Dhahbi AB, et al. 2017. The effect of variation of plyometric push-ups on force-application kinetics and perception of intensity. *Int J Sports Physiol Perform.* 12(2):190–197.

16   Kritz M, Cronin J, Hume P. 2010. Screening the upper-body push and pull patterns using bodyweight exercises. *Strength Cond J.* 32(3):72–82.

17   Welsch EA, Bird M, Mayhew JL. 2005. Electromyographic activity of the pectoralis major and anterior deltoid muscles during three upper-body lifts. *J Strength Cond Res.* 19(2):449–452.

PRACTICAL 7
THE SHOULDER AND ARM

Emma M. Beckman and Stephen D. Cousins

Introduction

In this practical session we will cover multi- and single-joint exercises of the shoulder and elbow commonly performed in resistance training. Primarily, the exercises will involve flexion or abduction of the glenohumeral joint as well as flexion and extension of the humeroulnar joint.

For most exercises that target the muscles of the shoulders and arms, individuals will be required to grip an implement and move either the shoulder or the elbow, or both, through a desired range of motion (ROM). There are common examples of poor technique that often occur when shoulder and arm exercises are instructed. Students should consider body position, breath holding and using momentum instead of muscle activation as three areas that provide a good basis to start observing and giving effective feedback to individuals as they exercise. It is important to recognise that while some cues are consistent across shoulder exercises, you may need to develop more than these listed to facilitate better technique. In addition to the instructional requirements, it is important that practitioners account for safety aspects in shoulder and arm exercises; for example, ensuring there is adequate floor-to-ceiling space prior to undertaking an overhead exercise.

A practical session on resistance training of the shoulder and arms would be incomplete without considering the role of the stabilisers that allow maximal force and strength to be obtained through the upper limbs.

Humeral Head Stability

During shoulder abduction, pectoralis major, teres major and latissimus dorsi will act to internally rotate the humerus which will act to turn the humeral head anteriorly. If one or more muscles such as the pectoralis major, teres major or latissimus dorsi are tight, they will inhibit rotation of the humerus and reduce stability. The rotator cuff muscles (subscapularis, supraspinatus, infraspinatus and teres minor) have key roles in keeping the humeral head centred in the glenoid fossa during movement of the upper limb. They also have active roles in abduction (supraspinatus), internal rotation (subscapularis) and external rotation (infraspinatus and teres minor).

Scapula Stability and Scapulohumeral Rhythm

The scapula is a bone that is placed on the posterolateral aspect of the thoracic cage and connects the humerus to the clavicle. As the rotator cuff muscles insert onto the scapula, this bone is intimately related to the stability of the humerus. The scapula can move in elevation, depression, protraction, retraction and rotation (upwards and downwards). The interaction between the movement of the scapula and humerus is referred to as scapulohumeral rhythm and describes the kinematic interactions between the degree of humeral elevation and degree of scapula rotation (commonly accepted as existing at a ratio of 2:1).

Included exercises:

- Shoulder press
- Upright row
- Lateral raise
- Front raise
- Shrug
- Rotator cuff curls
- Posterior raise/fly
- Triceps extension
- Triceps pushdowns
- Biceps curls

For each exercise, a primary variation will be presented with actions, starting position, finishing position, equipment set-up and execution of the exercise. This will be followed by a table of technique and cues and a table of variations for the exercise (if available).

Anatomy

The anatomy of the shoulder and the arm is shown in Figure 7.1 to provide a visual representation of the muscles of interest. The movements and muscles recruited are listed in Table 7.1.

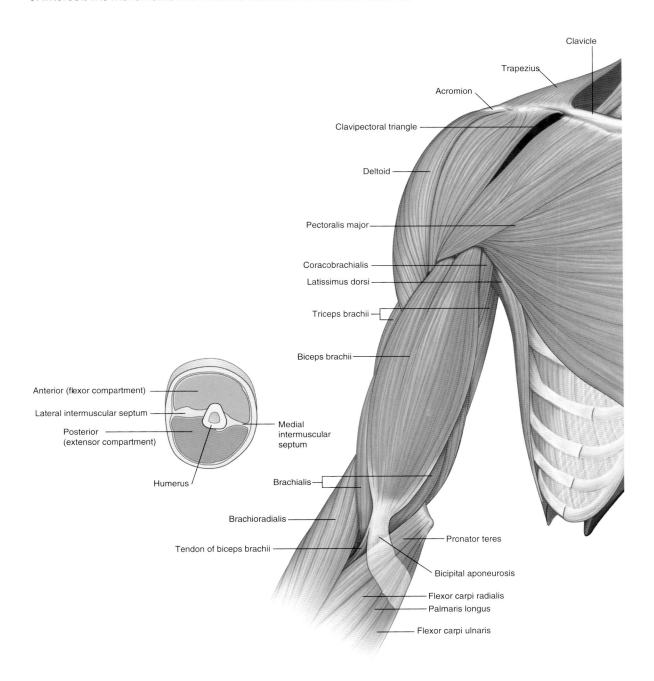

Figure 7.1 Muscles of the shoulder and arm
Source: Drake (2015).[1]

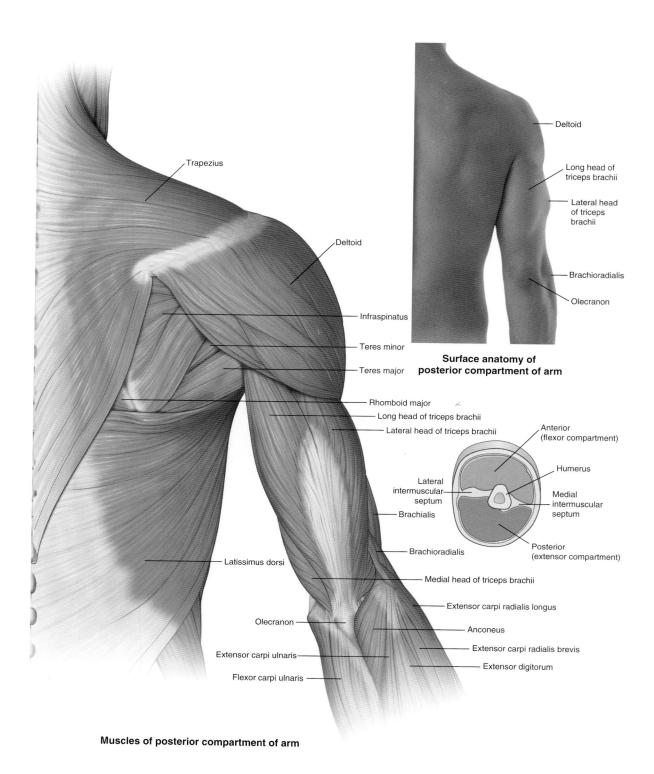

Muscles of posterior compartment of arm

Surface anatomy of posterior compartment of arm

Figure 7.1, cont'd

TABLE 7.1	Anatomy of the Shoulder and Arms
Movement	**Muscles Recruited**
Glenohumeral flexion	• Deltoid (anterior fibres) • Pectoralis major (clavicular fibres) • Coracobrachialis • Biceps brachii
Glenohumeral abduction	• Deltoid • Supraspinatus
Elbow extension	• Triceps brachii • Anconeus
Elbow flexion	• Biceps brachii • Brachialis • Brachioradialis
Humeral head internal rotation	• Pectoralis major • Latissimus dorsi • Teres major • Subscapularis (RC)
Humeral head external rotation	• Infraspinatus (RC) • Teres minor (RC)
Humeral head stabilisation	• Supraspinatus (RC) • Infraspinatus (RC) • Teres minor (RC) • Subscapularis (RC)
Lumbar spine stabilisation (deep)	• Transverse abdominis • Internal obliques • External obliques • Multifidus • Diaphragm • Pelvic floor
Lumbar spine stabilisation (superficial)	• Rectus abdominis • Iliocostalis (ES) • Longissimus (ES) • Spinalis (ES) • Quadratus lumborum
Scapular stabilisation	• Serratus anterior • Middle/lower fibres of trapezius

Mobilising and Stabilising the Shoulder: Pre-lifting Ideas

The shoulder is an inherently mobile joint that has the capacity to move in large ranges across a number of different planes. This mobility is essential for sports performance, as well as the successful achievement of many activities of daily living; however, the counter to mobility is often stability. It is therefore imperative that when loading the shoulders, care and preparation are taken to ensure that exercises are performed correctly and will achieve the desired outcomes. This section will give several pre-lift activities and a rationale for why they may be implemented. Table 7.2 shows several pre-lift activities.

TABLE 7.2	Mobilising and Stabilising Exercises for the Shoulder	
Activity	**Rationale**	
Windmills	Dynamic activities are an effective way of ensuring that the shoulder moves through full available active ROM prior to performing resistance exercises.	
Internal and external rotations	This involves recruitment activation of stabilising muscles in both an active and a stabilising way.	

TABLE 7.2 Mobilising and Stabilising Exercises for the Shoulder (continued)		
Activity	**Rationale**	
Body blade or Viper or end-range TheraBand	Stability is achieved when stabilisers are required to activate in the presence of perturbations. The body blade adds significant and variable perturbations to the shoulder to prepare the stabilisers to work during the session. This may also be used to simulate conditions of fatigue in the stabilisers if the session has a strong focus on rehabilitation.	
Flips	Kettlebells can be used as another source of perturbation at the shoulder and because of the weight distribution of the kettlebell may provide a more unpredictable stimulus than the repetitive actions in the body blade.	
Banded pull-aparts	Banded exercises are useful to activate muscles pre-lifting and will provide the greatest resistance generally at the end point of an exercise.	
Y-W-T	The scapular stabilisers are a group of muscles that stabilise the shoulder joint when moving your arm. Y-W-T exercises focus on these smaller supporting muscle groups and are known as scapular stabilisation exercises; importantly, they recruit the mid and lower trapezius, rhomboids and rotator cuff muscles.	

Exercise 7a: Shoulder Press

Basic Exercise

Primary actions:

- Shoulder flexion
- Elbow extension
- External rotation of the scapula

Exercise set-up:

- Seated in a stable position, maintain good posture with natural curvature of the spine.
- Avoid over-arching of the back.

Starting position:

- Grasp the bar with a closed pronated grip.
- The bar should be level with the clavicle, with elbow at full flexion (150°), under and slightly in front of the bar.
- The feet should be slightly wider than shoulder width, with the knees slightly flexed (if standing).

Finishing position:

- Elbows are fully extended with the bar above the head and shoulders, with the glenohumeral (GH) joint abducted.

Execution of exercise:

- Push the bar vertically until the elbows are fully extended during the concentric phase, ensuring the forearms are parallel to each other.
- Extend the neck slightly to allow the bar to pass by the face as it is raised and lowered.
- Avoid shrugging up with the shoulders.
- During the downward phase, allow the elbows to flex to lower the bar (under control) to touch the clavicles and anterior deltoids.

The primary variation of the shoulder press is shown in a seated position and using a barbell (Figure 7.2). This will be followed by technique and cues (Table 7.3) and variations for the exercise (Table 7.4).

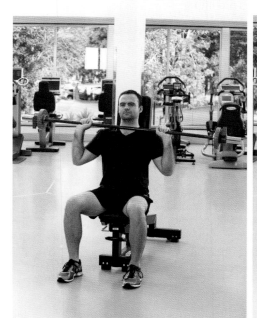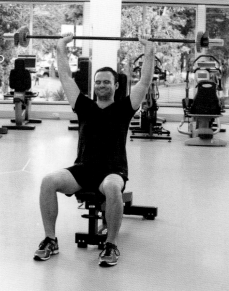

Figure 7.2 Primary variation of the shoulder press shown in a seated position and using a barbell; starting and finishing position (left) and middle position (right)

TABLE 7.3   Cues and Technique for the Shoulder Press

Poor Technique/Watch for	Good Cues
✖ Holding breath—this is likely to occur at heavier weights; however, with untrained individuals the Valsalva manoeuvre and breath holding is often unnecessary	✔ 'Inhale and hold during the lower (eccentric) phase and don't exhale until past the sticking point'
✖ Hyperextension of the lumbar spine, too much movement through the trunk during the exercise	✔ 'Keep your spine in a neutral position throughout the movement'
✖ Using the leg muscles to assist in moving load (i.e. rising up onto the toes)	✔ 'Try to use your arms on their own for this exercise' (if the individual cannot do this through effective cueing, it may be necessary to reduce the load)
✖ Poor ROM for shoulder flexion and abduction	✔ If this persists despite cues such as 'try to move through full range of motion', this issue may be a result of poor thoracic mobility
✖ Bouncing the load off the clavicle or shoulder muscles or locking the elbows	✔ Both of these alternate techniques are utilised by individuals in an attempt to get through more reps by effectively making the same resistance easier (by bouncing to move through the sticking point, or by locking elbows to allow the muscles to rest momentarily and taking the load through the skeletal system); if cues such as 'try not to make contact between the bar and the chest' do not address the issue, the load will have to be altered

TABLE 7.4   Variations of the Shoulder Press

Variation	Rationale		Considerations
Standing	This variation includes the challenge of controlling the core during the exercise.		As weight is added to this variation, individuals may start to bend the knees in a push press to increase the momentum of the body and make the exercise easier.

TABLE 7.4 Variations of the Shoulder Press (continued)

Variation	Rationale		Considerations
Dumbbells	The use of dumbbells will require more use of muscles that stabilise the shoulder such as the rotator cuff.		Individuals may choose to do this variation with a wider hand position, making the motion primarily shoulder abduction.
Medicine ball	The medicine ball can be used to make the shoulder press more dynamic and may include a throw and catch during the exercise.		This variation is most useful to develop power but it is important that correct technique is maintained even when velocity increases.
Variable hand spacing	When using a barbell, the positions of the hand will predominantly alter the action from pure shoulder flexion with a narrow grip to more shoulder abduction with a wider grip.		While all deltoid muscles will be recruited during the shoulder press, the contribution of each of the three heads may be altered slightly by these variations.

TABLE 7.4	Variations of the Shoulder Press (continued)		
Variation	**Rationale**		**Considerations**
Unstable surface	The standing (or kneeling) surface may be altered by using an unstable surface or wobble board or standing on one leg for the duration of the exercise. This will challenge the core and stabilising muscles.		Ensure the individual has the capacity to control the weights they are using in these variations. Consider decreasing weights considerably as the primary focus of the exercise is likely to be endurance, rather than maximal strength.

Activity 7.1 Research corner—overhead movements of the shoulder

Background

There has been considerable research interest over the years in the kinematics and kinetics of upper body exercises. This section provides a summary of some key studies that have added to our understanding of the shoulder. Overhead activities are often contentious in the literature due to the complexity of the shoulder and new practitioners should have a strong understanding of the biomechanics to allow them to optimise their exercise prescription. The studies presented below will be of use to those practitioners who wish to deepen their understanding of the movements involved.

- Ichihasni N, Ibuki S, Otsuka N, et al. 2014. Kinematic characteristics of the scapula and clavicle during military press exercise and shoulder flexion. *Journal of Shoulder and Elbow Surgery*. 23(5):649–657.
  - The authors reported the shoulder press produced greater upward rotation, external rotation and posterior tilting of the scapula and more protraction and elevation of the clavicle (in comparison to shoulder flexion exercises). They suggested that kinematic features of the shoulder press may make it a useful re-education exercise for patients with decreased scapular external rotation, upward rotation and posterior tilting.
- Moseley JB Jr, Jobe FW, Pink M, et al. 1992. EMG analysis of the scapular muscles during a shoulder rehabilitation program. *American Journal of Sports Medicine*. 20(2):128–134.
  - The authors studied the activities of the scapular muscles during the military press and other rehabilitation exercises and suggested that the military press is a useful exercise for the upper trapezius, middle serratus anterior and lower serratus anterior muscles.
- Paoli A, Marcolin G, Petrone N. 2010. Influence of different ranges of motion on selective recruitment of shoulder muscles in the sitting military press: an electromyographic study. *Journal of Strength and Conditioning Research*. 24(6):1578–1583.
  - The authors looked at ROM of the shoulder press and found employment of an incomplete ROM can reduce the involvement of the trapezius.

AIM:

- To be able to synthesise information from the literature and incorporate it into exercise programs

TASK:

- In small groups, consider how this research might impact your prescription of exercises of the shoulder.

Worksheet 7.1 Research Corner—Overhead Movements of the Shoulder

Question 1: Provide one clear example of how you would incorporate this evidence into your practice.

_____

_____

_____

_____

_____

Exercise 7b: Upright Row

Basic Exercise

Primary actions:

- Shoulder abduction
- Elbow flexion

Starting position:

- Grasp the bar with a closed, pronated grip with hands shoulder-width apart.
- Adopt a shoulder-width stance, with the knees slightly flexed, the elbows fully extended and with the bar level with the upper thigh.

Finishing position:

- The bar should be level with the clavicle, with the elbow in full flexion.
- Keep the elbows pointed out to the sides and at the highest bar position ensure they are level with or slightly higher than the shoulders and wrists.
- Keep the torso and knees in the same position throughout the exercise.

Execution of exercise:

- Lift the bar vertically with the torso until it reaches the level of the clavicle.
- Lead with the elbows and keep the bar close to the chest, ensuring the weight is lifted with an isolated effort from the upper body musculature.
- During the downward phase, slowly lower the bar to the start position, maintaining the position of the torso or knees.

The primary variation of the upright row is shown in standing position with an ezy curl bar (Figure 7.3). This will be followed by technique and cues (Table 7.5) and variations for the exercise (Table 7.6).

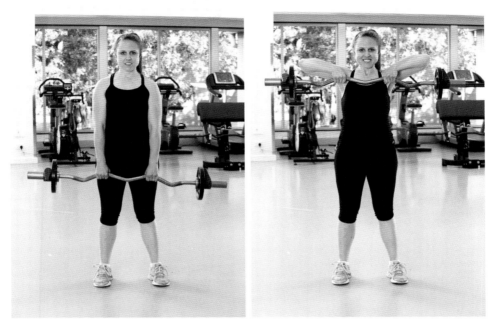

Figure 7.3 Primary variation of the upright row shown in a standing position with an ezy curl bar; starting and finishing position (left) and middle position (right)

TABLE 7.5 Cues and Technique for the Upright Row	
Poor Technique/Watch for	**Good Cues**
✘ Not leading with the elbows and trying to lift the weight up through the biceps in elbow flexion only	✔ 'Set your shoulders and lead with your elbows'
✘ Hyperextension of the lumbar spine, too much movement through the trunk during the exercise	✔ 'Keep your spine in neutral throughout the movement'
✘ Using the leg muscles to assist in moving load (i.e. rising up onto the toes) ✘ Swinging the bar upwards or using the lower body to generate momentum to lift the weight	✔ 'Try to use your arms on their own for this exercise' (if the individual cannot do this through effective cueing, it may be necessary to reduce the weight)
✘ Poor ROM for shoulder flexion and abduction	✔ If this persists despite cues such as 'try to move through full range of motion', this issue may be a result of poor thoracic mobility

TABLE 7.6   Variations of the Upright Row

Variation	Rationale		Considerations
Variable resistance	The use of TheraBands and tubing will change the resistance and make the end portion of the movement more challenging.		While this equipment is often utilised early in an individual's program to manage the resistance, it is important to observe their technique at end ROM and increase the length of the band if their technique falters at end of range.
Unilateral	Using one arm at a time or alternating between arms enhances the neural component of this exercise, requiring good coordination and core stability to remain in the correct position.		This exercise will challenge the lateral stabilisers of the trunk including the quadratus lumborum; instructors should watch for excessive trunk movement.
Hand spacing	Individuals may perform this exercise with a wide, medium or narrow grip. A narrow grip may challenge those with poor scapula control and reduce ROM.		Regardless of hand spacing, the position of the body should remain stable throughout the exercise, including neutral spine in both lumbar and thoracic regions.

TABLE 7.6   Variations of the Upright Row (continued)

Variation	Rationale		Considerations
Addition of a step up	Combining upper and lower body actions often increases the exercise's functionality and challenges the motor control of the exercise.		Ensure the exercises can be performed in isolation prior to adding together and only progress with weight when correct technique can be maintained.

Exercise 7c: Lateral Raise

Basic Exercise

Primary actions:

- Shoulder abduction

Starting position:

- Grasp two dumbbells with a closed, pronated grip in front of the hips with the elbows slightly flexed and pointing outwards and with the palms facing each other.
- Position the feet shoulder-to-hip-width apart, with the knees slightly flexed, back straight and shoulders back.

Finishing position:

- The dumbbells are raised until the elbows and wrists are parallel to the floor and in line with the shoulders.

Execution of exercise:

- Maintaining an erect upright body position, abduct the shoulders (humerus only) until the final position has been reached, ensuring the elbows and upper arms rise together, ahead of the forearms, hands and dumbbells, with the elbows remaining slightly flexed.
- Avoid externally rotating the humerus.
- During the downward phase and under control, allow the dumbbells to descend slowly back to the starting position.
- Raising dumbbells slightly forwards or backwards shall involve the anterior or posterior deltoids respectively.
- The contribution of the deltoids is reduced once dumbbells have been raised above 90° abduction. Trapezius and serratus anterior are working maximally at this point.

The primary variation of the lateral raise is shown in a standing position with dumbbells (Figure 7.4). This will be followed by technique and cues (Table 7.7).

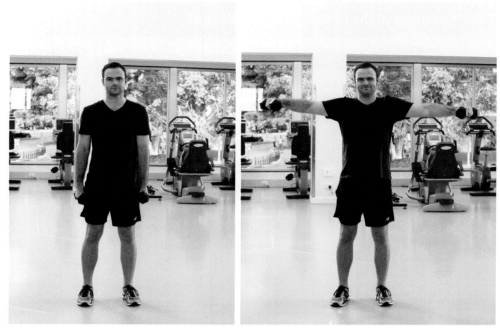

Figure 7.4 Primary variation of the lateral raise in a standing position with dumbbells; starting and finishing position (left) and middle position (right)

TABLE 7.7   Cues and Technique for the Lateral Raise

Poor Technique/Watch for	Good Cues
✗ Locking out elbows	✓ 'Keep a slight bend in your elbows throughout this exercise'
✗ Poor control of the scapula throughout the movement; may be seen by elevation in the initial phases of the exercise	✓ 'Set your shoulders' (keep your shoulder blades down; this may help if the issue is proprioceptive but if the issue is weakness and lack of endurance in the peri-scapular muscles, you may have to decrease the weight) ✓ 'Performing this activity in front of a mirror may help to ensure arms are straight and lifted to the correct height'
✗ Hyperextension of the lumbar spine, too much movement through the trunk during the exercise	✓ 'Keep your spine in neutral throughout the movement'

Exercise 7d: Front Raise

Basic Exercise

Primary action:

- Shoulder flexion

Starting position:

- Grasp two dumbbells with a closed, pronated grip in front of the hips with the elbows slightly flexed and pointing towards the body.

- Position the feet shoulder-to-hip-width apart, with the knees slightly flexed, back maintaining stable posture with natural curvature of the spine, shoulders back and eyes focused straight ahead.

Finishing position:

- The dumbbells are raised, with the elbows extended until the GH joint is flexed to 90°.

Execution of exercise:

- Maintaining an erect upright body position, flex the shoulders (humerus only) until the final position has been reached, ensuring the elbows and upper arms rise together, ahead of the forearms, hands and dumbbells, with the elbows remaining extended.
- Avoid externally rotating the humerus.
- During the downward phase and under control, allow the dumbbells to descend slowly back to the starting position.

The primary variation of the front raise is shown in a standing position with dumbbells (Figure 7.5). This will be followed by technique and cues (Table 7.8).

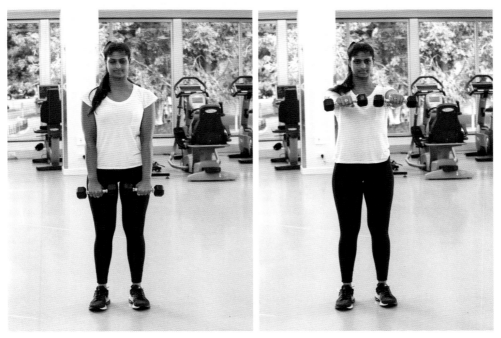

Figure 7.5 Primary variation of the front raise shown in a standing position with dumbbells; starting and finishing position (left) and middle position (right)

TABLE 7.8 Cues and Technique for the Front Raise	
Poor Technique/Watch for	**Good Cues**
✘ Holding breath, which is likely to occur with heavier weights; however, with untrained individuals the Valsalva manoeuvre and breath holding is often unnecessary and breathing throughout should be encouraged	✔ 'Inhale and hold during the lower (eccentric) phase and don't exhale until past the sticking point'
✘ Locking out knees and using the momentum of the body, swaying to lift the weights	✔ 'Have a slight bend in the knees and concentrate on keeping the body still while only moving the arms'

Exercise 7e: Shrug

Basic Exercise

Primary action:

- Scapula elevation

Starting position:

- Grasp two dumbbells with a hammer grip by the side of the body.
- Position the feet shoulder-width apart, with the knees slightly flexed, back maintaining stable posture with natural curvature of the spine, shoulders back and eyes focused straight ahead.

Finishing position:

- The arms remain straight and the shoulders are lifted towards the ears.

Execution of exercise:

- Maintaining an erect upright body position, elevate the scapula until the final position has been reached, ensuring the elbows remain extended.
- During the downward phase and under control, allow the dumbbells to descend slowly back to the starting position.

The primary variation of the shrug is shown in a standing position with dumbbells (Figure 7.6). This will be followed by technique and cues (Table 7.9).

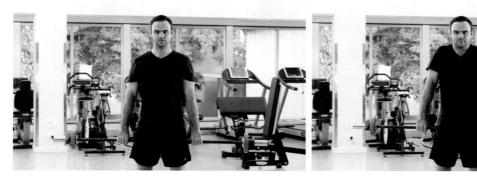

Figure 7.6 Primary variation of the shrug in a standing position with dumbbells; starting and finishing position (left) and middle position (right)

TABLE 7.9 Cues and Technique for the Shrug	
Poor Technique/Watch for	**Good Cues**
✗ Using too much weight and straining through the movement while holding breath	✓ 'Keep breathing throughout the exercise and pick a weight with which you can achieve full range of motion'

Activity 7.2 Research corner—monkey shrugs

Background

The monkey shrug is performed in a similar way to the classic dumbbell shrug; however, the start position is with the wrists approximately in line with the hips, which will therefore place the shoulders in approximately 30–45° of abduction (Figure 7.7).

The shrug is performed exactly as stated above; however, the emphasis becomes more on the upper traps than the levator scapulae. This was shown in a 2014 article by Pizzari and colleagues that assessed electromyography of the upper, middle and lower trapezius and the serratus anterior.[2] The upper traps have been shown to be effective in providing force closure at the sternoclavicular joint; therefore, this variation may be useful in individuals who need to take load way from the neck and optimise scapulohumeral rhythm, which is the movement of the humerus and scapula together.

AIM:

- To develop an understanding of when you may or may not use a variation of a shrug

TASK:

- Try this exercise in pairs. Discuss one context in which it might be useful to include it in your exercise prescription.

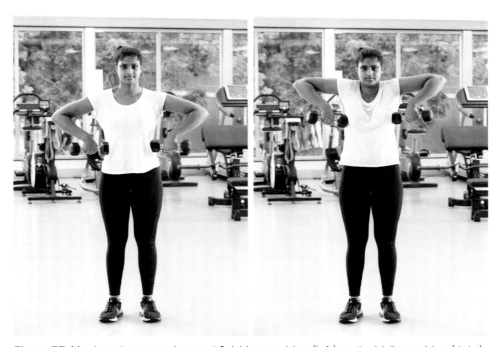

Figure 7.7 Monkey shrug starting and finishing position (left) and middle position (right)

Worksheet 7.2 Research Corner

Question 1: What is one context in which it might be useful to include monkey shrugs into your exercise prescription?

_____

_____

_____

_____

_____

Exercise 7f: Posterior Raise/Fly

Basic Exercise

Primary action:

- Horizontal shoulder extension

Starting position:

- Elbows are locked in a slightly bent position, the shoulder joint is neutral and the forearms are in a pronated position.

Finishing position:

- Shoulder joint is horizontally extended to 35°, with elbows remaining slightly flexed.

Body position:

- Sitting, leaning forwards at the waist (keeping back neutral/'straight'), shoulder blades neutral/'set' and chin neutral/'tucked in'.

Execution of exercise:

- Horizontally extend the shoulder joint to 35° (bilaterally).
- Maintain degree of elbow flexion.
- Do not externally rotate the humerus.
- Once the elbow joint has been brought up in line with the shoulder, it still needs to go another 35° behind the shoulder to strengthen the deltoids through the full ROM (assuming there is not a reduced ROM; e.g. due to a tight pectoralis major).

The primary variation of the posterior raise is shown in a standing position using dumbbells (Figure 7.8). This will be followed by technique and cues (Table 7.10) and variations for the exercise (Table 7.11).

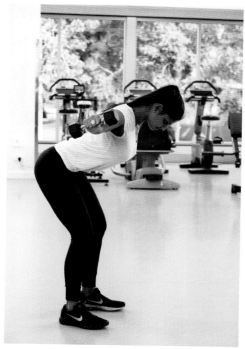

Figure 7.8 Primary variation of the posterior raise is shown in standing using dumbbells; this is the middle position of the exercise

TABLE 7.10   Cues and Technique for the Posterior Raise/Fly

Poor Technique/Watch for	Good Cues
✗ Not leaning over far enough, making this exercise predominantly shoulder abduction (like a lateral raise) rather than focusing on horizontal shoulder extension	✓ 'Keeping a nice straight back, bend a little more at the hips'
✗ Hyperextension of the shoulder or lumbar spine, too much movement through the trunk during the exercise	✓ 'Keep your spine in neutral throughout the movement'

TABLE 7.11   Variations of the Posterior Raise/Fly

Variation	Rationale		Considerations
Cables	When cables are able to be placed to allow pure horizontal extension in a standing position, the cable posterior fly can be a very effective exercise.		Low weights should be initially used to ensure the individual can maintain good neutral spine throughout the exercise.
Vary elbow angle	In the bent-over position, the position of the weights against gravity may initially be too advanced for the individual and the elbows can be bent to decrease the lever arm and ensure the exercise can be performed correctly.		If the individual cannot maintain appropriate spinal alignment when the elbows are straight, allowing the elbows to flex may allow the completion of the exercise without changing the body position.

Exercise 7g: Triceps Extension

Basic Exercise

Primary action:

- Elbow extension

Starting position:

- In a seated position, hold a dumbbell in both hands, with elbows fully flexed and GH joint in maximum flexion.

Finishing position:

- The GH joint remains in flexion with elbows fully extended.

Execution of exercise:

- Slowly extend the elbows until the finishing position is reached.
- Pause slightly at finishing position and lower the dumbbell to the starting position.

The primary variation of the triceps extension is shown in a seated position, using a dumbbell (Figure 7.9). This will be followed by technique and cues (Table 7.12) and variations for the exercise (Table 7.13).

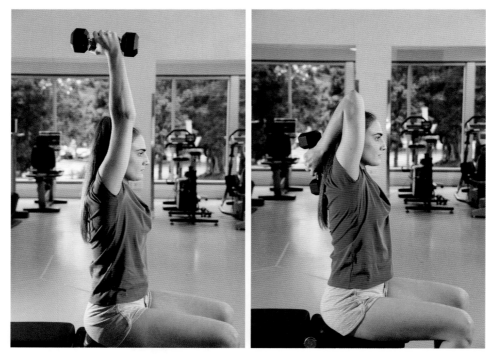

Figure 7.9 Primary variation of the triceps extension shown in a seated position, using a dumbbell; starting and finishing position (left) and middle position (right)

TABLE 7.12 Cues and Technique for the Triceps Extension	
Poor Technique/Watch for	**Good Cues**
✗ Straining forwards through cervical spine	✓ 'Keep a little tuck of the chin the whole way throughout the exercise'
✗ Difficulty getting full shoulder flexion, resulting in the weight not travelling directly against gravity, usually an issue with shoulder flexibility	✓ 'Look up straight' ✓ 'Performing this activity with a mirror may assist to keep the head up and the arms in line'

TABLE 7.13	Variations of the Triceps Extension		
Variation	**Rationale**		**Considerations**
Standing	To enhance the activation of stabilising muscles, this exercise can be performed in a standing position.		Ensure neutral spine is maintained throughout the exercise.
Bent over	This exercise is performed in a three-point kneeling position for enhanced stability or in a standing bent-over position to challenge the core.		Elbow should be kept against the side of the trunk throughout the exercise and the only movement should occur through elbow extension.
Triceps pushdown	By standing in a split stance during this exercise, the body position can remain stable. The use of the cable may be safer for untrained individuals as there is no risk of dropping the dumbbell.		Using a rope attachment to the cable machine can allow greater ROM and even incorporate shoulder extension in addition to elbow extension. To increase this ROM further, begin the exercise in a greater degree of shoulder flexion.

TABLE 7.13	Variations of the Triceps Extension (continued)		
Variation	**Rationale**		**Considerations**
Skull crusher	In a lying position, the individual grasps a dumbbell with both hands and positions the shoulder at 90° of flexion. The starting position is close to the forehead of the individual and the elbows are extended to lift the dumbbell.		This may be a safety risk for untrained individuals and should only be performed by competent individuals or with a spotter.

Activity 7.3 Triceps extension variation difficulty

AIM:

- To understand how changing the variation of the exercise can change the difficulty

TASKS:

- Perform 1 set of 15 reps of each of the variations listed for the triceps extension at a reasonable and similar weight/intensity.
- Report a rating of perceived exertion (RPE) that was reached for each exercise and make some notes about the difficulty of each exercise and any implications this might have on your prescription of this exercise in a program.

Worksheet 7.3 Triceps Extension Variation Difficulty		
Exercise	**RPE at End of Set of 15 Reps**	**Why You May or May Not include this Variation in a Program**
Standing		
Bent over		
Triceps pushdown		
Skull crusher		

Exercise 7h: Biceps Curl

Basic Exercise

Primary action:

- Elbow flexion

Starting position:

- Grasp the dumbbells with a supinated grip, with the elbows fully extended at the sides, keeping the GH joint and forearms in a neutral position.
- Seated with feet shoulder-width apart, maintain a stable posture with natural curvature of the spine and shoulders back.

Finishing position:

- Elbow should be fully flexed, with forearms in a supinated position, until the dumbbells are near the anterior deltoids.

Execution of exercise:

- Flex elbows slowly, either simultaneously or alternating each arm unilaterally.

The primary variation of the biceps curl is shown in a seated position with dumbbells (Figure 7.10). This will be followed by technique and cues (Table 7.14) and variations for the exercise (Table 7.15).

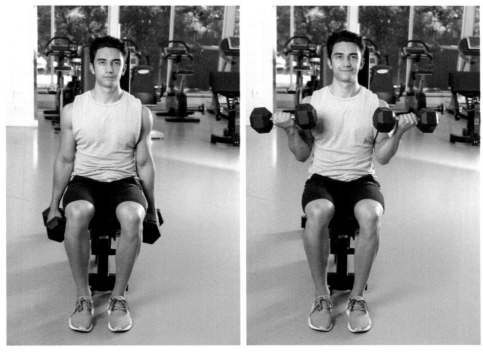

Figure 7.10 Primary variation of the biceps curl shown in a seated position with dumbbells; starting and finishing position (left) and middle position (right)

TABLE 7.14 Cues and Technique for the Biceps Curl	
Poor Technique/Watch for	**Good Cues**
✗ Jerking the body or swinging the weights upwards ✗ Do not bounce the weights on the thighs between repetitions	✓ 'Try to use your arms on their own for this exercise' (if the individual cannot do this through effective cueing, it may be necessary to reduce the load)

TABLE 7.15   Variations of the Biceps Curl

Variation	Rationale		Considerations
Standing	To enhance the activation of stabilising muscles, this exercise can be performed in a standing position.		Ensure neutral spine is maintained throughout the exercise.
Barbell	Using an EZ Curl Bar places the wrist in a more natural position than a straight bar.		Ensure cues are given to activate both arms equally to reduce the chance of one arm taking more load than the other.
Hammer curls	The curl is performed in a neutral grip with a greater emphasis on brachioradialis.		Ensure the wrists are maintained in a neutral position throughout the exercise and do not flex and extend.

TABLE 7.15	Variations of the Biceps Curl (continued)		
Variation	**Rationale**		**Considerations**
Preacher curl	This variation is performed using a bench that individuals place the upper arms on to ensure they remain still throughout the exercise, making it more difficult to use momentum and therefore it isolates biceps brachii.		Set up the equipment to ensure the shoulder and scapula can sit in a neutral position throughout this exercise.
Incline bench	Performing the biceps curl on an incline bench utilises the long head of the biceps brachii to a greater extent than when done normally as recruitment of the long head of the biceps brachii occurs through full ROM.		It is important to control the eccentric phase of this exercise to ensure the movement does not become a swinging movement.
Pronated versus supinated	Pronating the forearm recruits the brachialis for elbow flexion, whereas maintaining the forearm in supination throughout flexion is true flexion of the biceps brachii.		This may be more challenging as it focuses on smaller muscles, so a lighter weight than other variations might be necessary.

Activity 7.4 Research corner—exercises for the biceps

AIM:

- To deepen understanding of biceps exercises and muscle recruitment

TASKS:

- This section provides a summary of some key studies that have added to our understanding of biceps exercises and muscular recruitment.
- New exercise scientists should have a good understanding of the impact different variations of the exercise or different hand positions have on muscular recruitment to allow them to optimise their exercise prescription.
- The studies presented below will be of use to those students who wish to deepen their understanding of the exercises and the different muscles involved.
- You should read the studies (or the brief summaries provided below) and consider how it may influence your exercise prescription.

BACKGROUND:

- Oliveira LF, Matta TT, Alves D, et al. 2009. Effect of the shoulder position on the biceps brachii EMG in different dumbbell curls. *Journal of Sports, Science and Medicine*. 8(1):24–29.
  - The authors compared neuromuscular activity of the biceps brachii during different variations of the dumbbell curl (incline dumbbell curl, dumbbell preacher curl and the standard dumbbell biceps curl). The incline dumbbell curl and the dumbbell biceps curl resulted in considerable neuromuscular effort throughout the whole elbow range of motion. The incline dumbbell curl and the dumbbell biceps curl may be preferable for the improvement of biceps brachii force in training programs.
- Kleiber T, Kunz L, Disselhorst-Klug C. 2015. Muscular coordination of biceps brachii and brachioradialis in elbow flexion with respect to hand position. *Frontiers in Physiology*. 6:215.
  - The authors compared neuromuscular activity of the brachioradialis and biceps brachii in different hand positions (pronated, neutral and supinated). Significant differences in the contribution of brachioradialis were found in the pronated hand position compared to supinated and neutral hand position while the muscular activity of biceps brachii shows no significant changes in any hand position.

Worksheet 7.4 Research Corner—Exercises for the Biceps

Question 1: After reading the studies, how might this information influence your exercise prescription?

_____

_____

_____

_____

_____

Exercise 7i: Rotator Cuff Curl

Basic Exercise

Primary actions:

- Shoulder internal rotation
- Shoulder external rotation

Starting position:

- Standing, hold the TheraBand or cable, with the GH joint externally rotated and elbow flexed at 90° (for internal rotation).
- The elbow should be fixed against the body.

Finishing position:

- The GH joint should be internally rotated and the elbow flexed at 90°.
- The elbow should be fixed against the body.

Body position:

- Maintain stable posture with natural curvature of the spine.
- Scapular and thoracic spine should remain stabilised.

Motion:

- Internally rotate the arm, while keeping the elbow fixed by your side throughout the motion.
- The instructions above detail the internal rotator cuff curl and Figure 7.11 shows the start and finish position for an internal rotation. The starting position and finishing position are reversed for external rotator cuff curls.

Breathing:

- Exhale during the lifting motion, inhale during the lowering portion.

The primary variation of the rotator cuff curl is shown in a standing position with a cable (Figure 7.11). This will be followed by technique and cues (Table 7.16) and variations for the exercise (Table 7.17).

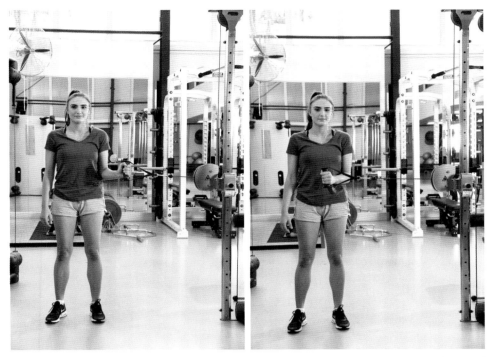

Figure 7.11 Primary variation of the rotator cuff curl shown in a standing position with a cable; starting and finishing position (left) and middle position (right)

TABLE 7.16 Cues and Technique for the Rotator Cuff Curl	
Poor Technique/Watch for	**Good Cues**
✘ Allowing the elbow to come away from the body	✓ 'Keep elbow against the torso' ✓ 'Use a towel between the elbow and the trunk and don't let it fall to the ground during the exercise'
✘ Using the leg muscles or the trunk muscles to assist in moving the load in standing variation	✓ 'Try to use the arms on their own for this exercise' (if the individual cannot do this through effective cueing, it may be necessary to reduce the load)

TABLE 7.17	Variations of the Rotator Cuff Curl		
Variation	**Rationale**		**Considerations**
Elbow position	Placing a towel between the elbow and the body can provide useful feedback as to whether the elbow is staying against the torso during the exercise. If the individual requires progression, the humerus can be abducted to 90° which will require significantly more stabilisation.		Shoulder abduction should only be added to the exercise if the individual has good scapula control.
Dumbbell	This variation is performed in a side-lying position with the bottom arm performing internal rotation and the top arm performing external rotation.		Ensure the correct movement plane for internal and external rotation to ensure each exercise is allowing the movement against gravity, not across it. If this movement is performed in standing the action against gravity is elbow flexion, not shoulder internal rotation.

Activity 7.5 Design a shoulder/arm exercise program

AIM:
- To provide shoulder exercises for specific goals and outcomes

TASK:
- Using the exercises presented in this chapter and your understanding of basic exercise prescription guidelines, detail a shoulder/arm exercise program for one of the following individual goals. (Consider the exercise order, difficulty and focus and give a brief justification for the program.)
    1. Powerlifter looking for maximal strength
    2. Body builder looking for muscular hypertrophy
    3. Endurance for an individual who does significant amounts of manual labour

Worksheet 7.5 Design a Shoulder/Arm Exercise Program		
Exercise	Sets/Reps	Other Information (repetitions in Reserve [RIR], Tempo, Rest, Justification)

References

1   Drake R 2015. *Gray's Atlas of Anatomy*. Churchill Livingstone.
2   Pizzari T, Wickham J, Balster S, et al. 2014. Modifying a shrug exercise can facilitate the upward rotator muscles of the scapula. *Clin Biomech*. 29(2):201–205.

PRACTICAL 8
THE BACK

Emma M. Beckman and Michael J. Dale

Introduction

This practical discusses exercises targeting the upper- and mid-back and active shoulder joint extension movements. We do not address exercises specifically targeting the maintenance of spinal neutral position. This distinction is not made to imply a lack of relevance of this capacity; indeed, the maintenance of a neutral spinal position is a prerequisite to all exercises discussed herein. Rather, we make this distinction to ensure that the focus of the work within this practical is maintained on the primary objective: to increase strength qualities of the muscles of the back. While the exercises presented here will indirectly challenge the neutral spinal position, this is not their first purpose. Their first purpose is to condition the musculature required for good scapulothoracic and glenohumeral articulation.

Due to their location, the muscles of the back can produce what are generally considered to be 'rowing' or 'pulling' movements; that is, a combination of scapular retraction, depression and/or shoulder joint extension or adduction. Training of the upper back generally centres around ensuring appropriate stability and mobility of the scapulae, and developing the capacity to exert extension and/or adduction force to move either the implement (barbell, dumbbell etc.) or the body (e.g. with a pull-up). Glenohumeral (GH) stability thus plays a prominent role in training the upper back. Given the intricate relationship between the movements that occur during exercises that train the back, this practical will have a significant focus on anatomy. Much of this anatomy will relate and refer to a number of other practicals, including the chest and shoulder and arms practicals; however, for ease of understanding and consistency of terminology it is dealt with in detail in this practical.

Exercises included in this practical are:

- seated row
- prone row
- one arm dumbbell row
- bent over row
- lat pull-down
- chin-up.

For each exercise, a primary variation will be presented with actions, starting position, finishing position, equipment set-up and execution of the exercise. This will be followed by a table of technique and cues and a table of variations for the exercise (as appropriate).

Anatomy

For movements that involve shoulder joint extension or horizontal extension, the scapula should move medially and inferiorly; that is, 'together and in'. The inferior border of the scapula should not rotate medially and the scapula should not rise off the rib cage (i.e. wing). The humeral head should stay fixed in the glenoid cavity, providing the pivot for the humerus to move around. Dynamic stability of the GH joint is partially maintained by the compressive force generated anteriorly, superiorly and posteriorly by the musculature of the rotator cuff (subscapularis, supraspinatus and both infraspinatus and teres minor, respectively). By virtue of their anterior and posterior humeral attachments, subscapularis and infraspinatus/teres minor also play a role in internal and external rotation respectively.

For movements that involve adduction of the GH joint from the extreme end range of abduction, the superior border of the scapula rotates laterally to maintain scapulohumeral rhythm as the humerus adducts.

Movement Categories

Movement of the scapulothoracic and GH joints can be broadly subdivided into three main categories.

1. Scapulothoracic movements. These movements occur where musculature originating on the torso (e.g. trapezius, rhomboids) act to control the position of the scapula. These muscles may move the scapula, causing adduction, abduction, elevation, depression or external/internal rotation of the scapulae. The lack of action of these muscles may also allow external forces or loads to cause some of these movements (i.e. poor rhomboid/middle trapezius function may allow undesired scapular abduction during movements). In most instances, if we are considering moving our scapulae, we will use musculature fixed to the torso (a generally stable base) to do so. We may in some circumstances fix the humerus via stabilising musculature and then move the scapula about the fixed humerus, but this is less common.

2. Scapulohumeral movements. These movements occur when musculature originating on the torso and/ or scapula (e.g. latissimus dorsi, deltoid, supraspinatus) act to control the position of the humerus on the scapula. We can conceive of these muscles and movements as those which directly control the position of the elbow joint in space. These movements include GH (or shoulder) joint flexion, extension, abduction and adduction. Again, movement of the elbow in space is the most common scenario; however, we may fix the position of the elbow in space via stabilising musculature and move the shoulder joint (and with it, the torso) about the elbow.

3. Scapulohumeral orientation control. These movements occur when musculature originating on the scapula and/or torso (but predominantly rotator cuff musculature of the scapula) acts to alter the orientation of the humerus on the scapula. Rather than changing the elbow (and thus the humeral) position in space, the degree of internal/external rotation of the humerus is changed. With a fixed elbow joint angle and position, this will result in the forearm and hand changing position in space.

The anatomy of the back is shown pictorially in Figure 8.1 to provide a visual representation of the muscles of interest. The movements and muscles recruited are listed in Table 8.1.

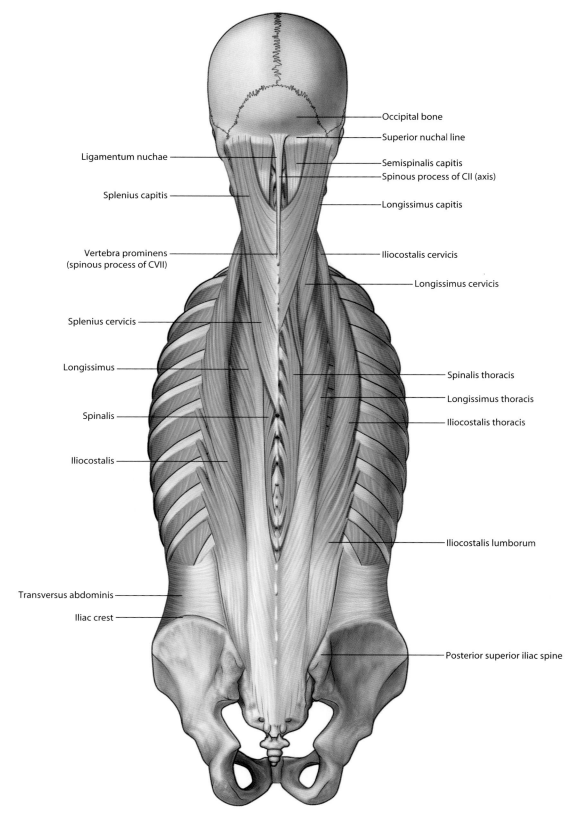

Figure 8.1 Key muscles of the back, both superficial and deep
Source: Drake (2015).[1]

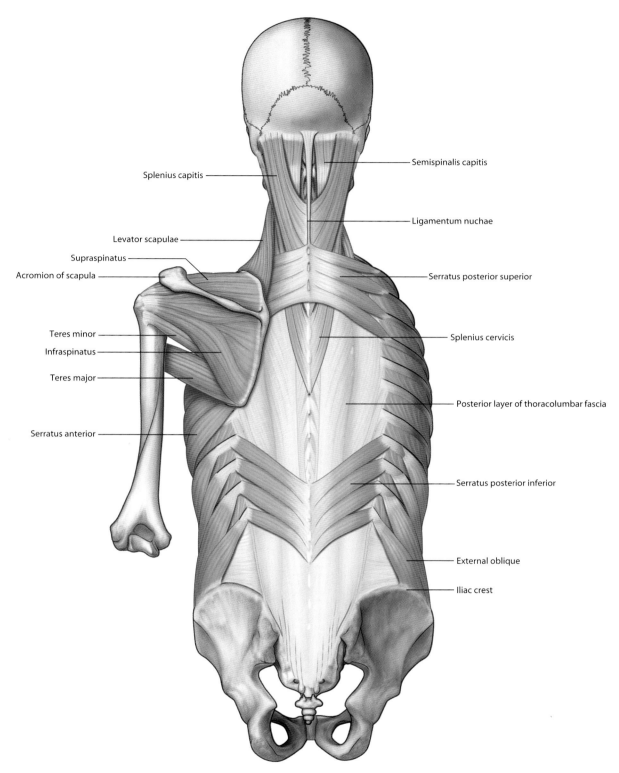

Splenius capitis

Levator scapulae

Supraspinatus

Acromion of scapula

Teres minor

Infraspinatus

Teres major

Serratus anterior

Semispinalis capitis

Ligamentum nuchae

Serratus posterior superior

Splenius cervicis

Posterior layer of thoracolumbar fascia

Serratus posterior inferior

External oblique

Iliac crest

Figure 8.1, cont'd

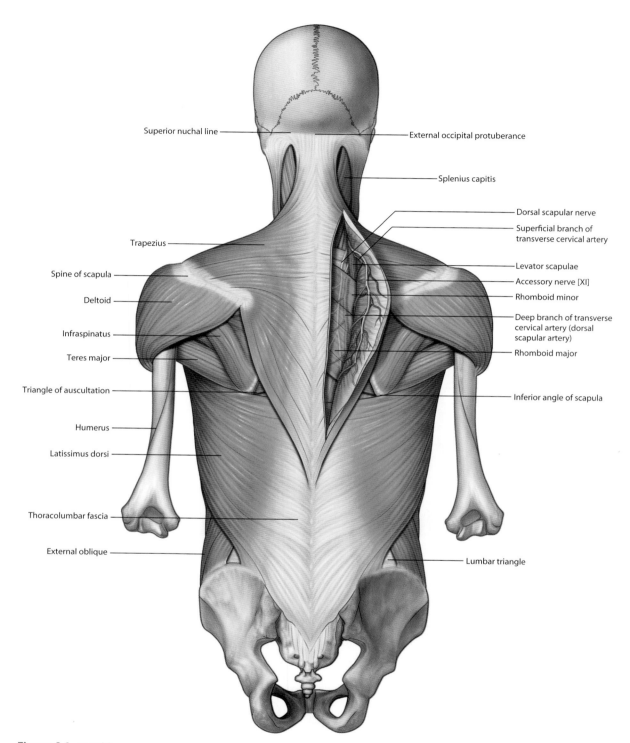

Figure 8.1, cont'd

TABLE 8.1	Anatomy of the Shoulder and Arms
Movement	**Muscles Recruited**
Scapulothoracic adduction	• Trapezius (middle) • Latissimus dorsi • Levator scapulae • Rhomboid major • Rhomboid minor
Scapulothoracic abduction	• Serratus anterior
Scapulothoracic elevation	• Trapezius (upper) • Levator scapulae • Rhomboid major • Rhomboid minor
Scapulothoracic depression	• Trapezius (lower) • Latissimus dorsi
Scapulothoracic internal rotation	• Levator scapulae • Rhomboid major • Rhomboid minor
Scapulothoracic external rotation	• Trapezius (upper and lower) • Serratus anterior
Scapulohumeral flexion	• Pectoralis major • Deltoid (anterior) • Coracobrachialis (weakly) • Biceps brachii (weakly) • Supraspinatus (weakly)
Scapulohumeral extension	• Pectoralis major • Latissimus dorsi • Deltoid (posterior) • Teres major
Scapulohumeral adduction	• Pectoralis major • Latissimus dorsi • Teres major • Triceps brachii • Coracobrachialis (weakly) • Teres minor (weakly)
Scapulohumeral abduction	• Deltoid (middle) • Supraspinatus • Infraspinatus

TABLE 8.1 Anatomy of the Shoulder and Arms (continued)	
Movement	**Muscles Recruited**
Scapulohumeral internal rotation	• Pectoralis major • Latissimus dorsi • Deltoid (anterior) • Subscapularis • Teres major
Scapulohumeral external rotation	• Deltoid (posterior) • Infraspinatus • Teres minor
Humeral head fixation/stabilisation	• Supraspinatus • Infraspinatus • Subscapularis • Teres minor

Exercise 8a: Seated Row

Basic Exercise

Primary actions:

- Glenohumeral extension
- Scapular retraction
- Elbow flexion

Starting position:

- Elbows are slightly flexed ($< 5°$), arms held out in front, holding with a neutral grip.

Finishing position:

- Elbows are flexed ($90°$), scapula retracted and depressed, and arms adducted.
- Hands are in line with the bottom of the rib cage.

Body position:

- Maintain isometric hip and knee flexion throughout motion.

Execution of exercise:

- Slowly pull the hands to the bottom of the rib cage.
- Execution consists of simultaneous elbow flexion, scapula retraction and GH extension.
- If biceps strength limits this exercise, straps may be utilised.

The primary variation of the seated row is shown with a cable row machine in long sitting position (Figure 8.2). This will be followed by technique and cues (Table 8.2) and variations for the exercise (Table 8.3).

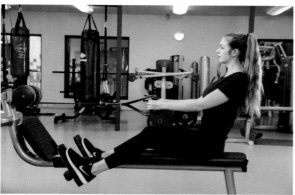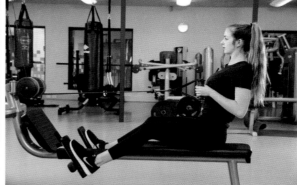

Figure 8.2 Primary variation of the seated row with a cable row machine in a long sitting position; starting and finishing position (left) and middle position (right)

TABLE 8.2 Cues and Technique for the Seated Row	
Poor Technique/Watch for	**Good Cues**
✗ Scapula wings	✓ Activate rhomboids by cueing 'pinch my finger' with finger placed on upper thoracic spine
✗ Upper fibres of the trapezius become overactive (shrugging)	✓ Activate lower traps with cue 'scaps in pockets'; creates depressive effect ✓ Relax upper traps by gently pushing down on shoulders and giving the cue 'relax out of the shrug'
✗ Rounded shoulders	✓ 'Chest up, shoulders back'
✗ Using erector spinae to extend lumbar spine to assist moving the weight (depends on goals)	✓ 'Think of the torso as a rigid segment'
✗ Extending the knees to assist moving the weight	✓ Cue 'pull with the back and arms' and 'no legs'
✗ Scapula does not move ✗ Moving the weight with only elbow flexion	✓ 'Squeeze shoulder blades together'; activate rhomboids by cueing 'pinch my finger' with finger placed on upper thoracic spine
✗ Holding breath	✓ Cue breathing by anchoring breath to phase of exercise: 'breathe out on the pull, breathe in on the return'

TABLE 8.3   Variations of the Seated Row

Variation	Rationale		Considerations
Supported	If an individual is struggling to maintain an appropriate lumbopelvic position during the exercise or it is difficult to initiate the pulling action, having the chest supported may allow the successful completion of this exercise.		The machine should be individually set up with the correct seat height and position of the chest plate to ensure an appropriate starting and finishing position.
Standing	When the individual has mastered the seated variation with optimal pelvic control, the exercise may be performed in standing which will generate greater stabilisation requirements. This exercise might be performed with the regular range of motion (ROM) but also might be amended to a face pull-type exercise. A split stance will provide the best base of support for the exercise.		The focus of the exercise in standing should be control and stabilisation rather than maximal strength; therefore, the weights may need to be reduced and a focus on slightly higher rep range taken to get the most out of the exercise.
Single arm	This variation can be performed in either seated or standing and is useful when training neuromuscular control and stabilisation for people who predominantly perform alternating activities of the upper limb rather than synchronous movements. This might make the activity more sports-specific for athletes who perform running as part of their training.		There is increased demand on the trunk in this exercise as it must resist rotation force to the contralateral side as the movement is performed.

TABLE 8.3 Variations of the Seated Row (continued)			
Variation	**Rationale**		**Considerations**
Wide grip	As the grip widens, different equipment such as a long bar might be required. The movement shifts from more pure GH extension to more horizontal extension as the humerus abducts to the width of the bar.		Tight pectoralis muscles may alter the desired position of the humerus and scapula as the grip widens. If there is considerable internal rotation of the humerus during any version of the seated row, the ROM may have to be restricted.

Activity 8.1 Key muscular anatomy—rhomboids

Background

The rhomboids originate from the spinous processes of the C7 and T1−5 vertebrae and insert along the medial border of the scapula, below the height of the medial portion of the spine of the scapula (Figure 8.3). Moving from origin to insertion, these fibres run diagonally inferolaterally. As a result of this orientation, the rhomboids function to cause adduction, elevation and internal rotation of the scapula. These muscles play an important role in setting the scapulae into a good retracted/adducted position and maintaining this position against external loads; that is, they act as important stabilisers of the scapulae.

Palpation

This activity and some of the following activities require you to palpate, or touch, your partner. Make sure you describe to your partner what you plan to do and ask for their permission before you touch them. This is of great importance when you are working in class but especially when you start working with clients.

Have your partner lie prone on an elevated bench or massage table, with one arm 'winged' (internally rotated with the forearm perpendicular to the spine and behind the back) as Figure 8.4. Find the medial border of the scapula and then move medially, palpating superiorly to inferiorly and vice versa. The fibres of rhomboid major and minor will run obliquely upwards at a shallow angle, with the medial end of the fibres superior to the lateral end. In contrast, middle and lower fibres of the trapezius, which lie superficial to the rhomboids, will run medially horizontally and downwards (trapezius fibres will fan out from the height of the spine of the scapula, with lower fibres angled more steeply downwards). Ask your partner to push their 'winged' arm elbow towards the ceiling. You should feel the superficial trapezius fibres contract, but may also be able to identify the deeper rhomboids contracting as well.

AIM:
- **Palpate the rhomboids on a partner**

TASKS:
- Follow the above steps to palpate the rhomboids of your partner while they are in the prone position.
- Have your partner perform the seated row exercise and palpate the rhomboids during this exercise.
- Encourage strong scapular retraction at the end of the ROM by using a cue such as 'squeeze my fingers'.
- After completing this exercise, discuss with another student the difficulty of palpating specific muscles (especially deep ones) throughout active exercises.

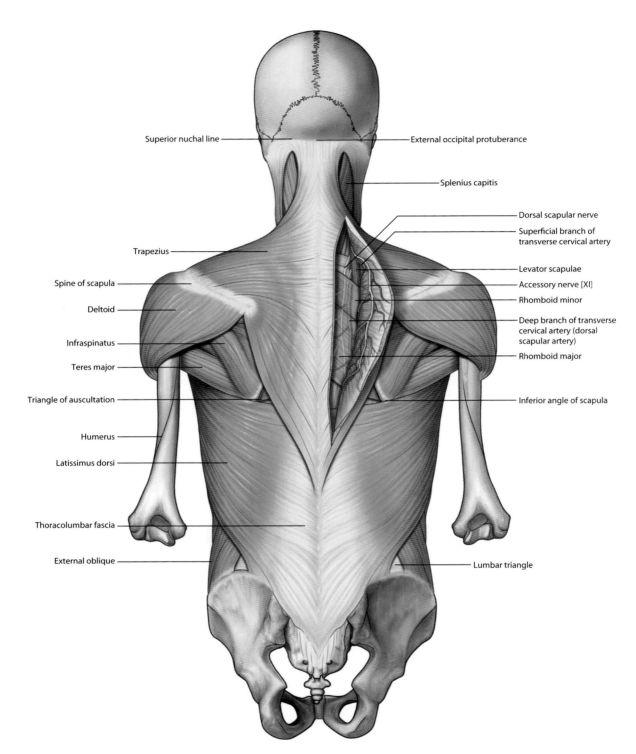

Figure 8.3 The rhomboids shown in relation to other muscles of the back
Source: Drake (2015).[1]

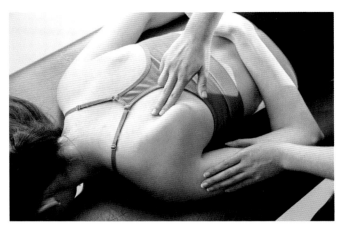

Figure 8.4 Position for palpation exercise

Activity 8.2 Seated row variations

AIM:
- Understand how variations of the same exercise can change muscle contraction

TASK:
- Conduct the seated row under the following conditions:
    1. chest unsupported, narrow neutral grip and arms adducted (elbows close to ribcage)
    2. chest unsupported, wide pronated grip on a long bar and arms abducted (elbows flared high, away from the ribcage at approximately 90°).

Worksheet 8.2 Seated Row Variations

Question 1: Compare the sensation of contraction at the end of the range. Do these two variations feel different in any way? Why might this be so? _____

_____

_____

_____

Exercise 8b: Prone Row

Basic Exercise

Primary actions:
- Glenohumeral extension
- Scapular retraction
- Elbow flexion

Starting position:
- Elbows are slightly flexed (< 5°), arms held below holding the bar vertically in line with shoulders.
- Note that a high bench is required to achieve an ideal start position; a low bench (i.e. one that might be used for bench press) will not allow the ideal arm extension start position to be achieved.

Finishing position:

- Elbows are flexed and the bar lifted as high as possible.
- Scapulae are retracted and hands are in line with the bottom of the rib cage.

Body position:

- Lie prone on the bench while maintaining neutral spinal alignment.

Execution of exercise:

- Slowly pull the bar up to the bottom of the rib cage.
- Execution consists of simultaneous elbow flexion and scapula retraction and depression.

The primary variation of the prone row is shown using a prone row bench and a barbell (Figure 8.5). This will be followed by technique and cues (Table 8.4) and variations for the exercise (Table 8.5).

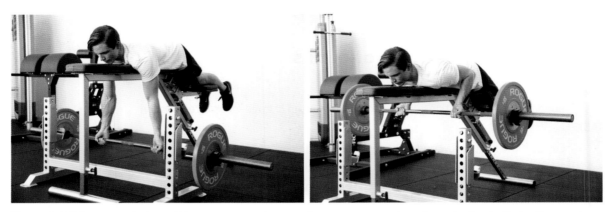

Figure 8.5 Primary variation of the prone row shown using a prone row bench and a barbell; starting and finishing position (left) and middle position (right)

TABLE 8.4 Cues and Technique for the Prone Row	
Poor Technique/Watch for	**Good Cues**
✗ Rounded shoulders	✓ 'Shoulders back'
✗ Using erector spinae to extend lumbar spine to assist moving the weight (depends on goals)	✓ 'Think of the torso as a rigid segment'
✗ Neck is extended with each repetition	✓ 'Keep neck in neutral position throughout the exercise, avoiding actively extending it on each repetition'

TABLE 8.5	Variations of the Prone Row			
Variation	**Rationale**			**Considerations**
Hand spacing	A wide hand spacing and including an instruction to pull the bar towards the upper chest will result in greater horizontal extension in this exercise.			The length of the bench and the position of the client may impact on their cervical spine position. Ensure this is kept as neutral as possible given equipment restrictions.
Elbow tracking	Even with a relatively narrow grip and/or a final position with the hands (and bar) at the lower ribcage, it is possible to execute this movement with a bias towards horizontal abduction if the elbows are allowed to flare out. Keeping the elbows tracking close to the ribcage will ensure shoulder extension is achieved.			When viewed from above, the final position should involve a relatively small angle between the long axis of the body and the humeri. As this angle increases (i.e. moves towards 90°), the movement becomes horizontal abduction and therefore the contribution of the posterior deltoid is emphasised.

Activity 8.3 Key muscular anatomy—posterior deltoid

Background

This large triangular muscle originates at the insertion of the trapezius—the lateral one-third of the clavicle, the acromion process, and the spine of the scapula in a similar horseshoe or U-shaped format—and inserts onto the humerus at the deltoid tuberosity as shown in Figure 8.6. Generally considered to have anterior, medial and posterior fibres, the contribution to the rowing action considered here is predominantly borne by the medial fibres (which are responsible for the degree of abduction and therefore the elbow position in the frontal plane). The posterior fibres, as the arm abducts towards 90°, become more optimally oriented to deliver horizontal extension of the humerus, as opposed to pure extension when abduction is absent or minimal. Note, however, that the contribution of posterior deltoid to extension is generally exceeded by the role played by the larger and more mechanically advantaged latissimus dorsi, particularly when extending from a more flexed shoulder joint position.

Palpation

Have your partner sit on a low bench or chair. Locate the origins of the deltoid: the lateral clavicle, the acromion process and the lateral spine of scapula. Palpate from these structures down the arm and identify superficial fibres converging towards a point approximately one-third of the way down the humerus. These fibres belong to the deltoid muscle. Have your partner attempt to abduct their arm while you resist this motion; you should feel these fibres contract. Now allow your partner to abduct their arm to 90°, and have them horizontally extend the arm against resistance. You should be able to move from the middle fibres of the deltoid, which will be contracted to hold the arm at 90° abduction, to the posterior fibres of the deltoid, which you will feel becoming more active during resisted extension. Try alternately palpating latissimus dorsi and posterior deltoid during resisted horizontal extension and compare the difference.

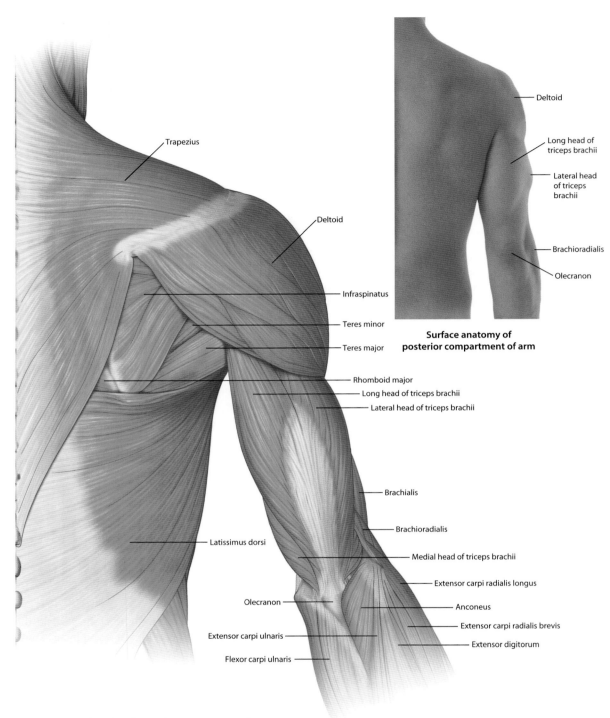

Muscles of posterior compartment of arm

Figure 8.6 Trapezius shown in relation to other muscles of the back
Source: Drake (2015).[1]

AIM:

- Palpate the posterior deltoids on a partner

TASKS:

- Follow the above steps to palpate the posterior deltoid on a partner in a seated position.
- Conduct this palpation exercise during the execution of the prone row. Particularly focus on palpation towards the finishing position of this exercise.

Activity 8.4 Prone row execution

AIM:

- Understand how variations of the same exercise can change muscle contraction to properly execute the prone row and change difficulty

TASK:

- With a partner, follow the instructions in the worksheet below and answer the questions.

Worksheet 8.4 Prone Row Variations

Question 1: With a moderate load, have your partner practise 'setting' the shoulder girdle into neutral by retracting against the load before initiating the pull phase of the prone row exercise. Hold the neutral position with an isometric contraction of the rhomboids and trapezius for an extended period. Watch for unwanted elevation of the scapulae later in the hold. What does this tell you about relative strength between the upper and lower fibres of the trapezius? How might we use cues to avoid this?

_____

_____

_____

_____

_____

Question 2: Against a moderate to heavy load, conduct repetitions of the prone row with the arms adducted (elbows close to the ribcage, pulling towards the lower sternum). Then, after adequate rest, repeat this task with the elbows abducted (elbows flared away from the ribcage at approximately 90°), pulling towards the upper sternum. Have your partner do the same but in reverse (elbows flared first). In which condition can you complete more repetitions? Why?

_____

_____

_____

_____

_____

Exercise 8c: One-arm Dumbbell Row

Basic Exercise

Primary actions:

- Glenohumeral extension
- Scapular retraction
- Elbow flexion

Starting position:

- One knee is placed on the bench while the ipsilateral arm supports the upper body on the same bench. The other leg supports the body on the ground.
- The elbow is slightly flexed ($<5°$) and the dumbbell is held with a neutral grip in line with the shoulder.
- Alternative set-up: Stand to the side of the bench with the body perpendicular, rather than parallel to the bench. Position the feet approximately shoulder-width apart and flex the knee joints slightly. Flex at the hip joint towards a torso parallel to the floor position. Support the torso with the non-loaded hand on the bench. This set-up may be beneficial if the bench height is inappropriate to the anthropometry of the individual and/or if the person performing the exercise is having difficulty assuming the correct position with both the knee and the hand on the bench.

Finishing position:

- The elbow is flexed (approximately 135°) and the scapula is retracted and depressed.
- The dumbbell is in line with the bottom of the rib cage.
- The arm is adducted.

Body position:

- Maintain a neutral spine (postural alignment).
- Ensure that the shoulders are square (i.e. both are the same height from the bench).
- Ensure that the hips are square (i.e. both are the same height from the bench).

Execution of exercise:

- Lift the dumbbell vertically to the finishing position.
- Do not drop the dumbbell in the lowering phase or allow the shoulders to deviate from their square position (the temptation will be to allow the loaded side to drop towards the floor).
- This position with the aid of gravity adds a postural holding element to the rowing action, which increases the emphasis placed on scapula and humeral head stabilisation, lumbar spine stabilisation and the pelvis during exercise. More importance should be given to maintaining correct body position and movement than to weight lifted during the exercise.

The primary variation of the one arm dumbbell row is shown using a dumbbell and a bench (Figure 8.7). This will be followed by technique and cues (Table 8.6) and variations for the exercise (Table 8.7).

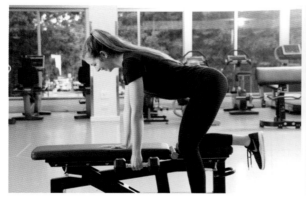 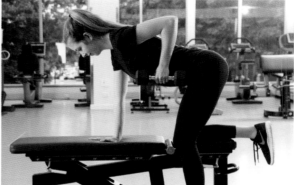

Figure 8.7 Primary variation of the one-arm dumbbell row shown using a dumbbell and a bench; starting and finishing position (left) and middle position (right)

TABLE 8.6   Cues and Technique for the One-arm Dumbbell Row

Poor Technique/Watch for	Good Cues
✘ Scapula wings	✔ Activate rhomboids by cueing 'pinch my finger' with finger(s) placed on upper thoracic spine
✘ Rounded shoulders	✔ 'Chest up, shoulders back'
✘ Poor lumbar spine position with exaggerated lordosis	✔ 'Keep a neutral spine position throughout the exercise'
✘ Scapula does not move	✔ 'Squeeze shoulder blades together'
✘ Moving the weight with only elbow flexion	✔ Activate rhomboids by cueing 'pinch my finger' with finger placed on upper thoracic spine

TABLE 8.7   Variations of the One-arm Dumbbell Row

Variation	Rationale		Considerations
Elbow tracking	It is possible to execute this movement with a bias towards horizontal abduction if the elbow is allowed to flare out. Keeping the elbow tracking close to the ribcage will ensure shoulder extension is achieved.		When viewed from above, the final position should involve a relatively small angle between the long axis of the body and the humerus. As this angle increases (i.e. moves towards 90°), the movement becomes horizontal abduction and therefore the contribution of the posterior deltoid is emphasised.
Level of support	Lower levels of support are progressions within this exercise, but note that they are not solely progressions of the upper back musculature. Changing the level of support also impacts on (i.e. progresses the challenge for) the ability of the lumbar spinal stabilisers to maintain the required body position.		As the individual moves from more to less support (i.e. from kneeling on the bench, to standing with one arm supported on the bench, to no support), continuously monitor both the back angle to the floor and the lumbar spinal curve (if either the back angle to the floor changes to a more vertical position, or the lumbar spinal neutral position is lost, the lumbar spinal stabilisers are likely to be fatiguing). Terminate the set and allow for recovery or provide more support, and consider lower-back stability endurance work to enhance the capacity to row in less-supported environments.

Activity 8.5 Positioning the one-arm dumbbell row

AIM:

- Set up a partner in the correct position to complete the one-arm dumbbell row exercise

TASK:

- Figure 8.8 shows an individual with poor technique performing this exercise.
- Consider cues you might use to improve the positioning and execution of the exercise.
- Consider the use of higher, lower, wider benches or additional equipment such as steps if you feel this may also improve the execution of the exercise.

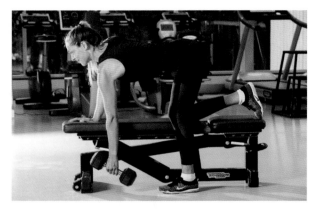

Figure 8.8 Example of poor positioning in the dumbbell row

Worksheet 8.5 Positioning the One-arm Dumbbell Row

Question 1: What cues would you use to help your client position properly?

_____

_____

Question 2: How does changing the equipment help improve execution of the exercise?

_____

_____

Activity 8.6 Comparing techniques

AIM:

- Compare two different techniques to perform the one-arm dumbbell row

TASKS:

- Select a dumbbell that represents a moderate load. Conduct repetitions with one arm focusing on good technique—not allowing spinal rotation at either end of the ROM. You should attempt to go to failure (i.e. when you feel yourself begin to lose 'good form').
- Swap to the other arm and conduct repetitions, but this time, allow (carefully) spinal rotation at the bottom (towards the floor) and top (away from the floor) of the range. Continue until fatigued.

Worksheet 8.6 Comparing Techniques

Question 1: On which side can you complete more repetitions?

_____

Question 2: On which side does form 'feel' better?

_____

Question 3: At the moment of fatigue, were you fatigued in the same musculature when comparing side to side? Why might there be differences?

_____

_____

_____

_____

_____

Exercise 8d: Bent-over Row

Basic Exercise

Primary actions:

- Glenohumeral extension
- Scapular retraction
- Elbow flexion
- Spinal stabilisation (anti-flexion)

Starting position:

- From the standing position with a loaded barbell, slightly flex the knees.
- Now flex at the hip, maintaining a neutral spine and a small degree of knee joint flexion. Aim for the torso to be approximately parallel to the floor. Allow the bar to hang at full elbow extension, under the shoulders. Do not allow the load (i.e. the plates) to touch the floor—adjust the knee and hip joint flexion to prevent this. All repetitions begin from this position.

Finishing position:

- Elbow is flexed (approximately 135°) and the scapula is retracted and depressed.
- The bar is in contact with the torso.
- The arms will be adducted if the grip is narrow, abducted if the grip is wide.

Body position:

- Maintain a neutral spine (postural alignment).
- Do not alter the degree of knee joint flexion from the start position.
- Do not alter the degree of hip joint flexion from the start position.

Execution of exercise:

- Pull the bar upwards towards the torso.
- Forearms and wrists should remain vertical; do not curl the bar up towards the torso.
- The bar should touch the torso at the lower sternum/upper abdomen height. The elbows should be above the back at this position.

The primary variation of the bent over row is shown in a standing position with a barbell (Figure 8.9). This will be followed by technique and cues (Table 8.8) and variations for the exercise (Table 8.9).

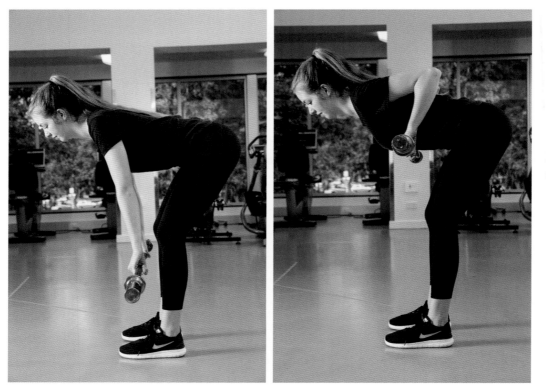

Figure 8.9 Primary variation of the bent-over row shown in a standing position with a barbell; starting and finishing position (left) and middle position (right)

TABLE 8.8 Cues and Technique for the Bent-over Row	
Poor Technique/Watch for	**Good Cues**
✕ Rounded shoulders	✓ 'Chest up, shoulders back'
✕ Extending the knees and the trunk to assist moving the weight	✓ Cue 'pull with the back and arms' and 'no legs' ✓ 'Keep your back parallel to the floor'

TABLE 8.9   Variations of the Bent-over Row

Variation	Rationale		Considerations
Narrow grip width versus wider	Narrow focuses on shoulder joint extension (biasing towards latissimus dorsi involvement), wider promotes SJ horizontal extension (biasing towards posterior deltoid involvement).	 	Ensure that the appropriate elbow tracking behaviour occurs during narrow grip execution (i.e. ensure that the angle between the humeri and the long axis of the torso is kept low if the objective is SJ extension).
Varying anthropometries and flexibility will limit the ability to assume a 'horizontal' torso	As repetitions continue, often a more upright posture is taken, indicating fatigue of the spinal stabilisers. However, note that hamstring flexibility, rather than lumbar stabilising strength endurance, may also limit the degree to which the near-parallel position can be obtained and maintained.		Back orientation changes within a set can indicate spinal stabiliser fatigue. If this occurs early in the set, consider a more supported and less challenging variation (such as the seated or prone row).

TABLE 8.9 Variations of the Bent-over Row (continued)			
Variation	**Rationale**		**Considerations**
Overhand versus underhand grip	The underhand grip forces a supinated forearm orientation that allows for greater contribution of the biceps brachii musculature to this movement.		Ensure that the individual does not 'curl' the bar to the chest; shoulder joint extension to the point where the elbows are beyond the dorsal surface of the trunk is still a requirement.

Activity 8.7 Bent-over row posture correction

AIM:
- To position a partner to execute the bent-over row correctly

TASK:
- Follow the instructions in the worksheet below and answer the questions.

Worksheet 8.7 Bent-over Row Variations

Question 1: Set up: Ask three or four students to get into the start position. Note the varying final angle of the torso to the floor of each one and the most common comment from those who struggle to approximate the torso parallel to the floor position. Allow these individuals a greater degree of knee joint flexion. Does this allow a better (i.e. lower) position? Why might this be so?

_____

_____

_____

_____

_____

Question 2: Against a moderate load, conduct repetitions until technical failure. Have your partner observe these repetitions, with particular attention to the orientation of the torso with reference to the floor and any change in spinal posture. What stabilising musculature is heavily stressed by this exercise?

_____

_____

_____

Question 3: How might we train the stabilisers to allow us to conduct a full set of bent-over rows without losing control of our start position? What comments did your partner make during your execution of the bent-over row? Does this indicate a need for training the stabilising musculature?

_____

_____

_____

_____

Exercise 8e: Latissimus (lat) Pull-down

Basic Exercise

Primary action:

- Glenohumeral adduction OR extension

Starting position (wide grip):

- Elbows are slightly flexed ($< 5°$), arms above the head, holding the bar with a wide pronated grip.

Starting position (narrow grip):

- Elbows are slightly flexed ($< 5°$), arms above the head, holding the bar with a narrow, pronated or supinated grip.

Finishing position (wide grip):

- Arms are adducted with elbows flexed, pulling the bar down to upper chest level in front of the head.
- The scapula rotates internally, and retracts and depresses.

Finishing position (narrow grip):

- Arms are extended with elbows flexed, pulling the bar down to upper chest/collarbone level in front of the head.
- The scapula rotates internally, and retracts and depresses.

Body position:

- Maintain stable posture with neutral spine, while seated with approximately $90-100°$ hip flexion. Allow only sufficient additional hip flexion beyond $90°$ as is required to allow the bar to travel safely past the face to the upper chest.

Execution of exercise:

- Pull the bar down in the vertical plane until finishing position is reached.
- Elbows stay in the frontal (wide grip) or sagittal (narrow grip) planes throughout.
- Do not allow alteration of the hip angle as a strategy to allow more weight to be lifted.

The primary variation of the lat pull-down is shown in a machine using a cable with a long bar (Figure 8.10). This will be followed by technique and cues (Table 8.10) and variations for the exercise (Table 8.11).

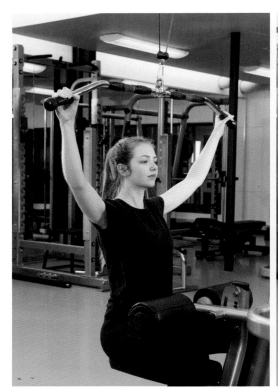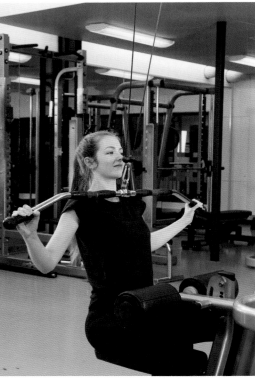

Figure 8.10 Primary variation of the lat pull-down shown in a machine using a cable with a long bar; starting and finishing position (left) and middle position (right)

TABLE 8.10 Cues and Technique for the Lat Pull-down	
Poor Technique/Watch for	**Good Cues**
✘ Extending trunk in exaggerated lumbar lordosis with each repetition	✓ 'Keep the core engaged and trunk as a solid unit throughout each set'
✘ Not controlling the speed of the bar in the eccentric phase	✓ 'Control the weight on the way back up to the starting position'
✘ Pulling the bar too far down, resulting in internal rotation of the shoulder	✓ 'Only pull the bar to the collarbone'

TABLE 8.11	Variations of the Lat Pull-down		
Variation	Rationale		Considerations
Grip width	**Wide grip** • The elbows travel in the frontal plane • Recruitment of lower fibres of the pectoralis major • Targets arm/SJ adduction • Commonly executed with pronated grip and thus less utilisation of biceps brachii and greater reliance on brachioradialis and brachialis **Narrow grip** • The elbows travel in the sagittal plane • Greater utilisation of biceps brachii if grip is supinated; more reliance on brachioradialis and brachialis if grip is pronated • Targets arm/SJ extension		• Inappropriate ROM—end point: the bar should approximate the mid-chest height to ensure scapular retraction and depression is complete • Inappropriate ROM—start point: more than minimal ($<5°$) elbow joint flexion at top/start of movement • Changing hip joint angle throughout lift (typically increasing hip joint angle)—creating a more 'horizontal' row action • Altering head position—reaching to the bar with the chin: this error is often associated with inappropriate ROM (end point, above)

Activity 8.8 Key muscular anatomy: latissimus dorsi

Background

This broad (latissimus) back (dorsi) muscle originates in the lower back from the spinous processes of T7–12, and via the thoracolumbar fascia to the lumbar and sacral vertebrae and the posterior one-third of the iliac crest (Figure 8.11). Some fibres also arise from the 9th to the 12th ribs. The latissimus dorsi inserts into the bicipital groove of the humerus. Latissimus dorsi fibres rotate such that the lower originating fibres insert highest, and vice versa. This muscle is a powerful adductor and extensor of the arm at the shoulder joint. The latissimus dorsi also internally rotates the humerus.

Palpation

Have your partner lie prone on an elevated bench or massage table, with one arm hanging off the edge of the bench/table. Locate the inferior angle of the scapula by palpating the medial border inferiorly until the inferior angle becomes obvious. If the inferior angle is difficult to locate, 'wing' the arm by internally rotating the arm to place the forearm perpendicular to the spine and behind the back. The scapula (and the inferior angle particularly) will become more prominent. Having found the inferior angle, now palpate along the lateral border of the scapula, and then grasp the thick mass of muscle tissue immediately lateral to the lateral border. This mass of tissue is the latissimus dorsi (and possibly also the teres major, which lies superiorly to the latissimus dorsi and acts to assist it). If you cannot tell if you have raised muscle tissue, maintain pressure on the structure you have grasped but allow it to slowly slip between your fingers. Muscle will have a distinct fibrous and dense feel; skin tissue (and subcutaneous fat) will be dramatically easier to compress. Now ask your partner to extend their arm towards their hip. Resist this motion with your other hand, causing your partner to have to contract the latissimus dorsi more strongly. You should feel this contraction. Have your partner repeat this process and explore inferiorly and superiorly, palpating high into the axilla and as low as possible along the lateral trunk, identifying as much of the latissimus dorsi as possible.

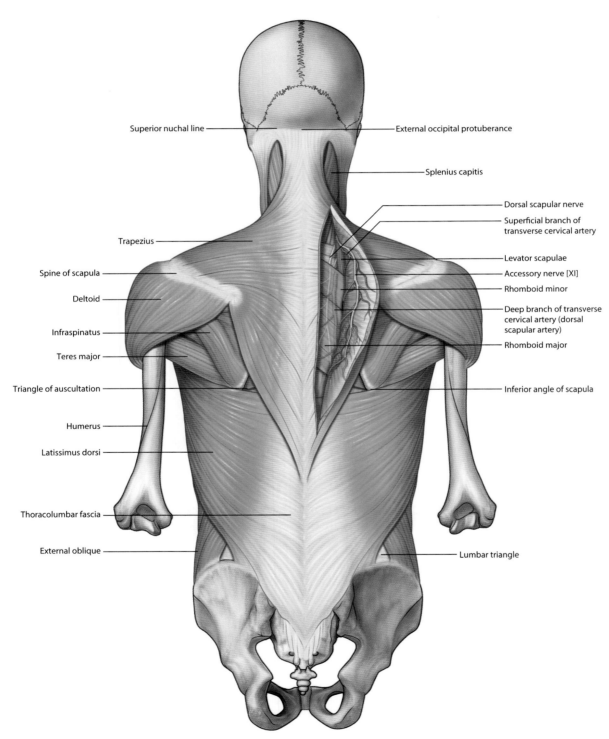

Figure 8.11 Latissimus dorsi in relation to other muscles of the back
Source: Drake (2015).[1]

AIM:
- Palpate the latissimus dorsi

TASKS:
- Follow the steps above to palpate the latissimus dorsi.
- Have your partner conduct several lightly to moderately loaded repetitions of the lat pull-down exercise and repeat your palpation, identifying the activity of the latissimus dorsi.
- Ask your partner to change between narrow and wide grip variations during your palpation.

Activity 8.9 Lat pull-down variations

AIM:
- Understand how different variations of the lat pull-down exercise may affect the muscle fibres

TASKS:
- Try the lat pull-down using four different methods:
  1. wide grip, pronated
  2. wide grip, supinated
  3. narrow grip, supinated
  4. using a light weight and a middle-width grip, pull the bar to the level of the forehead and then internally rotate at the SJ (causing the bar to arc forwards and down to mid-chest height).
- Using the anatomical and functional descriptions above, consider the activity of the latissimus dorsi in these movements.
- Palpate the latissimus dorsi while your partner performs repetitions of the exercise.

Worksheet 8.9 Comparing Techniques	
Question 1: What benefit is there to the rotation of fibres that the latissimus dorsi undergoes?	

Variation	Your Comments/Personal Experience
1	
2	
3	
4	

Can you feel the latissimus dorsi active during the full ROM?

In variation 4, can you feel the latissimus dorsi acting to cause internal rotation?

Exercise 8f: Chin-up/Pull-up

Basic Exercise

Primary action:

- Glenohumeral adduction or extension

Starting position:

- Elbows are slightly flexed ($< 5°$), arms above the head, holding the bar with a pronated grip.

Finishing position:

- GH joint is adducted with elbows fully flexed, with the bar in line with the clavicle in front of the head.
- Scapulae internally rotate, retract and depress.

Body position:

- Maintain stable posture with a neutral spine.

Execution of exercise:

- Lift the body in a vertical plane until the finishing position is reached.

The primary variation of the chin-up is shown using a chin-up bar and unassisted (Figure 8.12). This will be followed by technique and cues (Table 8.12) and variations for the exercise (Table 8.13).

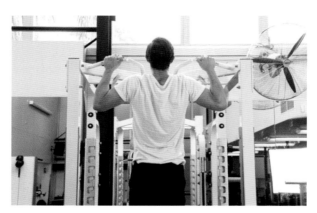

Figure 8.12 Primary variation of the chin-up shown using a chin-up bar and unassisted; this is the middle position

TABLE 8.12	Cues and Technique for the Chin-up/Pull-up
Poor Technique/Watch for	**Good Cues**
✗ Only going through partial ROM; this may indicate that the exercise is too challenging for the individual and should be changed	✓ 'Try and let your arms go almost completely straight before starting the next pull'
✗ Swinging the body and using momentum to pull upwards	✓ 'Keep the body straight and focus on driving the elbows towards the body'
✗ Holding breath	✓ Cue breathing by anchoring breath to the phase of the exercise: 'breathe out on the pull, breathe in on the return'

TABLE 8.13	Variations of the Chin-up/Pull-up		
Variation	**Rationale**		**Considerations**
Hand width	Hand width alters the plane of movement of elbows from sagittal (narrow grip) to frontal (wide grip) and SJ movement from extension (narrow grip) to adduction (wide grip).		Choice of width should be made with a goal in mind, rather than 'defaulting' to a standard without consideration. Think about whether a wide or narrow grip would be appropriate for specificity or emphasising a particular muscle.
Pronated, supinated, neutral	Hand position changes the elbow joint flexor involvement: supinated biases towards biceps brachii, pronated towards brachioradialis and brachialis.		Minor hand position changes can be used as progressions/ regressions.

TABLE 8.13   Variations of the Chin-up/Pull-up (continued)

Variation	Rationale		Considerations
Assisted chin-ups (machine or bands)	This allows execution of the full ROM even in conditions of insufficient strength-to-body-mass ratio. Stabilisers will be challenged as well as prime movers if a band-assisted chin-up is conducted.		When using either assistance method, the tendency to flex at the hip should be avoided. The same long 'planked' position through the hips as in a full chin-up or pull-up should be encouraged. Flexed hip positions encourage hip extension against the assistance method to achieve the final, high position. This 'final boost' will not be present in the full, unassisted version of the exercise and so should not be relied on. When band assisting, longer band distraction (i.e. looped around the feet), while providing more assistance, is more likely to encourage sway under the bar due to the greater distance from the point of force application to the axis of rotation (feet to hands) than when shorter band distraction is used (band looped around the knees). In either case, the student should be watchful for uncontrolled sway and be prepared to minimise this by limiting the sway manually.

TABLE 8.13	Variations of the Chin-up/Pull-up (continued)		
Variation	**Rationale**		**Considerations**
Body-weight row	Use a Smith machine or something where the feet are fixed on the floor.		Using a Smith machine or any position where the feet are fixed allows the use of some leg muscles to assist in this variation. By changing the distance the feet are away, you can change the intensity. The straighter the legs, the more difficult the exercise.

Activity 8.10 Key muscular anatomy—brachioradialis

Background

Arising from the upper two-thirds of the lateral supracondylar ridge of the humerus, and inserting on the base of the styloid process, the brachioradialis runs the length of the forearm; however, the bulk of the muscle is at the elbow rather than the wrist joint (Figure 8.13). A key forearm flexor, the role of the brachioradialis is often ignored in favour of the biceps brachii. Neutral grip elbow joint flexion is where the brachioradialis is emphasised.

Palpation

Flex your elbow to 90°, with the wrist in neutral (neither pronated nor supinated). Have your partner place their hand over your wrist and push down on it. Push up against your partner's hand (i.e. do not allow their downward force to extend your elbow joint). You should see your brachioradialis 'pop' up on the superior aspect of your forearm. Allow your partner to palpate the belly of this muscle to confirm the location of the brachioradialis.

AIM:
- Palpate the brachioradialis

TASK:
- Conduct a set of narrow, neutral grip chin-ups to fatigue. Immediately afterwards, repeat the palpation exercise above with your partner. Can you feel fatigue in your brachioradialis?

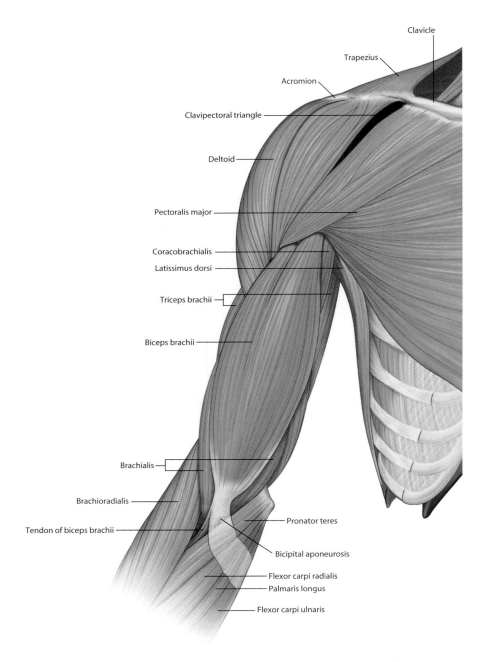

Figure 8.13 Brachioradialis shown compared to other muscles of the arm
Source: Drake (2015).[1]

Activity 8.11 Band-assisted chin-ups

AIM:

- To understand how bands may assist in chin-up execution

TASKS:

- Loop a strong (i.e. thick) powerband over the chin-up bar.
- Have the trainer pull the band down and apart, creating a stirrup to place both feet into as shown in Figure 8.14.
- Ensure that the individual assumes a good chin-up position (i.e. a long, 'planked' torso with the hip extended to neutral).
- Using a narrow, underhand grip (i.e. the strongest and therefore 'easiest' position), explore the difference between a high position where the chin is at the level of the bar, and a high position where the chest is at the level of the bar.

Worksheet 8.11 Band-assisted Chin-ups

Question 1: Based on muscle activation, what are the differences you notice between the high position and the low position?

_____

_____

_____

Question 2: Which position is likely to be of most benefit to the individual?

_____

_____

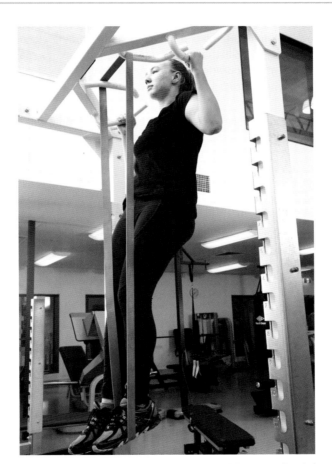

Figure 8.14 Shows the positioning of the band assisting the chin-up, using it looped around one leg

Reference

1   Drake R 2015. *Gray's Atlas of Anatomy*. Churchill Livingstone.

PRACTICAL 9
THE LEGS

Emma M. Beckman and Justin W. L. Keogh

Introduction

The legs arguably contain the most important muscle groups of the entire body. This region generates large forces that are then transferred along the kinetic chain and expressed distally. Routine tasks such as rising from a seat and walking up stairs through to complex athletic manoeuvres such as sprinting, jumping, kicking and tackling are largely the result of the coordinated production of muscular forces originating from the lower body musculature. As such, the lower body is often the primary focus of training plans for improving performance, reducing the risk of injury or injury rehabilitation for many athletic groups as maintaining adequate balance, leg muscle mass, strength, power and endurance is important to maintain overall health, functional ability and minimise the risk of falls with ageing. Lower body strengthening exercises are also highly recommended for middle-aged and older adults.

There are a variety of exercises used to train the lower body, each with multiple variations. While the performance of multi-joint lower body exercises such as squats, lunges and deadlifts by asymptomatic individuals has less injury risk than most team sports, the most common injuries associated with these exercises are to the knee and lumbar spine. The risk of these injuries may be decreased by emphasising good technique and a full range of motion (ROM) prior to large external loads (barbells and dumbbells) being utilised. In particular, the risk of injury to the knee may be reduced by minimising excessive anterior or medial tibial translation, with the risk of lumbar injury reduced by maintaining a neutral spine and a more vertical trunk position where possible.

The ability to maintain a neutral spine and to minimise medial deviation of the knee will often become more challenging with increased depth of leg exercises (predominantly determined via knee joint ROM), load applied or the complexity of the exercise. Therefore, assessment of general movement competency and the effect of ROM, load and exercise complexity on the ability to maintain a neutral spine is important. A variety of factors may affect this including:

- anthropometrics
- mobility
- intermuscular coordination
- strength
- experience with a specific exercise
- physical and/or cognitive fatigue.

While it is outside the scope of this practical to go into each of these in depth, it is important for students who intend to instruct exercises of the lower limbs to consider each of these in relation to their exercise prescription and each client. This practical will provide some guidance as to how effective instruction may assist to individualise exercises of the legs. Links are made to additional reading that can further the understanding of these factors.

Included exercises are:

- squat
- lunge
- deadlift
- leg press
- hip extension
- knee extension
- knee flexion
- calf raise.

For each exercise, a primary variation will be presented with actions, starting position, finishing position, equipment set-up and execution of the exercise. This will be followed by a table of technique and cues and a table of variations for the exercise (if available).

Anatomy

The hip, knee and ankle are the primary joints of interest in this practical. Most of the exercises deal with movement predominantly in the coronal and sagittal plane. These will often involve flexion and extension of the hip, knee and ankle, with hip adduction and abduction also featured. The importance of training the body in all planes of movement is recognised and a subsequent practical on neuromuscular control will introduce the importance of multi-planar movement and training the coordination of the body. Table 9.1 lists the primary movements and muscles responsible for these actions.

The anatomy of the legs is shown in Figure 9.1 to provide a visual representation of the muscles of interest. The movements and muscles recruited are listed in Table 9.1.

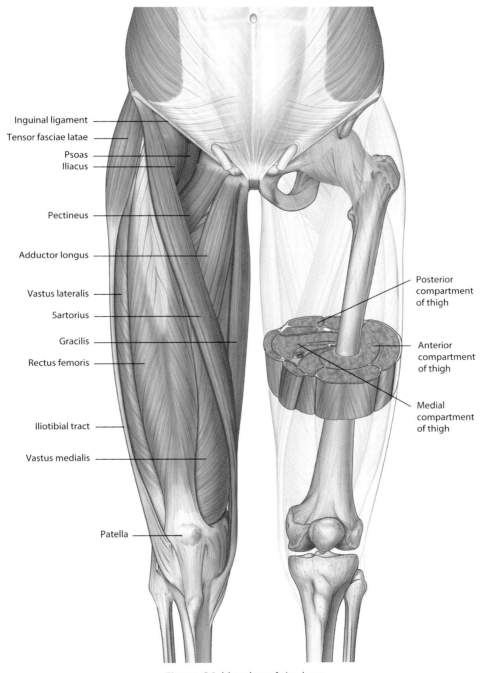

Figure 9.1 Muscles of the legs
Source: Drake (2015).[1]

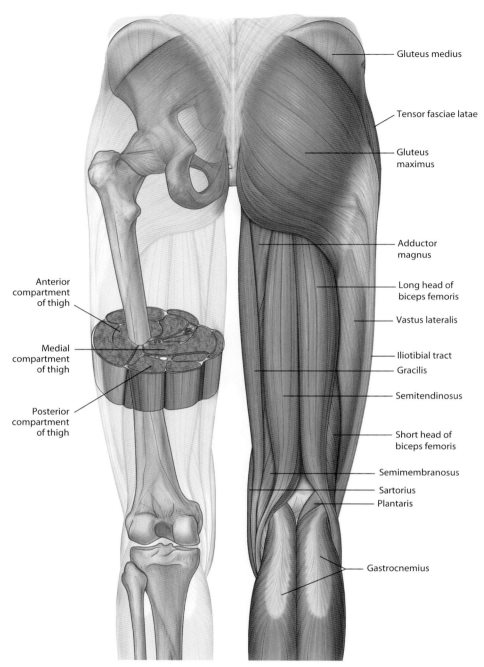

Figure 9.1, cont'd

TABLE 9.1 Anatomy of the Legs	
Movement	**Muscles Recruited**
Hip extension	• Gluteus maximus • Gluteus medius (posterior fibres) • Adductor magnus (posterior fibres) • Biceps femoris (long head) • Semitendinosus • Semimembranosus
Hip adduction	• Adductor magnus • Adductor longus • Adductor brevis • Pectineus • Gracilis
Hip abduction	• Gluteus medius • Gluteus minimus • Tensor fasciae latae • Sartorius
Knee extension	• Rectus femoris • Vastus lateralis • Vastus intermedius • Vastus medius
Knee flexion	• Biceps femoris • Semitendinosus • Semimembranosus • Gracilis • Sartorius • Popliteus • Gastrocnemius
Plantar flexion	• Gastrocnemius • Soleus • Tibialis posterior
Lumbar spine stabilisation (deep)	• Transverse abdominis • Internal obliques • External obliques • Multifidus • Diaphragm • Pelvic floor
Lumbar spine stabilisation (superficial)	• Rectus abdominis • Iliocostalis (ES) • Longissimus (ES) • Spinalis (ES) • Quadratus lumborum

TABLE 9.1 Anatomy of the Legs (continued)	
Movement	**Muscles Recruited**
Pelvic and femoral head stabilisation	• Gluteus medius • Gluteus minimis • Piriformis

Exercise 9a: Squat

Squats are one of the three lifts involved in the sport of powerlifting (along with the bench press and deadlift) and are therefore one of the most commonly prescribed exercises for increasing lower body muscle mass, strength and power. The barbell back squat will be described in depth below as it is the most commonly performed squat variation. Additional detail on alternative squat exercises will be provided in the variation table.

Basic Action

Primary actions:

- Knee extension
- Hip extension
- Plantar flexion

Equipment set-up:

- The bar is positioned in a squat rack approximately at armpit height.
- Safety bars are positioned just below the required depth.

Starting position:

- Feet are shoulder width or slightly wider apart, feet flat on the floor.
- Arms are fully flexed with the bar over the shoulders.
- Stand with knees and hips slightly flexed.

Finishing position:

- Knees and hips are flexed to a required range.

Execution of exercise:

- Hips initiate movement (sit back, not down) resulting in some forward inclination of the trunk (while maintaining a neutral spine), accompanied by concurrent knee flexion and dorsiflexion until the required depth is reached.

Safety and spotting

- Spot from either behind (one spotter) or from the side (two spotters preferred) of the client.
- As a spotter, you must be in a position to rapidly assist the lifter if needed.

The primary variation of the squat is shown as a barbell squat (Figure 9.2). This will be followed by technique and cues (Table 9.2) and variations for the exercise (Table 9.3).

Squat Variations

Table 9.3 shows the most common squat variations, and provides some rationale or description of these variations along with some notes on common issues with each variation. In general, the cues listed in the instruction section will be highly relevant to all of the variations; however, when there are important variation-specific considerations, they have also been included.

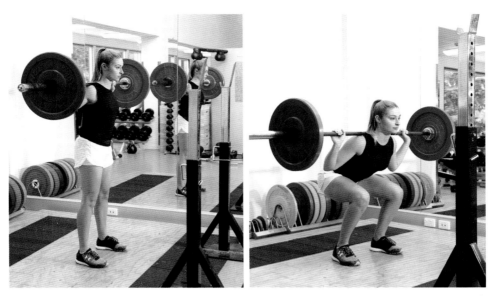

Figure 9.2 Primary variation of the squat shown as a barbell squat; starting and finishing position (left) and middle position (right)

TABLE 9.2 Cues and Technique for the Squat	
Poor Technique/Watch for	**Good Cues**
✗ Lack of control at the pelvis, may present as: • lateral instability of pelvis • too much anterior and posterior movement • bouncing at the bottom of range • inability to control the knees tracking over the feet throughout the exercise	✓ 'Core tight: control the back and pelvis'
✗ In standing exercises, unwanted flexion of the spine or posterior pelvic tilt may occur, especially when looking down at the floor and as the individual approaches the lowest position of the exercise	✓ 'Look straight ahead and think about keeping your spine in a neutral position'
✗ Knee extension completed too early in relation to hip extension	✓ 'Lead with the hips; push hips through to finish off'
✗ Heels rising off the ground and the individual pushing through the toes	✓ 'Push through your heels'

TABLE 9.3   Variations of the Squat

Variation	Description and Rationale		Considerations
Back squat depth	Considered the most common variation; bar positioned anywhere between upper trapezius and posterior deltoids		The depth of this exercise may vary from a quarter squat depth (with knees moving through 45° of flexion), to a half depth (knees flexed at 90°), to parallel (thigh to ground) and then to a full-depth squat whereby the gluteals may make contact with the calf musculature.
Front squat	Bar placed in front of shoulders; this forward placement of the load means that the trunk remains more upright throughout and therefore more emphasis is on the knee extension action than the ROM in the hips		Wrist flexibility could hinder the achievement of the correct position. Be sure to cue the individual to keep their elbows up. There are grip alternatives such as placing the bar across the deltoids and stabilising the bar with the arms crossed in front. The use of specific front squat harnesses can assist the lifter with inadequate flexibility or control.

TABLE 9.3   Variations of the Squat (continued)

Variation	Description and Rationale		Considerations
Single leg	Increases the need for gluteus medius and minimus to control pelvis position to ensure the maintenance of a neutral pelvic position throughout the exercise		The gluteus medius controls the stability in this exercise by providing isometric hip abduction. If this is weak, consider strengthening hip abduction in isolation before progressing this exercise to a single leg squat. Another option is to perform the single leg squat through the ROM in which the stability can be controlled, using cables or handles as pictured, and over time work to increase this range.
Swiss ball wall squat	Reduces the requirement of the core to control the movement and allows focus on the ROM. Often seen as a regression from a free-standing squat		This variation doesn't strictly replicate the squat due to the restriction of centre of mass moving vertically. This variation may also be more difficult to load, as barbells typically can't be used. This squat variation may be useful for untrained (especially older) individuals or for those who experience back discomfort during regular squats.

TABLE 9.3	Variations of the Squat (continued)		
Variation	**Description and Rationale**		**Considerations**
Jump squat	The addition of a plyometric component utilises the stretch-shortening cycle and emphasises power development	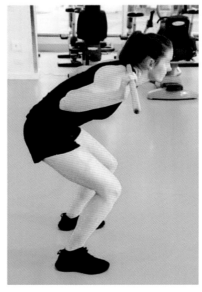	The ability to perform body-weight squats through a full ROM with good control is suggested before progressing to the jump squat. Typically, the individual should not flex their knees past 90° during jump squats if they wish to maximise jump height and minimise ground contact time.

Activity 9.1 Combining effective instruction with good feedback—what is wrong with this picture?

Background

You are an accredited exercise scientist. A 22-year-old female with no previous training experience comes to you wishing to learn to squat with the aim of building some lower body muscle mass. You initially teach her regressions of the squat, moving from a simple standing squat, using a bench for some proprioceptive feedback onto the squat rack with a light weight. The picture below (Figure 9.3) is taken during her first set. She reports feeling some strain in her back during and after completing the full set. You have concerns that her technique does not coincide with what you know to be typical or ideal and decide to give her some augmented feedback that will hopefully improve her technique and reduce the lower back strain across her second and third set. Table 9.4 lists options to try and some considerations for each. The cues provided may be enough to improve her technique to a point where you are comfortable with her continuing the exercise.

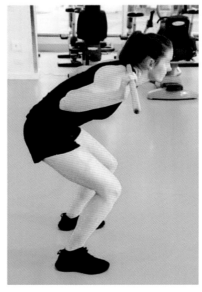

Figure 9.3 Example of poor squat position

TABLE 9.4	Possible Concerns and Cue Strategies for the Poor Squat Position in Figure 9.3	
Concern	**Additional Exercise Cues**	**Result**
Is she leaning too far over and might just not realise how horizontal her trunk is at the bottom of the squat?	'On the next rep, just try and lift your chest. Stick out your chest a little.'	The movement might come from the lumbar spine, not the hips, and exaggerate her lumbar curve or she might start to fall backwards with the position of her centre of mass behind her feet.
Her feet might be too narrow, meaning that she is relying on pure dorsiflexion to get the range required to perform the exercise.	'Just make your feet a little bit wider and slightly turn your feet out.'	This may mean that she starts collapsing at the foot and overpronating to achieve more range. At this point it is useful to check how much dorsiflexion she has in a bent knee position as this could be a structural issue limiting her overall technique.
There doesn't seem to be too much dorsiflexion available.	'Heel on the weight plate (about 2 cm raise).' Although not a cue, stretching the calf prior to the next set might assist.	Raising the heel is never a permanent solution. Restricting the full depth of the squat should be considered (depending on your training goals) until more dorsiflexion can be achieved.
The heel raise helps but she is losing that sensation of pushing through the heels and finds it difficult to load with the heels up.	Try a front squat position.	The front squat might allow her to be more upright depending on the depth; at the very least it shows her what you mean by the movement of the trunk/hips.

Activity 9.2 Research corner—the safety of the squat exercise

Background

Historically there has been a concern regarding injury risk to the knee joint during the squat; however, these concerns are generally unfounded when dealing with healthy populations or even athletes competing in strength sports. The relatively low rates of knee injury during these strength sports is highlighted by a recent systematic review of the injury epidemiology of weightlifting, powerlifting, bodybuilding, strongman, Highland games and CrossFit by Keogh and Winwood.[2] The following factors are important to consider.

Knee ligament failure loads[3]

- A healthy posterior cruciate ligament (PCL) can tolerate approximately 4000 N of force (400 kg).
- Peak posterior shear forces during a squat are < 3000 N.
- A healthy anterior cruciate ligament (ACL) can tolerate 1725 to 2160 N.
- Peak anterior shear forces during a squat are < 500 N.

Knee injury and increasing squat depth[4]

- A higher risk of injury was once hypothesised for deep squats; however, there is strong contemporary evidence to suggest that this is not the case.
- The highest retropatellar compressive forces and stresses occur at 90° of knee flexion. As knee flexion increases past 90°, there is greater load distribution and force transfer across knee structures that results in reduced retropatellar compressive forces and stresses.

- Heavier loads have a tendency to be lifted through a reduced knee ROM (quarter or half squat). Quarter and half squats performed with supramaximal loads may result in the trunk musculature being the limiting factor and increase knee loading.

It is important to consider that like skeletal muscle, training adaptations occur in the mechanical properties of bone, tendons and ligaments as well as the participant's mobility and intermuscular coordination. As such, cautious application of the progressive overload principle should be applied when teaching the squat and improving depth. This should also be done in consideration of the primary factor of squat technique, which is maintenance of a neutral spine.

AIM:
- Gain an understanding of why squatting to full depth may be difficult for some people

TASK:
- In pairs, practise squatting without load to full depth. If neither partner has difficulty with the squat, pairs should come together to form bigger groups to see more variations in squat technique.

Worksheet 9.2 Research Corner—Safety of the Squat Exercise

Question 1: Observe the squat technique of each group member. What might be limiting full depth?

_____

_____

Question 2: What does the group member report is limiting their ability to go to full depth?

_____

_____

Exercise 9b: Lunge

Similar to the squat movement pattern, many variations of the lunge exercise exist. The body-weight static split squat will be described in detail below (and shown in Figure 9.4) as it is the most commonly performed lunge variation. Common cues are shown in Table 9.5. Additional detail on more advanced lunge exercises, including options to increase the external load by dumbbells and barbells, will be provided in the variation table (Table 9.6). Stepping lunges will also be described given the important functional parallels with common human movement.

Basic Action

Primary actions:
- Knee extension
- Hip extension
- Plantar flexion

Starting position:
- Feet are shoulder-width apart, with the front leg positioned so that the rear knee is underneath or just in front of the hips at the bottom of the repetition.
- Stand tall with a neutral spine.
- Arms are hanging by the sides or crossed over the chest.

Finishing position:
- Knees and hips are flexed to a required range.

Execution of exercise:
- Back knee flexes allow the hips to drop downwards and the front knee to flex until the required depth is reached. It is generally recommended that the back knee does not forcibly make contact with the ground and that the trunk remains relatively vertical.

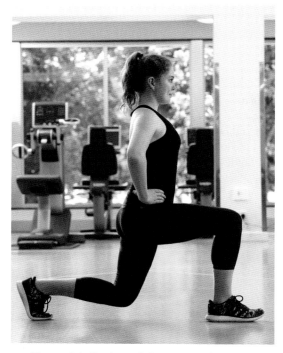

Figure 9.4 Body-weight static split squat

TABLE 9.5 Cues and Technique for the Lunge	
Poor Technique/Watch for	**Good Cues**

✗ Lack of control at the pelvis may present as:
  • lateral instability of pelvis
  • too much anterior and posterior movement
  • bouncing at the bottom of range
  • inability to control the front knee tracking over the feet throughout the exercise
	✓ 'Core tight: control the back and pelvis'

✗ Heels rising off the ground and individual is pushing through toes when the activity is a closed chain exercise	✓ 'Push through your heels'

Lunge Variations

There are many variations of the lunge that relate to the body position, the execution of the exercise and the equipment that can be utilised as shown in Table 9.6. It is important that the goal of the exercise is taken into account when a variation is being considered. For example: Is strength in a functional split position important? Is the primary focus to improve balance in different directions and positions?

TABLE 9.6   Variations of the Lunge

Variation	Rationale		Considerations
Bulgarian squat	The lifted position of the back leg in a Bulgarian squat increases the stability challenge and the load through the front leg.		Individuals with tight hip flexors will find this variation difficult. Assess whether too much rotation or pelvic movement has to occur to achieve the starting position in order to determine if this variation is appropriate. Lowering the height of the bench in which the back leg is positioned or slightly reducing the horizontal distance between the front and back feet may assist.
Dumbbell overhead	Use of dumbbells increases the load in the lunge but the placement of the load overhead can be used to challenge total body balance and joint stability requirements, especially of the shoulder and its connection to the opposite hip.		Watch for too much posterior pelvic tilt in this variation, especially if the individual has tight latissimus dorsi muscles that make it difficult to achieve a correct overhead position.
Short step versus long step	Altering the length of step may alter the relative muscle recruitment and loading of some of the knee ligaments. A shorter step may increase quadriceps activation and patella tendon loading. A longer step may increase gluteal activation and PCL loading.		The ability to alter the length of the regular lunge step may be affected by joint ROM. When performing short steps, the individual will require greater dorsiflexion range on their front foot. When performing long steps, the individual will require greater hip flexion range on their back leg. The long step lunge is not recommended during early phases of PCL rehabilitation.

TABLE 9.6	Variations of the Lunge (continued)		
Variation	**Rationale**		**Considerations**
Walking lunges	Lunges may be performed stationary or progressively with alternate steps taken. This will increase specificity for any activity that required the forward progression of the centre of mass.		Stability is challenged in this variation and it is important to cue individuals to place the front foot in line with the width of the shoulders as individuals may lose balance and increase medial/lateral shear knee forces if the step is too narrow or wide.
Step anterior/ posterior/ medial/lateral	While lunges are often considered to be sagittal plane activities, they can be done by stepping to the side to challenge the abductors and adductors of the hip.		Careful instruction is required when moving into new planes that are less trained in a number of individuals. Ensure stability is achieved prior to each step taken.

Activity 9.3 So many variations! How do you use them?

AIM:

- Understand variations of the lunge

TASKS:

- An athlete comes to you with the primary goal of improving their high jump performance as they have made the state team for the high jump event.
- Detail six progressions you would make starting from a standing stationary lunge and justify each change in relation to specificity and loading principles.

Worksheet 9.3 So Many Variations! How Do You Use Them?	
Exercise	**Rationale**
For example, standing, stationary lunge	For example, it will be important for this athlete to ensure they have sufficient ROM and strength available to perform the standard lunge with reps performed in one plane, prior to moving towards more difficult exercises.

Exercise 9c: Deadlift

As one of the three lifts involved in the sport of powerlifting, the deadlift is one of the most commonly prescribed exercises for increasing overall body muscle mass, strength and power. The conventional barbell deadlift (Figure 9.5) will be described in depth below as it is the most commonly performed deadlift variation. Additional detail on alternative deadlift exercises will be provided in the variation table (Table 9.9). Common cues for teaching the deadlift are provided in Table 9.7.

Basic Action
Primary actions:

- Hip extension
- Knee extension
- Plantar flexion

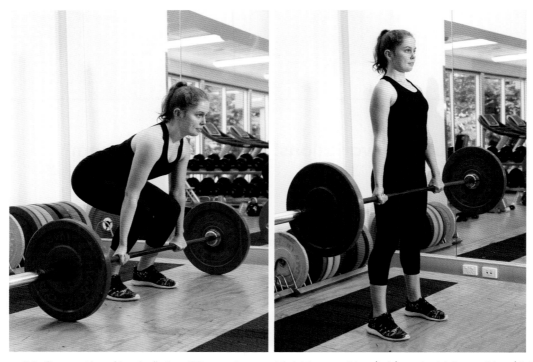

Figure 9.5 Conventional barbell deadlift; starting and finishing position (left) and middle position (right)

TABLE 9.7   Cues and Technique for the Deadlift

Poor Technique/Watch for	Good Cues
✘ Excessive or prolonged breath holding. This is likely to occur at higher weights; however, with untrained individuals the Valsalva manoeuvre and breath holding is often unnecessary and should be avoided	✓ 'Inhale and hold the breath during the latter stage of the lower (eccentric) phase and don't exhale until past the sticking point during the upward (concentric) phase'
✘ Lack of control at the pelvis, may present as: • lateral instability of pelvis • too much anterior and posterior movement • bouncing at the bottom of range • inability to control the knees tracking over the feet throughout the exercise	✓ 'Core tight: control the back and pelvis'
✘ Unwanted flexion of the spine or posterior pelvic tilt may occur, especially when looking down at the floor and as the individual approaches the lowest position of the exercise	✓ 'Look straight ahead and think about keeping your spine in a neutral position'
✘ Knee extension completed too early in relation to hip extension	✓ 'Lead with your hips and push your hips through to finish off'
✘ Heels rising off the ground and individual is pushing through toes	✓ 'Push through your heels'

Equipment set-up:
• The bar is positioned at the appropriate depth for the client (floor, squat rack or lifting blocks).

Starting position:
• Feet are flat on the floor, hips and knees flexed, holding the bar at shoulder width.
• Position the bar close to the shins ('over the shoelaces').
• Hold the bar with mixed grip (one pronated and one supinated), maintaining a straight arm position achieving a neutral spine posture just prior to initiating the concentric phase.

Finishing position:
• Stand upright with the knees and hips extended so that the bar rests across the thighs with the arms straight.

Execution of exercise:
• 'Take the slack with the bar' or 'stiffen up'
• Initial movement is hip extension, followed by knee extension.
• Concurrent hip and knee extension continues until the body is brought to an upright position.
• The bar follows (almost touches) the legs throughout the lift.

Grip Variations

The ability to perform this exercise may be limited by poor grip strength. There are three key variations that may assist the individual in overcoming this (Table 9.8).

Deadlift Variations

The key action of the deadlift remains the same regardless of the variation used. The primary similarities across all deadlifts are the importance of keeping a neutral spine, maintaining straight arms and keeping the weight close to the shins and thighs. However, during the lift, a number of variations emphasise particular aspects of the movement and therefore load or deload various anatomical structures that may be important considerations when ensuring the exercise prescription meets the individual's goals. Variations are shown in Table 9.9.

TABLE 9.8   Grip Variations of the Deadlift

Grip	
Hook grip: This grip involves placing the thumb between the barbell and the remaining fingers. It is typically used by weightlifters in training and competition.	
Mixed grip: The placement of one hand in overhand and one in underhand grip has been shown to increase the lifting strength when compared to an overhand grip and is typically used by powerlifters in training and competition.	
Lifting straps: When weights get significantly heavier, lifting straps allow the load to be lifted through the arms rather than relying on the grip strength in isolation.	

TABLE 9.9   Variations of the Deadlift

Variation	Rationale		Considerations
Romanian deadlift	Focus on the hip hinge as the majority of movement is hip extension while the knees and lumbar spine remain relatively neutral.		Given the emphasis on the gluteus maximus and hamstrings, it is important to ensure that the spine is kept neutral in this variation. Individuals with tight hamstrings may use pelvic movement and posterior tilt to achieve the required range. Therefore, individuals should perform this exercise through the ROM in which they can maintain a neutral spine.

TABLE 9.9	Variations of the Deadlift (continued)		
Variation	**Rationale**		**Considerations**
Single leg deadlift	This variation greatly challenges the stability of the standing leg and emphasises the hip and pelvic stabilisers. Dumbbells and barbells are effective for this variation when the individual's balance is improved.		The lateral movement of the pelvis will be the key technique issue in this variation and students should take care to ensure the exercise is performed safely. If balance is poor, this variation will not be effective.
Sumo deadlift	This variation has the knees positioned considerably wider than the conventional deadlift. This wider stance may increase recruitment of the adductors and medial hamstrings as well as the joint moments at the ankle and knee. The resistance force will typically be closer to the lumbar spine than seen in conventional deadlifts, especially for those individuals who adopt a more upright trunk position in the sumo deadlift.		Bar displacement (thus mechanical work and estimated energy expenditure) is greater in the conventional position than this variation. Knee tracking will be an important element to observe and cue in this variation. This position will place greater stress on hip external rotation which has been suggested to lead to hip impingements (especially as stance width increases).

TABLE 9.9	Variations of the Deadlift (continued)			
Variation	**Rationale**			**Considerations**
Hex bar deadlift	This variation allows the lifter to maintain a more vertical trunk position and to position the resistance force closer to the lumbar spine than conventional deadlifts. Compared to a conventional deadlift, the hex bar version may allow the lifter to utilise their quadriceps to a greater extent and to deload the lumbar spine.			This is useful for individuals who have difficulty keeping the bar close to the shins in a conventional deadlift.

Activity 9.4 Combining effective instruction with good feedback—what's wrong with this picture?

Background

You are working as an accredited exercise scientist with a young woman in her mid-20s. She is hoping to start a popular high-intensity gym-based group fitness class soon but has come to you for a few sessions to make sure she has good technique and isn't going to injure herself in the group exercise environment. The photo in Figure 9.6 shows her position during the concentric phase of the deadlift. It will be absolutely imperative to correct her technique in order to be confident that she can safely perform this exercise with load under limited supervision in the near future. Table 9.10 lists strategies to try and improve your concerns with her technique, along with a number of cues or instructional techniques that may be effective. The third column of the table details what you are observing or looking for in order for her to progress to conventional deadlifts effectively.

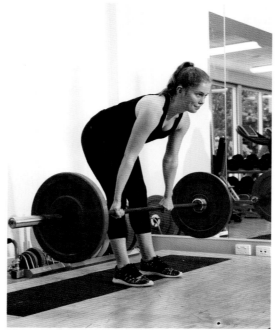

Figure 9.6 Position during concentric phase of the deadlift

TABLE 9.10   Strategies and Suggestions to Improve Technique When You Observe Something of Concern

Concerns	Changes to Technique	How to Progress or Regress the Exercise
The lack of neutral spine at the start of the deadlift could simply be related to poor proprioception and limited prior training.	'Stick your glutes out a little, like you're sitting back in a chair (possibly use a mirror for visual feedback)'	Cues to retain neutral spine may be effective throughout the full range of the exercise. If these are unsuccessful, you may wish to limit the ROM, whereby the barbell starts at mid/upper shin height by placing it on safety racks, in a squat rack or on blocks. As the individual is able to control their spinal position with the partial deadlift, the ROM can be increased until the bar starts on the floor.
It is possible that limitations in hamstring flexibility mean she is unable to achieve neutral spine in full range.	'Let's check your hamstring length, maybe do a few stretches before our next set?'	Change to limitations in hamstring length will take time to achieve, so initially you may have to reduce the ROM for this exercise.
Poor gluteal muscle activation and control may be responsible for the poor technique.	'Let's try a rack pull activity where we concentrate on pushing through those glutes!'	A rack pull is a restricted-range deadlift and may be a way to train gluteal activation and eccentric control prior to increasing load and range. Optimal position may be with the bar starting resting just above the knee. Activating glutes in this activity prior to a full conventional deadlift may also assist in future sets performed immediately after.

AIM:
- Practise using various cues to improve deadlift technique

TASK:
- In pairs, practise deadlifts using a conventional technique.

Worksheet 9.3 Combining Effective Instruction with Good Feedback—What's Wrong with This Picture?

Question 1: What cues did you use that were most effective in correcting deadlift technique?

_____
_____
_____
_____
_____

Exercise 9d: Leg Press

The leg press is perhaps the most common machine exercise for developing the muscles of the lower body. There are many commercially available leg press machines (an example of which is shown in Figure 9.7), with each machine offering some minor differences in exercise set-up and performance. The most common leg press performed is the incline seated version, which is detailed below. Cues are shown in Table 9.11. Additional detail on alternative leg press exercises will be provided in the variation table (Table 9.12).

Basic Action

Primary actions:

- Knee extension
- Hip extension
- Plantar flexion

Equipment set-up:

- Ensure the platform is positioned sufficiently high enough so that the client can easily position their feet on the platform with approximately 10° to 20° of knee flexion.
- Ensure the bottom safety pin is positioned at the required depth.
- Sit on the apparatus, holding the hand rests.
- The upper body remains stationary and supported throughout.

Starting position:

- Knees are slightly flexed and feet are in the middle of the platform at shoulder-width apart so that the heels will remain in contact with the platform throughout the ROM.

Finishing position:

- Knees and hips are flexed (90° to 80°) with heels remaining flat on the platform.

Execution of exercise:

- While maintaining pressure on the heels, slowly lower the platform to finishing position and then extend legs back to starting position.

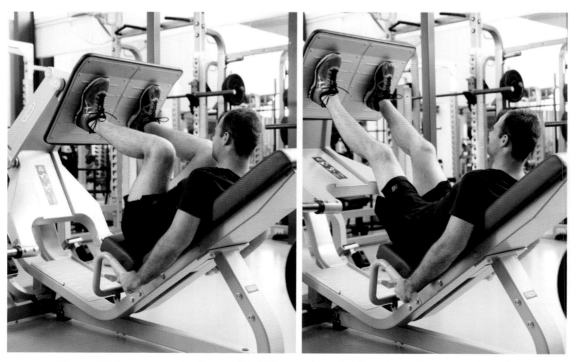

Figure 9.7 Leg press; starting and finishing position (left) and middle position (right)

TABLE 9.11 Cues and Technique for the Leg Press	
Poor Technique/Watch for	**Good Cues**
✗ Lack of control at the pelvis, may present as: • lateral instability of pelvis • too much anterior and posterior movement • bouncing at the bottom of range • inability to control the knees tracking over the feet throughout the exercise	✓ 'Core tight: control back and pelvis'
✗ Heels rising off the plate and individual is pushing through the toes	✓ 'Push through your heels'

TABLE 9.12 Variations of the Leg Press			
Variation	**Rationale**		**Considerations**
Feet low on platform	This involves a greater utilisation of the vastus knee extensors muscle group.		It may be difficult for people with restrictions in ankle ROM (dorsiflexion) to keep their heels on the plate. This version may also contribute to additional anterior knee pain or discomfort in some individuals.
Externally rotated foot position	By externally rotating the feet and having a wider stance, more emphasis is placed on the adductor group of muscles (medial thigh).		Knees should still track over the toes, so instructors should be careful to watch the position of the knees through the ROM.
Horizontal seat equipment set-up	The horizontal leg press set-up will allow greater ease of access for older populations.		It is often more difficult to load the horizontal leg press to the same degree as an incline set-up so if large loads are required for an individual this should be considered when deciding which versions of the leg press to perform. If insufficient loads are available, you may perform the leg press with a single leg at a time. Due to the stability provided by the leg press machine, single leg presses are much easier to perform than single leg squats or lunges.

Exercise 9e: Hip Extension—Supine Bridge

Basic Action

Primary action:

- Hip extension

Starting position:

- Lie supine on the floor with knees flexed at approximately 75° and feet flat on the floor.

Finishing position:

- Knees, hips and shoulders are in a straight line with only the feet, shoulders and head in contact with the ground.

Execution of exercise:

- Lift the pelvis until finishing position is achieved and either hold the end position for a length of time or move between starting and finishing positions to make the exercise more dynamic.
- Cues to assist in correct execution will include instructing the individual to squeeze through the glutes and tuck in the ribs so as to maintain a neutral or even posterior pelvic tilt.

The primary variation of the hip extension supine bridge is shown in supine on the floor using body weight (Figure 9.8). This will be followed by technique and cues (Table 9.13).

Variations—Hip Thrust

The basic supine bridge may be modified to target greater loading capacity by moving the shoulders onto a bench and placing weights or TheraBands across the hips to increase the resistance. The middle position of this exercise under load is shown in Figure 9.9 where the hips are level.

The hip thrust may also be performed with a single leg in contact with the ground. This single leg version increases the loading on the exercising leg's hip extensor (gluteal and to a lesser extent hamstring muscles), hip abductor and external rotator muscles due to the tendency of the unsupported leg's hip to drop downwards. When sufficient control is demonstrated and strength is developed, this single legged hip thrust may also be performed with additional loading from a dumbbell or TheraBands.

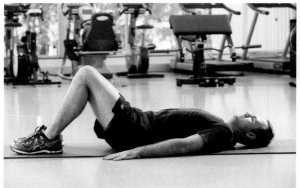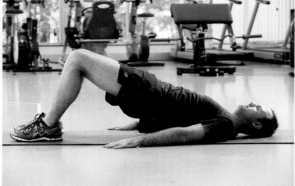

Figure 9.8 Primary variation of the hip extension supine bridge is shown in supine on the floor using body weight; starting and finishing position (left) and middle position (right)

TABLE 9.13 Cues and Technique for the Hip Extension—Supine Bridge	
Poor Technique/Watch for	**Good Cues**
✗ Lack of control at the pelvis, may present as too much anterior and posterior movement	✓ 'Core tight—control back and pelvis'
✗ Heels rising off the ground and individual is pushing through toes	✓ 'Push through your heels'

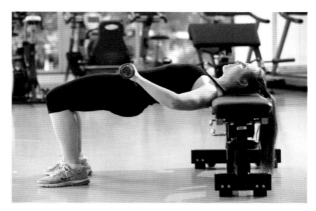

Figure 9.9 Middle position for the hip thrust

Exercise 9f: Knee Extension

Basic Action

Primary action:

- Knee extension

Equipment set-up:

- Be seated on the apparatus with hands holding the hand rests.
- The upper body remains stationary and supported throughout.

Starting position:

- Knees are flexed with the legs correctly aligned with the apparatus.

Finishing position:

- Knees are in full extension.

Execution of exercise:

- Slowly extend the leg to finishing position and then slowly return legs back to starting position. Depending on the equipment this may require both legs to work together or each may be done independently. If the shin pads roll up and down the tibia during the exercise, this indicates that it is positioned incorrectly and adjustments should be made before the next set. This can be achieved by aligning the knee joint centre with the axis of rotation of the knee extension machine and placing the shin pads on the distal portion of the anterior shin.

The primary variation of the knee extension is shown using a leg extension machine (Figure 9.10). This will be followed by a table of technique and cues (Table 9.14).

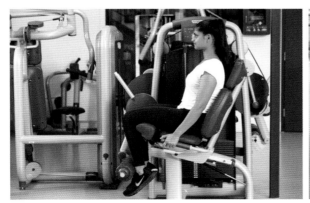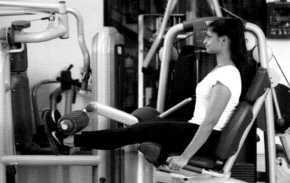

Figure 9.10 Primary variation of the knee extension shown using a leg extension machine; starting and finishing position (left) and middle position (right)

TABLE 9.14 Cues and Technique for the Knee Extension	
Poor Technique/Watch for	**Good Cues**
✗ Excessive or prolonged breath holding is likely to occur at higher weights; however, with untrained individuals the Valsalva manoeuvre and breath holding is often unnecessary	✓ 'Inhale and hold the breath during the latter stage of the lower (eccentric) phase and don't exhale until past the sticking point during the upward (concentric) phase'

Exercise 9g: Knee Flexion—Lying Leg Curl

Basic Action

Primary action:

- Knee flexion

Equipment set-up:

- Lie prone on the apparatus, with the hand holding the hand rests.
- The upper body remains stationary and supported throughout.

Starting position:

- Knees are extended with the legs correctly aligned with the apparatus.

Finishing position:

- Knees are in full flexion.

Execution of the exercise:

- Slowly flex the legs to finishing position and then slowly return legs back to starting position.

The primary variation of the knee flexion exercise is shown in a knee flexion machine in prone position (Figure 9.11). This will be followed by technique and cues (Table 9.15) and variations for the exercise (Table 9.16).

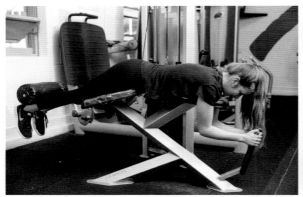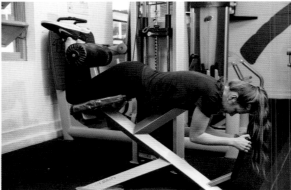

Figure 9.11 Primary variation of the knee flexion exercise shown in a knee flexion machine in prone position; starting and finishing position (left) and middle position (right)

TABLE 9.15 Cues and Technique for the Knee Flexion—Lying Leg Curl	
Poor Technique/Watch for	**Good Cues**
✗ Using the lumbar spine to move the load	✓ 'Push your hips into the bench and concentrate on bending through the knee'

TABLE 9.16	Variations of the Knee Flexion—Lying Leg Curl		
Variation	**Rationale**		**Considerations**
Seated leg curl	Seated machine is useful for individuals who find lying in prone positions uncomfortable. It requires the hamstrings to produce force at a longer muscle length. This version may also offer additional advantages in reducing the risk of hamstring strain injury.		If there is movement of the shank pad during the exercise, this is usually an indication of incorrect placement and adjustments may need to be made before commencing another set.
Fitball leg curl	In a supine position with shoulders on the floor and feet on the ball, this variation provides an element of challenge due to the stability component. It also requires an additional contribution of the gluteus maximus muscle to provide the required hip extension.		Ankle position should stay in neutral throughout. Some individuals will feel this variation in their calves due to the downward action on the ball. Some individuals will also be unable to reach a fully extended hip position due to weak gluteals and/or tight hip flexors.
Nordic curl	Research has shown that the eccentric challenge of this exercise results in adaptations that exceed many other common hamstring exercise variations. This makes it an excellent high-performance variation for athletes doing repeated sprints and kicking actions.		It is important to perform this variation safely and ensure neutral pelvic position is maintained as far as possible. It requires significant hamstring strength and will be too challenging for many beginners to perform correctly.

Exercise 9h: Calf Raise

Basic Action

Primary action:

- Ankle plantar flexion

Equipment set-up:

- Sit on the leg press apparatus with hands holding the hand rests.
- The upper body, hips and knees remain stationary and supported throughout.

Starting position:

- Ankles are in dorsiflexion with the ball of the foot in contact with the press plate, shoulder-width apart.
- Knees are slightly flexed (5°).

Finishing position:

- Ankles are in full plantar flexion.

Execution of exercise:

- Slowly plantar flex the ankle, lifting the press plate to finishing position and then lowering it to starting position.

The primary variation of the calf raise is shown seated in the leg press machine (Figure 9.12). This will be followed by technique and cues (Table 9.17) and variations for the exercise (Table 9.18).

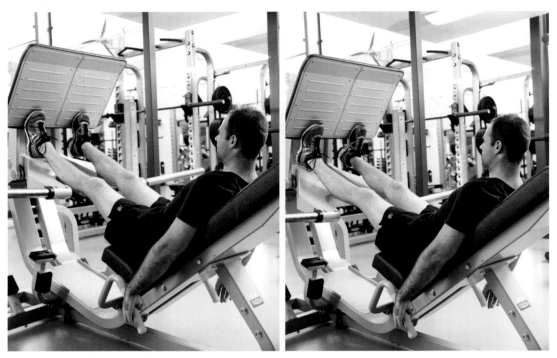

Figure 9.12 Primary variation of the calf raise shown seated in the leg press machine ; starting and finishing position (left) and middle position (right)

TABLE 9.17 Cues and Technique for the Calf Raise	
Poor Technique/Watch for	**Good Cues**
✗ Individuals often fail to go through complete ROM throughout	✓ 'Move your ankle all the way through the movement and pull your toes all the way back towards you'

TABLE 9.18	Variations of the Calf Raise		
Variation	Rationale		Considerations
Seated	During the seated calf raise, the gastrocnemius is placed in a shortened position as a result of knee flexion, resulting in greater isolation of the soleus.		This action puts the calf in a position of active insufficiency (shortened) and individuals may be more prone to experiencing calf cramps in this position.
Standing	When this exercise is performed standing on a box or a step, it allows a greater ROM than simply standing on the floor as the starting position is full dorsiflexion.		Dumbbells can be used to increase load in this variation; however, holding them will take away the opportunity to stabilise. The variation can be progressed by using one leg at a time with a dumbbell held in the alternate hand, or specially designed standing calf raise machines.

Activity 9.5 Case study—lower limb exercise programming

You have a new client who is a state-level 22-year-old female squash player. She experienced a grade 2 PCL strain in her right leg 3 months ago when she collided with an opponent while lunging for a shot during a game of squash. As she initially had moderate pain in her knee even during activities of daily living such as bending down, walking and climbing stairs, she has been quite inactive over the last 3 months. She experiences no pain during regular activities of daily living and body-weight squats and there is no current injury; however, she feels that she has lost some strength and muscle mass in the injured limb. She has asked you to write her a strength and conditioning program to assist in her rehabilitation from this injury.

Your discussions with the client and your understanding of the sport of squash highlight the importance of her being able to perform lunges in multiple directions and over varying distances to reach the ball.

AIM:
- To progress exercises of the lower limb

TASK:
- Based on the data provided in the review by Escamilla,[3] address the questions in the worksheet.

Worksheet 9.4 Lower Limb Exercise Programming

Question 1: Use this space to make notes or diagrams regarding the exercise.

_____

_____

_____

_____

_____

Question 2: What would be your general progression model that you would have this athlete do over the next 6 to 8 weeks in relation to the following two aspects of the exercise prescription?
a.   type of exercise (knee (leg) curl, knee extension, lunges, leg press and squats)?
b.   range of motion (0 to 50° or 50–100° of knee flexion)

_____

_____

_____

_____

_____

Question 3: When you feel the squash athlete is ready to perform lunges again, please describe the progressions you would have them do based on the following factors:
a.   direction of step (anterior, lateral and anterolateral)
b.   length of step (short or normal)

_____

_____

_____

_____

_____

_____

Activity 9.6 Making the most of equipment—bands

Background

While TheraBands have been traditionally used to provide low-level resistance for rehabilitative exercises, they are now used in many areas of the health, sports and exercise industries. Examples of these new applications include strength and conditioning for high-level athletes as well as for strength athletes including powerlifters, with both these groups typically utilising TheraBands and barbells in the same exercise. In rehabilitative and high-performance contexts, TheraBands are generally used to provide additional resistance to a movement, but they can also be used to provide assistance. In the following sections, we provide examples of how TheraBands may be used to provide resistance and assistance respectively for common multi-joint lower body exercises.

Using Therabands as a Form of Resistance

TheraBands can be looped around the end of the barbell (outside of the weight plate as shown in Figure 9.13 is safest to avoid the TheraBand slipping at the bottom of the ROM) and specialty pegs of more recent squat racks.

If specialty pegs are not available on the squat rack, you can attach the other end of the TheraBand to a heavy dumbbell and/or plates on the ground or even the safety bars. The individual can then perform exercises such as a back squat or deadlift with barbell and TheraBand loads. As the TheraBands stretch during the upward (concentric) phase, the total resistance increases throughout the concentric phase, and decreases during the descent (eccentric) phase as the barbell is lowered. The increased resistance near the top of the movement better replicates the strength curve for ascending exercises such as the squat, deadlift and bench press. The selection of the appropriate TheraBand resistance to utilise with barbell loads and how this may differ for taller and shorter individuals may take some trial and error. For example, shorter individuals may need to utilise double or triple loops of the TheraBands about the barbell in order to get the same degree of extra resistance that a tall individual will experience. The manufacturers of many TheraBands provide general recommendations on the most appropriate TheraBand size based on the barbell loads lifted in particular exercises.

You can also attach the TheraBands above the individual (e.g. at the top of a squat rack) so they provide assistance rather than resistance. The use of TheraBands in this context is particularly relevant to the teaching of single leg exercises such as the single leg squat and lunge variations. In these exercises, the other end of the TheraBands can be positioned on the end of a barbell (as used for resisted exercises) or positioned under the individual's armpits or attached to a harness that the individual wears. The primary benefit of using TheraBands to assist the single leg exercises is that they reduce the magnitude of the resistance load and provide greater stability, particularly at the bottom of the ROM, which is typically the hardest position in these exercises. By reducing the magnitude of resistance load and providing additional stability, beginners (even those of limited lower body strength and balance) can still perform a sufficient volume of training to elicit muscular adaptations and improve overall coordination and balance. As the athlete progresses, the magnitude of assistance can be reduced by using one instead of two TheraBands, using smaller TheraBands and/or reducing the degree of stretch on the TheraBands.

AIM:

- To develop experience in using bands to change resistance

TASK:

- In small groups create one exercise using bands to either increase or decrease resistance of a leg exercise. Present this exercise to the class with some scientific reasoning related to what type of client it might be best suited.

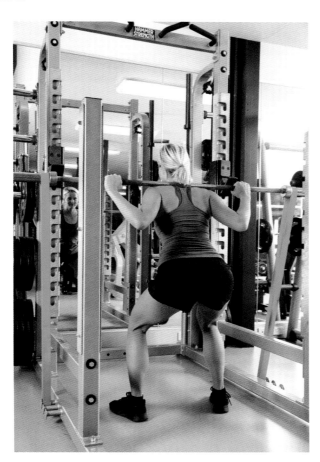

Figure 9.13 Using TheraBands as a form of resistance

References

1   Drake R 2015. *Gray's Atlas of Anatomy*. Churchill Livingstone.
2   Keogh JWL, Winwood PW. 2017. The epidemiology of injuries across the weight training sports: a systematic review. *Sports Med.* 47(3):479–501. doi: 10.1007/s40279-016-0575-0
3   Escamilla RF. 2001. Knee biomechanics of the dynamic squat exercise. *Med Sci Sports Exerc.* 33(1):127–141.
4   Hartmann H, Wirth K, Klusemann M. 2013. Analysis of the load on the knee joint and vertebral column with changes in squatting depth and weight load. *Sports Med.* 43(10):993–1008.

PRACTICAL 10
EXERCISE FOR MAXIMAL STRENGTH, POWER AND SPEED

G. Gregory Haff, Lachlan P. James and Emma M. Beckman

Introduction

Maximal strength is an important quality that has a direct impact on sports performance and the prevention of injuries[1,2] as well as activities of daily living with non-athletes. In fact, increasing strength may be one of the most important training goals as maximal strength levels have a significant impact on movement speed and the capacity to express a high-power output.[3] This is particularly important when working with novice or weaker individuals as it has been consistently shown that directing training towards the development of maximal strength can have a significant impact on the ability to produce force rapidly and express high-power outputs. With stronger individuals, the use of ballistic or explosive exercises designed to increase the ability to produce high amounts of force in relatively short periods of time, which is referred to as the rate of force development (RFD), becomes increasingly important.[3] Ultimately, stronger individuals are able to express higher RFD and power outputs than their weaker counterparts.[2]

An individual's ability to express high levels of power, or perform work rapidly, can be improved by using various resistance training methods. Many of these methods have been covered in previous practicals. This practical is divided into three parts that will expand on those methods by introducing the following training modalities.

- Part A: Weightlifting exercises and their derivatives
- Part B: Plyometric, ballistic and medicine ball training
- Part C: Speed, agility and change of direction

Weightlifting-based exercises and their derivatives as well as more ballistic movements such as the jump squat or bench throws are commonly used to improve speed and power. The amount of emphasis placed on high-velocity versus high-force movements varies depending on the individual's training age, training history and maximal strength levels. In general, speed and power training should be carried out in a non-fatigued state, particularly if these elements are a training priority. With this in mind, a training cycle should be set up in order to avoid attempting speed or power training with delayed-onset muscle soreness (DOMS) or general fatigue from a heavy session the previous day. Finally, given the ballistic and explosive nature of power training, these types of exercises should not be conducted without a comprehensive warm-up.

Part A: The Weightlifting Derivatives

One of the most effective training methods for maximising power output is the use of training exercises derived from the sport of weightlifting, which is often referred to as Olympic lifting. The term 'Olympic lifts' is often used incorrectly to describe the exercises contained in this sport. In reality, this is a misnomer as only the sport of weightlifting is contested in the Olympics. The sport of weightlifting consists of two competition exercises: the snatch and the clean and jerk. In addition to the competitive exercises these athletes often use weightlifting derivatives which can include exercises such as the power snatch, power clean, clean/snatch pull, power jerk, push press or the jump shrug exercises in their training.[4] These exercises are beneficial to athletes because they require total body coordination, are ground-based multi-joint exercises and are able to allow for the development of power across the force–velocity spectrum.[5] Ultimately, these exercises have been shown to optimise the expression of power in sporting settings because they allow for the maximisation of the RFD and increase power-generating capacity, which more readily transfers to sporting performance.[3] Both novice and experienced lifters see excellent improvements in athletic performance after incorporating these lifts into a training plan.[6] However, the transfer of training adaptation tends to occur at a fast rate in those who are stronger.[7] As such, these exercises are often the foundation of sound strength and conditioning programs.

In this practical the student will be exposed to the teaching progression for the power snatch and power clean. The power snatch requires the athlete to lift the barbell from the floor to arms-length overhead in one continuous movement. The power clean requires the athlete to lift the barbell from the floor to the shoulders in one continuous movement.

Basic Phases of the Power Snatch and Power Clean

These lifts are often broken into key phases.

- **First Pull:** This occurs when the barbell is raised from the floor and lifted to roughly the patellar tendon (i.e. knee level). This is best accomplished by straightening the knee.
- **Transition:** This is initiated from the end of the first pull and ends when the barbell is elevated to high-thigh (power snatch) or mid-thigh (power clean). This phase of the lift involves a re-bending of the knees, which is known as the double knee bend. This technique is easily learned when an appropriate teaching progression is used.
- **Second pull:** This involves an explosive extension of the knees and hips, followed by ankle plantar flexion and a shrugging motion. This movement pattern is often referred to as the triple extension. Effectively this is a jump shrug type movement pattern.
- **Catch:** This is when the bar is received either at arms-length overhead (power snatch) or on the shoulders (power clean).

Safety

Weightlifting is a safe activity with a very low incidence of injury when instructed by qualified professionals. It is important that these exercises are only taught after a fundamental movement literacy is established and basic strength training exercises are mastered (i.e. squatting, deadlifting and pressing). If an appropriate teaching progression is utilised, not only are these exercises safe to perform they are generally easy to learn. Recent research has shown that the hang power clean, one of the weightlifting derivatives, can be learned in as little as 4 weeks of training and result in meaningful performance gains in the same time period.[8]

Anatomy

Weightlifting uses a significant number of muscles in the lower body, the trunk and the upper body. Figure 10.1 shows some of the key muscles for weightlifting and their locations in the body. Table 10.1 shows key movements and muscles recruited during weightlifting.

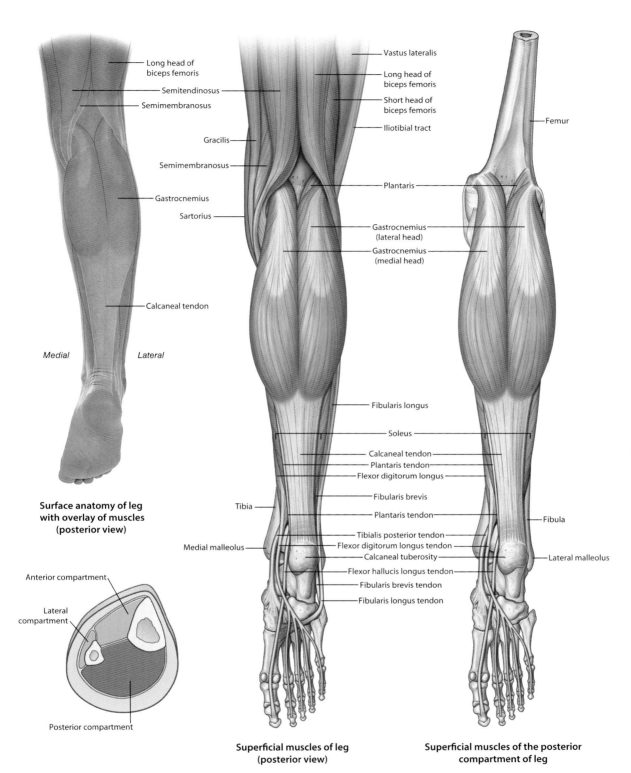

Surface anatomy of leg with overlay of muscles (posterior view)

Superficial muscles of leg (posterior view)

Superficial muscles of the posterior compartment of leg

Figure 10.1 Some of the key muscles for weightlifting
Source: Drake (2015).[9]

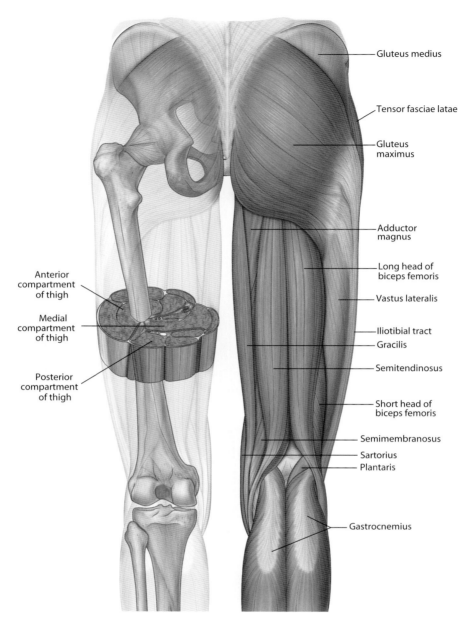

Figure 10.1, cont'd

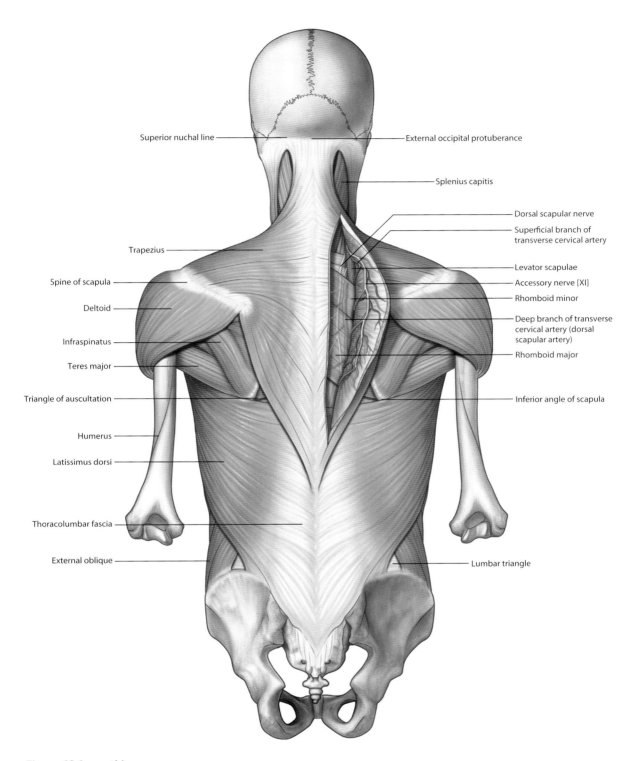

Figure 10.1, cont'd

TABLE 10.1   Anatomy

Movement	Muscle Recruited
Hip extension	• Gluteus maximus • Gluteus medius (posterior fibres) • Adductor magnus (posterior fibres) • Biceps femoris (long head) • Semitendinosus • Semimembranosus
Knee extension	• Rectus femoris • Vastus lateralis • Vastus intermedius • Vastus medius
Plantar flexion	• Gastrocnemius • Soleus • Plantaris • Peroneus longus • Peroneus brevis • Tibialis posterior • Flexor digitorum longus • Flexor hallucis longus
Pelvic and femoral head stabilisation	• Gluteus medius • Gluteus minimus • Piriformis
Scapular elevation	• Upper trapezius • Levator scapulae
Scapular stabilisation	• Serratus anterior • Middle/lower fibres of trapezius
Humoral head stabilisation	• Supraspinatus (RC) • Infraspinatus (RC) • Teres minor (RC) • Subscapularis (RC)
Lumbar spinal stabilisation (deep)	• Transverse abdominis • Internal obliques • External obliques • Multifidus • Pelvic floor
Lumbar spine extension	• Rectus abdominis • Iliocostalis (ES) • Longissimus (ES) • Spinalis (ES) • Quadratus lumborum

Exercise 10a: Power Snatch

The power snatch is a dynamic movement pattern which requires the athlete to move the barbell from the floor in one continuous movement to a fixed position overhead.[10]

Determining the Grip Position

The power snatch requires a wide grip which can be determined by measuring: 1. the distance between the first to opposite shoulder or 2. the elbow to elbow distance as shown in Figure 10.2.

Basic Movement

Table 10.2 describes the phases of the power snatch. This is followed by a teaching sequence to make it easier to instruct the complex movements that comprise the power snatch. Cues and techniques are then explained in Table 10.3 with examples of poor technique and some examples of cues that may assist to improve the movements.

Power Snatch Teaching Sequence

The best method for teaching the power snatch is to use a top-down teaching progression:

- determine snatch grip
- snatch grip behind neck press
- overhead squat
- snatch balance
- snatch pull (from power position)
- power snatch (from power position)
- snatch grip Romanian deadlift
- snatch pull (from below knee)
- power snatch (from below knee)
- snatch pull to knee
- snatch pull
- power snatch from floor.

Variations: Snatch, hang snatch, hang power snatch, split snatch, one-arm power snatch, snatch pulls and snatch grip jump shrug

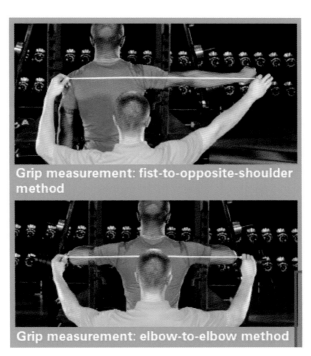

Figure 10.2 Determining the grip for a power snatch
Source: Photos from Caulfield and Berninger (2016).[10]

TABLE 10.2   Phases of the Power Snatch

Phase	
Starting position: • Feet should be flat on the floor about shoulder-width apart with the toes pointed slightly outwards. • Squatting down with the hips lower than the shoulders, the bar is grasped evenly with the use of a pronated snatch grip and with the arms fully extended. • The bar should be close to the shins and over the balls of the feet. • The body should be positioned so that the back is neutral or slightly arched, the scapulae are depressed and retracted, the chest is held up and out, the shoulders are over or slightly in front of the bar and the eyes are focused straight ahead.	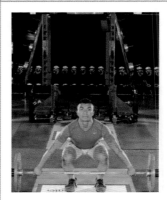
First pull: • The knees and hips are forcefully extended in order to lift the bar off the floor. • The torso-to-floor angle should be kept constant and the hips should not rise before the shoulders. • The spine should remain in a neutral or slightly arched position while the arms are fully extended and the shoulders are over or slightly ahead of the bar. • As the bar is raised from the floor, it should remain as close to the shins as possible. • The photo to the right represents the end of the first pull.	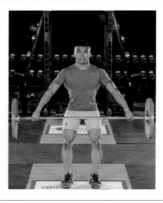
Transition: • As the bar is raised to above the knees, the knees flex and move under the bar while it remains in contact with the thigh and the hips move slightly forwards. • The back should remain in a neutral or slightly arched position with the elbows being fully extended. • The photo to the right represents the end of the transition and the start of the second pull.	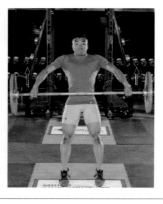
Second pull: • The knees, hips and ankles are rapidly extended while keeping the bar as close to the body as possible. • The back should remain in a neutral position with the elbows remaining straight. • After the completion of the triple extension, the shoulders should be shrugged upwards elevating the bar as high as possible. • The photo to the right represents the end of the transition and the start of the second pull.	

TABLE 10.2 Phases of the Power Snatch (continued)	
Phase	
Catch: • When the bar reaches its highest elevation, the arms pull the body under the bar and rapidly extend, fixing the bar overhead in a position slightly behind the ears as the athlete simultaneously flexes the hips and knees while moving the feet outwards into a quarter squat position.	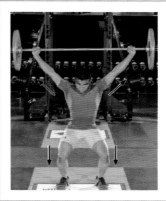
End position: After the bar is fixed overhead the athlete extends the hips and knees until they are standing in a fully erect position with the bar overhead.	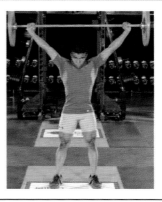

Source: Photos from Caulfield and Berninger (2016).[10]

TABLE 10.3 Cues and Technique for the Power Snatch	
Poor Technique/Watch for	**Good Cues**
✗ Lateral instability of pelvis ✗ Failure to maintain neutral spine or slightly arched position ✗ Knees move laterally or medially ✗ Ankle eversion ✗ Bar drifts forwards away from the shin during first pull ✗ Shoulder drops behind bar during first pull ✗ Hips rise faster than the knees during first pull ✗ Elbows bend early during first, transition or second pull (i.e. flex before full body extension) ✗ Incomplete extension at the end of the second pull ✗ Feet do not shuffle outwards into a squat stance during the lift ✗ Knees and hips do not flex upon receiving bar overhead ✗ Bar is caught in front of the head	✓ 'Focal point straight ahead' ✓ 'Maintain torso-to-floor angle during first pull' ✓ 'Maintaining neutral or slightly arched position' ✓ 'Keep arms extended until shrug is complete' ✓ 'Finish the pull' ✓ 'Stay tight when catching the bar' ✓ 'Keep bar close to body'

Activity 10.1 Teaching weightlifting derivatives to experienced and novice lifters

AIM:

- Understand how to modify your teaching techniques for a novice versus a more experienced lifter

TASKS:

- From the group, select one individual with limited experience in weightlifting and one individual with prior experience in either weightlifting derivatives or at least considerable experience in squat and deadlift movements.
- These two individuals should be coached to perform the starting position and the first pull of the power snatch by at least two other members of the group.
- Complete Worksheet 10.1.

Worksheet 10.1 Teaching Weightlifting Derivatives to Experienced and Novice Lifters

Question 1: What was the most significant challenge for the novice lifter in terms of achieving good technique?

_____

_____

_____

_____

Question 2: What were the differences in communication styles necessary to instruct the novice compared to the more experienced lifter?

_____

_____

_____

_____

Question 3: What were the most effective cues that were ideal in fixing elements of the novice lifter's technique?

_____

_____

_____

_____

_____

Activity 10.2 Teaching the power snatch

AIM:

- Understand how to teach the power snatch

TASKS:

- Find a partner and apply some observation analysis to each step of the power snatch sequence. Briefly, these stages of analysis are as follows.

1. Introduce the exercise. (Have they done it before? What does it do? How does it relate to the client's goals?)
2. Demonstrate the exercise and identify the critical features.
3. Observe the client perform the exercise and provide appropriate cueing.
4. Give feedback after the set is completed.
5. If necessary, repeat stages 2 to 4 before moving on to the next step of the sequence.

- Once your partner has completed the power snatch from the floor with a relatively light weight, sensibly increase the weight until a working set is reached. Repeat this process with your partner now instructing you.

Worksheet 10.2 Teaching the Power Snatch

Question 1: Reflect on your own performance instructing the power snatch. Identify and describe three factors that need improvement in your teaching technique for this exercise.

1. _____

   _____

2. _____

   _____

3. _____

   _____

Exercise 10b: Power Clean

The power clean is a dynamic movement pattern which requires the athlete to move the bar in a single movement from the floor to a position on the front of the shoulders.[10]

Table 10.4 covers the movements of the power clean from the starting position, through the pull phases and into the catch. Examples of poor technique and some helpful cues are provided in Table 10.5.

Variations: Clean, hang clean, hang power clean, split clean and clean pulls.

Power Clean Teaching Sequence

The best method for teaching the power clean is to use a top-down teaching progression:

- front squat
- clean pull (from power position)
- power clean (from power position)
- clean grip Romanian deadlift
- clean pull (from below knee)
- power clean (from below knee)
- clean pull (to knee)
- clean pull
- power clean from floor.

TABLE 10.4   Movements of the Power Clean

Phase	
Starting position: • Feet should be flat on the floor about shoulder-width apart with the toes pointed out slightly. • Squat with the hips lower than the bar while the bar is grasped evenly with a pronated grip. • The hands should be slightly wider than shoulder-width apart, outside the knees and the elbow should be fully extended. • The bar should be close to the shin and over the balls of the feet. • The body should be positioned so that the back is neutral or slightly arched, the scapulae are depressed and retracted, the chest is held up and out, the shoulders are slightly in front of or over the bar and the eyes are focused straight ahead.	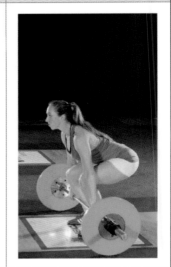
First pull: • The knees and hips are forcefully extended in order to lift the bar from the floor to approximately the knees. • The torso-to-floor angle should remain in a neutral or slightly arched position while the arms are fully extended and the shoulders are over or slightly ahead of the bar. • As the bar is raised from the floor, it should remain as close to the shins as possible. • The photo on the right is of the end of the first pull and the start of the transition.	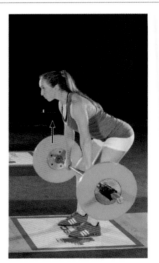
Transition: • As the bar is raised to the knees, the knees flex and move under the bar while it remains in contact with the thigh, and the hips move slightly forwards. • The back should remain in a neutral or slightly arched position with the elbows being fully extended. • The photo on the right is of the end of the transition and the start of the second pull.	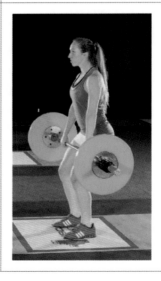

TABLE 10.4   Movements of the Power Clean (continued)

Phase	
Second pull: • The knee, hips and ankles are rapidly extended (triple extension) while keeping the bar as close to the body as possible. • The back should remain in a neutral position with the elbows remaining straight. • After completion of the triple extension the shoulders should be shrugged upwards, elevating the bar as high as possible. • The photo on the right is of the end of the second pull.	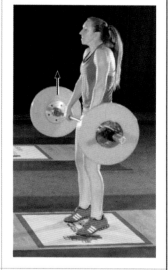
Catch: • When the bar reaches its highest elevation, the arms pull the body under the bar while rotating the arms around and under the bar. • The hips and knees are simultaneously flexed to a quarter squat position. • As the arms rotate under the bar, the elbows are lifted to a position in which the upper arm is parallel to the floor.	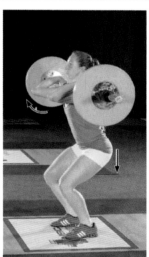
End position: The torso should remain erect while the athlete extends the knees and hips to move to a fully erect standing position.	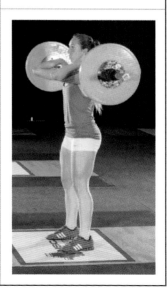

Source: Photos from Caulfield and Berninger (2016).[10]

TABLE 10.5 Cues and Technique for the Power Clean	
Poor Technique/Watch for	**Good Cues**
✗ Lateral instability of pelvis ✗ Failure to maintain neutral spine or slightly arched position ✗ Knees move laterally or medially ✗ Ankle eversion ✗ Bar drifts away from shin during first pull ✗ Shoulders drop behind bar during first pull ✗ Elbows bend early during first, transition or second pull (i.e. flex before full body extension) ✗ Incomplete extension at the end of the second pull ✗ Feet do not shuffle outwards into squat stance ✗ Knees and hips do not flex upon receiving the bar on the shoulders ✗ Elbows do not rotate into a position parallel to the floor while holding the bar on the shoulders	✓ 'Focal point straight ahead' ✓ 'Maintain torso-to-floor angle during first pull' ✓ 'Keep back tight, maintaining neutral or slightly arched position' ✓ 'Keep arms extended until shrug is complete' ✓ 'Torso remains tight when catching the bar' ✓ 'Upper arm is parallel to the floor when catching the bar on the shoulders'

Activity 10.3 Teaching the power clean

AIM:

- Understand how best to teach the power clean

TASKS:

- Find a partner and apply the stages of observation analysis to each step of the power clean sequence. Briefly, these stages of analysis are as follows.
  1. Introduce the exercise. (Have they done it before? What does it do? How does it relate to the client's goals?)
  2. Demonstrate the exercise and identify the critical features.
  3. Observe the client perform the exercise and provide appropriate cueing.
  4. Give feedback after the set is completed.
  5. If necessary, repeat stages 2 to 4 before moving on to the next step of the sequence.
- Once your partner has completed the power clean from the floor with a relatively light weight, sensibly increase the weight until a working set is reached. Repeat this process with your partner instructing you. Complete Worksheet 10.3 once the exercise is complete.

Worksheet 10.3 Teaching the Power Clean

Question 1: Reflect on your own performance instructing the power clean. Identify and describe three factors that need improvement in your teaching technique for this exercise.

1. _____

   _____

2. _____

   _____

3. _____

   _____

Part B: Plyometrics and Ballistic Training

Plyometrics involve a broad range of exercises that allow for the application of maximal force in the shortest possible amount of time.[11] Fundamentally, the stretch shortening cycle (SSC), which combines mechanical and neurophysiological mechanisms, provides the foundation for all plyometric exercise. SSCs occur when an activated muscle is stretched eccentrically and then immediately performs a concentric muscle action. The SSC is comprised of three phases: eccentric, amortisation and concentric.[11] During the eccentric phase, elastic energy is stored in the series elastic components and the muscle spindles are stimulated. This elastic energy is then released during the concentric muscle action. The amortisation phase is the linking phase and should be kept as short as possible in order to maximise the benefits of the plyometric exercise.[11]

While plyometric exercises are ballistic, they differ from specific ballistic exercises in the way that overload is applied to them. Specifically, plyometrics alter the stretch rate, stretch duration and stretch magnitude to increase the demands of the action. For example, to overload a depth jump (plyometric exercise) the box height used can be increased (stretch rate and magnitude) or the contact time can be shortened (stretch duration). Conversely, with ballistic exercises such as the loaded jump squat or weightlifting exercises, the resistance is generally increased to overload the athlete. In this practical activity, plyometric and ballistic exercises also encompass medicine ball exercises and sprinting drills.

Example Exercises

- **Jumps in place:** These involve jumping and landing in the same place. Typically, these exercises emphasise the vertical component of jumping. Examples of jumps in place are the squat jump, tuck jump and split jump. Double-leg jumps are considered to be lower intensity than single-leg jumps. The purpose is often repetition compared to a maximal effort although single jumps may be used.

- **Standing jumps for height or distance:** Emphasise either horizontal or vertical aspects of the jump. Standing jumps are maximal-effort jumps so rest periods should be given between efforts. Examples of standing jumps are jumps for distance or over barriers. Double-leg jumps are considered to be lower intensity than single-leg jumps.

- **Multiple hops and jumps:** These involve repeated movements and typically are combinations of jumps in place or standing jumps. Examples of multiple jumps are the zigzag hop or jumps over hurdles as seen in Figure 10.3.

- **Bounds:** These involve multiple exaggerated movements emphasising horizontal speed and tend to cover distances about 30 m. They can include single- and double-leg bounds in addition to alternate leg bounds. Examples of bounding exercises are skipping and power skipping.

- **Box drills:** These are used to increase the intensity of multiple jumps and hops. The box can be jumped onto or off of and may involve one, both or alternating legs. The box jump seen in Figure 10.4 is done with both legs.

- **Depth jumps:** Gravity and the athlete's body mass are used to enhance intensity of the eccentric portion of the exercise. These exercises require the athlete to step off a box and jump vertically, horizontal or to another box. These exercises can be done with one or both legs. Figure 10.5 shows an example with both legs.

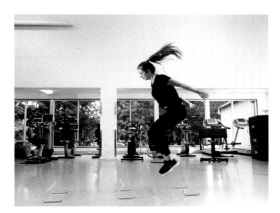

Figure 10.3 Multiple hops can be performed over mini hurdles

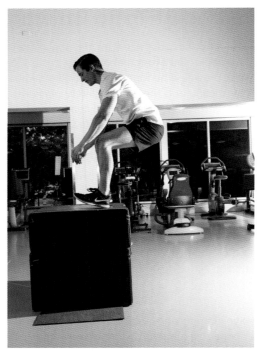

Figure 10.4 Box jumps for height

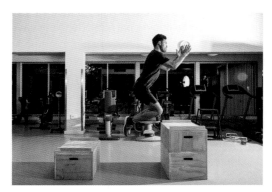

Figure 10.5 Box depth jumps with two legs

Activity 10.4 Movement competency

Background

Plyometrics involve significant velocity and therefore require a good movement base to be performed safely. It is important for students to use key basic movements to make observations about the readiness of an individual to engage in high-load and high-speed movements. One example is if you observe a squat and there is a lack of control in the eccentric phase; this individual may not be ready for a jump squat. Alternatively, they might have sufficient strength and control in a bilateral squat jump but be unable to perform single-leg exercises to the correct depth to allow progression to an exercise such as single-leg bounds.

AIM:

- Understand screening for movement competency and why it is important to establish an adequate degree of movement competency before progressing to plyometric training

TASKS:

- In small groups, develop a movement screen containing 3 to 4 movements that will give the instructor a good indication of the client's preparedness to undertake plyometric training.
- Include some key technical features to focus on for each movement.

- Once completed, each group can demonstrate a chosen movement to the larger group until all have been covered.
- Movements used may include a variety of submaximal jumping tasks such as a single jump and land, a long jump and land, rebound jumps, and jump and land on a single leg. Additional movements include a basic squat and single-leg squat.
- Complete Worksheet 10.4.

Worksheet 10.4 Movement Competency	
Movement	Critical Features

Activity 10.5 Plyometric exercises

AIM:
- Complete plyometric exercises and understand common movement errors and how to address them

TASKS:
- In groups of two or three rotate through the plyometric exercises listed in Worksheet 10.5.
- For each exercise, note the common errors, the teaching cues that you found most effective, the intensity and the complexity (out of 10).
- Complete Worksheet 10.5.

Worksheet 10.5 Plyometric Exercises				
Exercise	Common Errors	Teaching Cues	Intensity (/10)	Complexity (/10)
Jumps in place				
Standing jumps				
Multiple hops and jumps				
Bounds				
Box drills				
Depth jumps				

Activity 10.6 Considerations for plyometric exercises

AIM:

- To understand considerations of prescribing plyometric exercises

TASK:

- Complete Worksheet 10.6.

Worksheet 10.6 Considerations for Plyometric Exercises

Question 1: What effects does the type of training surface have (e.g. sand versus grass versus tartan track versus cement)?

_____

_____

Question 2: What safety considerations should be put into place before undertaking plyometric jump training?

_____

_____

Question 3: Among the general population, is there a minimum strength threshold that must be reached before they can be taught how to safely perform ballistic exercises?

_____

_____

Alternative Equipment: Medicine Ball Training

Plyometric and ballistic training can also be undertaken with the use of medicine balls. Medicine balls can be used to enhance the transfer of strength gains from traditional resistance training to more applied speed and power movements.[12] Medicine balls come in a wide variety of shapes, sizes, densities and weights which can be used with a variety of exercises depending on requirements. Typically, medicine balls are thrown explosively when used for plyometric exercises. There are numerous exercise variations that can be constructed to use a medicine ball. Globally, these exercises can fall under the following categories: 1. total body exercises; 2. combination jumps and medicine ball work; 3. core exercises; and 4. upper body exercises. Examples of these exercises are presented in Table 10.6.

TABLE 10.6 Example Exercises for Different Categories of Medicine Ball Training	
Total Body Exercise	**Combination Jumps and Medicine Ball Work**
<ul><li>Lunge squat with toss</li><li>Underhand throw</li><li>Overhead throw</li><li>Backward throw</li></ul>	<ul><li>Catch and pass with jump-and-reach</li><li>Bound with chest pass</li><li>Multiple jump with chest pass</li><li>One jump and overhead throw</li></ul>
Core Exercise	**Upper Body Exercise**
<ul><li>Overhead sit-up toss</li><li>Russian twist</li><li>Trunk rotation</li></ul>	<ul><li>Chest pass (Figure 10.6)</li><li>Two-hand side-to-side throw</li><li>Single-arm throw</li><li>Medicine ball power drop</li><li>Explosive push-up (Figure 10.6)</li></ul>

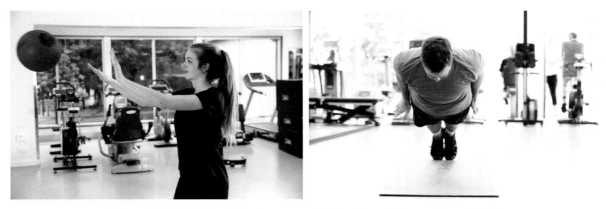

Figure 10.6 Medicine ball chest pass (left) and explosive push-up (right)

Activity 10.7 Medicine ball exercises

AIM:
- Prescribe exercises for different types of athletes using medicine balls

TASK:
- Form small groups and from Table 10.6 (or based on your own creativity and knowledge) list three exercises using a medicine ball that are designed to improve performance in one of the following cases:
  - 100 m sprinter
  - pole vaulter
  - water polo player
  - netballer.
- Each group should present their exercises to the whole class, with a strong justification for their inclusion.
- Complete Worksheet 10.7.

Worksheet 10.7 Medicine Ball Exercises	
Athlete chosen: _____	
Exercise 1:	
Description of exercise with justification	
Effective teaching cues	
Common errors	
Rank the intensity and complexity (/10)	
Exercise 2:	
Description of exercise with justification	
Effective teaching cues	
Common errors	
Rank the intensity and complexity (/10)	

Worksheet 10.7 Medicine Ball Exercises (continued)	
Exercise 3:	
Description of exercise with justification	
Effective teaching cues	
Common errors	
Rank the intensity and complexity (/10)	
Exercise 4:	
Description of exercise with justification	
Effective teaching cues	
Common errors	
Rank the intensity and complexity (/10)	
Exercise 5:	
Description of exercise with justification	
Effective teaching cues	
Common errors	
Rank the intensity and complexity (/10)	

Part C: Speed, Agility and Change of Direction

Acceleration Training

The ability to accelerate and achieve high movement velocities (i.e. speed) and then change direction are foundational skills for most team sports athletes.[13] All of these abilities are interrelated and are somewhat dependent upon the athlete's maximal strength levels.[13,14] The ability to rapidly change direction in response to a sport-specific stimulus (i.e. agility) is foundational to successful sporting performance in most team sports. To maximise speed, agility and change of direction training should occur when fatigue is minimal and full recovery occurs between repetitions.

Acceleration, or increasing an object's velocity, is a critical skill needed in most team sports where sprints are seldom longer than 20 m. A central component of being able to accelerate is a high level of relative lower body strength.[13] The ability to accelerate can be maximised by employing specific training drills.

Important Considerations for Acceleration Training

The following are important considerations when providing acceleration training.

- **Fundamental acceleration drills:** These are used to improve body mechanics during acceleration activities. For example, wall push drills (where the athlete drives the upper body with arms outstretched against a wall and performs the running action with the lower limbs) can be used to teach the athlete to contact behind the centre of gravity in the first few steps in order to reduce braking forces and enhance forward propulsion.

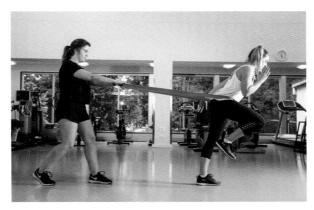

Figure 10.7 Resisted speed training drill

- **Acceleration drills:** These are performed as 5–40 m sprints designed to emphasise the ability to accelerate the body to full speed in as short a time as possible. Example drills are beach starts and three-point starts where the athlete is given a stimulus and required to accelerate as quickly as possible to a specific target or distance.
- **Resisted speed training drills:** These are performed with the athlete pulling or pushing against an implement that provides an external resistance.[13] No more than a 10% decrease in the athlete's standard speed should be allotted when using this type of training to enhance acceleration and speed. Example exercises are light-sled pulling or dragging a tyre for a distance between 10 and 40 m.[15] An example of a resisted speed training drill is presented in Figure 10.7.

Speed Training

The ability to express high forces in sprinting is a key requirement of increasing movement speed. As such, the development of high levels of strength is necessary to increase maximal relative strength when attempting to maximise movement speed.[13] While strength is very important, the addition of speed-specific training methods is also necessary in order to optimise this performance characteristic.

Important considerations for training speed

- **Fundamental speed drills:** These are used to develop proper form and technique. Ideally, they should be performed when the athlete is not fatigued from other types of training.[15] Example drills are arm-swing drills, straight-leg running, fast-clawing drills, butt kicks and high-knee drives.
- **Assisted speed training drills:** These use implements, such as a sport cord (i.e. bungy cord), or running down an incline to help the athlete run faster than normal. Sometimes this type of training is termed over-speed training. It is often recommended when performing assisted speed training that the athlete not exceed 100% of their normal running speed.[13,15]

Note: Some assisted speed training drills are not appropriate for athletes who do not possess excellent sprint technique. Often when athletes are pulled in speeds in excess of their current capacity, they tend to overstride which increases the breaking forces and if done regularly may lead to the development of an ineffective motor pattern at maximum velocity. Additionally, devices such as bungy cords can make it particularly difficult for the athlete to control velocity and maintain a constant amount of assistance.

Activity 10.8 Developing speed drills

Background

Research is consistently identifying ways of optimising speed. A number of studies have identified drills and activities that are related to developing speed. Complete the drill activities provided in Worksheet 10.8.

AIM:
- To obtain, understand and apply information about the different mechanisms of speed and how to apply them in drills

TASKS:

- Following completion of an instructor-led warm-up, form pairs and attempt the sprinting activities presented in Worksheet 10.8.
- In the worksheet, circle whether the emphasis of the drill is on maximal speed, technical development or acceleration.
- After each student has performed the drill, give each other feedback with respect to performance.

Worksheet 10.8 Developing Speed Drills

Drill 1. Perform a gradual submaximal acceleration (rolling start) before reaching maximal speed. Hold this top speed for 10–30 m.

    maximal speed   technical development   acceleration

Drill 2: Over a distance of 60–150 m alternate periods of maximal effort (10–30 m) and periods of near maximal effort considering technical factors such as:

- arm swing with elbows at 90°, moving from hip height to shoulder height
- neutral head alignment
- relaxed upper body
- upright trunk
- neutral spine and level hips
- arms and legs do not cross the midline of the body.

    maximal speed   technical development   acceleration

Drill 3: Over a distance of 5–20 m accelerate at maximal effort from a stationary start. Initiate with a relatively low centre of mass and gradually rise upright in the later stages.

    maximal speed   technical development   acceleration

Change-of-direction Training

Agility is defined as a rapid, whole-body change of direction or speed in response to a specific stimulus.[14] Agility requires the optimal integration of sensory systems involved in neuromuscular control. In addition, it includes perceptual and decision-making factors, visual scanning, anticipation, pattern recognition, situation awareness and movement confidence. As a result, agility is characterised by a high degree of cognitive demand. In this manual, agility should be considered in the context of sporting performance but also the agility of non-sporting participants (e.g. older individuals).

Agility requires an individual to be able to coordinate several activities including the ability to start and react quickly, accelerate, decelerate, move in the proper direction and change direction as rapidly as possible while maintaining balance and postural control.[16] Given these requirements, there is an obvious overlap with neuromotor exercises that address coordination and balance. This practical will concentrate on the ability of an individual to react quickly to a stimulus and adjust their movement patterns safely and effectively. Reaction time refers to an individual's ability to react to a stimulus. Reaction time is influenced by the individual's vision, hearing, anticipation and resultant neuromuscular response. Reaction time is a component of agility, but it is also a skill that can be trained individually. The ability to react quickly is maximised by including exercises that encourage maximal body movement speed. The training of agility can be optimised by task constraint manipulation. Examples of this may include changes in pitch size, changes in player number, changes in game rules, changes in fatigue level or changing the role of the player.

Important Considerations for Agility Training

Agility exercises can be classified into three types.

1. Programmed: Pre-planned, the individual is aware of the movements required prior to beginning the exercise.
2. Reactive: Not pre-planned, the individual reacts as quickly as possible to information provided during the exercise.
3. Quick exercises: Designed to produce fast movements characterised by quick foot motion that can be programmed or reactive.

Beginner agility training programs should focus on higher repetitions of fundamental skills being completed in short timeframes in order to optimise motor development and learning. Modifications of agility-based activities include reducing the time taken to complete the exercise without a reduction in accuracy (e.g. ensuring an individual focuses on remaining as close to the cones as possible in a figure-eight drill while progressively decreasing the time taken to complete the lap). Progression of agility-based exercises can also be facilitated by increasing the demands of the task and the speed; for example:

- transitioning from foundation skills to functional specific movements (e.g. moving from a figure-eight exercise to changing direction in response to a defensive player's actions)
- increasing the difficulty of the exercises (e.g. including a reactive component, decreasing the distance between direction changes)
- changing the plane of movement in which the activity is completed in multiplanar movements (e.g. jumping sideways)
- introducing environmental challenges (e.g. changing the surface)
- introducing an additional task during the completion of the overall task (e.g. a cognitive element such as counting backwards in threes from 100).

Examples of additional agility exercises and considerations around their use in programs are given in Table 10.7.

TABLE 10.7 Agility Exercises with Their Rationale and Considerations	
Exercise	**Rationale and Considerations**
Star/compass exercise where an individual stands in the middle of a star or compass pattern and is asked to step to different directions (e.g. north, south-east)	This exercise is designed to improve the ability to change direction quickly. Progressions of this activity could include moving from a programmed series of direction changes, to a reactive series of direction changes in response to verbal cues, to reactive quick drills requiring participants to change direction quickly. Mastering this task would allow individuals to be able to change direction quickly in response to verbal cues (e.g. having to change direction after being made aware of an unseen hazard).
Moving star/compass exercise with change in directions due to verbal prompts	This exercise progresses from the star/compass exercise in that the individual completes the direction change while in motion. This requires an increased emphasis on neuromuscular coordination and balance.
Bouncing balls in different directions requiring the individual to move forwards and catch them	This exercise challenges agility as it is reactive, requires a multiplanar movement and requires the coordination of joints to complete. Alternating the speed of the bounces, the physical distance between the bounces and the height of the bounce increases the difficulty of the movement and requires increased agility to respond to the changes in the task demands.

TABLE 10.7 Agility Exercises with Their Rationale and Considerations (continued)	
Exercise	**Rationale and Considerations**
Moving between cones; progressions: • distance between cones and number of cones (in order to increase the number of direction changes required) • reaching down to touch cones before moving back to starting position	Progressions are designed to increase the difficulty of the pattern of movement required. • Shorter distances between cones and increasing the number of direction changes increases the complexity of the pattern of movement. • Adding positional changes into the movement changes the plane of movement in which the activity is performed and requires coordination of multiple joints in order to complete the movement. • The addition of an accuracy component while completing the task increases the difficulty of executing the movement.
Basic movements: forwards, backpedalling, side shuffling, drop-steps, crossover steps and diagonal steps T-drill: running forwards, shuffling right, shuffling left and running backwards	• Basic movement drills require individuals to transition between movement types which requires a change in the coordination of the muscles needed to produce the movement. Progression of this activity could include a programmed series of transitions from one movement to the next or reactive changes to a verbal or visual prompt. • T-drills progress the basic movement drills by incorporating a combination of movements and changes to the movement direction which requires rapid muscle response (e.g. a forward run with a sideways shuffle and backward run to move from one point to another).
Ladder drills	Ladder drills are used to develop foot speed, balance and coordination in order to produce quick and agile movement between the ladder rungs. Ladder movements can start with a basic forward movement and progress by changing body and foot positions, including lateral and backward movements and including a reactive time-based element.
Shadow (following an individual) and mirror (facing an individual) drills	Shadow drills require a reactive response to a visual stimulus. The drill requires the quick processing of visual information and the formulation of an appropriate muscular response. Mirror drills increase the difficulty of the task as they require the individual to replicate the movement using their opposite limb (e.g. moving their left arm in response to someone moving their right arm).

Activity 10.9 Agility exercises

AIM:

- To complete agility exercises and understand how modifications may increase the difficulty

TASKS:

- Complete the agility exercises in Worksheet 10.9 and rate each for the level of difficulty by placing a X on the scale.
- Provide a modification to each exercise and rate this exercise for level of difficulty.

Worksheet 10.9 Agility Exercises	
Agility exercise	**Difficulty Rating**
Star/compass exercise Modification: _____ _____	Very easy Easy Difficult Very difficult Very easy Easy Difficult Very difficult
Moving star/compass exercise Modification: _____ _____	Very easy Easy Difficult Very difficult Very easy Easy Difficult Very difficult
Moving between cones Modification: _____ _____	Very easy Easy Difficult Very difficult Very easy Easy Difficult Very difficult
Moving between cones and reaching down to touch cones before moving back to starting position Modification: _____ _____	Very easy Easy Difficult Very difficult Very easy Easy Difficult Very difficult

Activity 10.10 Designing agility drills

Background

The contemporary body of scientific literature defines agility as a rapid, whole-body change of direction or speed in response to a sports-specific stimulus.[13,14] Perceptual-cognitive factors can affect an athlete's ability. This capacity can be maximised through using agility-based drills as part of a comprehensive athlete training plan.

AIM:

- To understand what is required for a movement to be classed as 'agility' and be able to design agility drills appropriate for the athlete

TASK:

- Design an agility drill that could be used in training to achieve the outcomes in Worksheet 10.10.
- Present your drill, detail the equipment required and, if available, run the group through the drill.

Worksheet 10.10 Designing agility drills		
Outcome	Overview of drill	Equipment required
Change of direction in response to a moderately predictable visual stimulus with fairly reasonable reaction time demands (to replicate an activity such as changing direction in rugby league in response to a teammate's change of direction or to a tennis ball return shot)		
Reaction time and change of direction in response to an auditory stimulus (to replicate an activity such as a beach sprint start in surf lifesaving)		
Change of direction in response to a completely unpredictable stimulus with fast reaction time (e.g. demands of playing netball)		

References

1   Gabbett TJ. 2016. Influence of fatigue on tackling ability in rugby league players: role of muscular strength, endurance and aerobic qualities. *PLoS One.* 11(10):e0163161.

2   Suchomel TJ, Nimphius S, Stone MH. 2016. The importance of muscular strength in athletic performance. *Sports Med.* 46(10):1419–49. doi:10.1007/s40279-016-0486-0

3   Haff GG, Nimphius S. 2012. Training principles for power. *Strength Cond J.* 34(6), 2–12.

4   Suchomel TJ, Comfort P, Stone MH. 2015. Weightlifting pulling derivatives: rationale for implementation and application. *Sports Med.* 45(6):823–39. doi:10.1007/s40279-015-0314-y

5   Suchomel TJ, Comfort P, Lake JP. 2017. Enhancing the force–velocity profile of athletes using weightlifting derivatives. *Strength Cond J.* 39(1):10–20.

6   James LP, Comfort P, Suchomel TJ, Kelly VG, Beckman EM, Haff GG. 2018. Influence of power clean ability and training age on adaptations to weightlifting-style training. *J Strength Cond Res.* 33(11):2936–44.

7   James LP, Haff GG, Kelly VG, Connick M, Hoffman B, Beckman E M. 2018. The impact of strength level on adaptations to combined weightlifting, plyometric and ballistic training. *Scand J Med Sci Spor.* 28(5):1494–1505.

8   Haug WB, Drinkwater EJ, Chapman DW. 2015. Learning the hang power clean: kinetic, kinematic and technical changes in four weightlifting naive athletes. *J Strength Cond Res.* 29(7):1766–79.

9   Drake R 2015. *Gray's Atlas of Anatomy.* Churchill Livingstone.

10 Caulfield S, Beringer D. 2016. Exercise technique for free weight and machine training. In GG Haff & N Triplett (Eds.), *Essentials of Strength Training and Conditioning* (4th ed, pp. 351–408). Champaign, IL: Human Kinetics.

11 Potach DH, Chu DA. 2016. Program design and technique for plyometric training. In GG Haff & N Triplett (Eds), *Essentials of Strength Training and Conditioning* (4th ed., pp. 471–520). Champaign, IL: Human Kinetics.

12 Earp JE, Kraemer WJ. 2010. Medicine ball training implications for rotational power sports. *Strength Cond J.* 32(4):20–5.

13 DeWeese BH, Nimphius S. 2016. Program design and technique for speed and agility training. In GG. Haff & N Triplett (Eds), *Essentials of Strength Training and Conditioning* (4th ed., pp. 521–548). Champaign, IL: Human Kinetics.

14 Sheppard JM, Young WB. 2006. Agility literature review: classifications, training and testing. *J Sports Sci.* 24(9):919–32.

15 Hoffman JR, Graham JF. 2012. Speed training. In JR Hoffman (Ed.), *NSCA's Guide to Program Design* (pp. 165–184). Champaign, IL: Human Kinetics.

16 Ratamess N. 2012. *ACSM's Foundations of Strength Training and Conditioning.* Philadelphia: Wolters Kluwer Health/Lippincott Williams & Wilkins.

PRACTICAL 11
FLEXIBILITY EXERCISES

Emma M. Beckman and Jemima G. Spathis

Introduction

Flexibility can be considered as the arc of movement through which a joint can move or be moved. Flexibility is direction specific. In cases where multiple muscle groups cross a joint, a single stretching exercise may influence a number of muscles. The instruction of flexibility exercises is important and is often an underutilised component of an exercise session. This practical aims to consolidate a student's knowledge of the types of stretches that are available for inclusion and to give practical guidance on how to implement them in an exercise session. The terms 'flexibility' and 'stretching' will be used interchangeably throughout this practical. The practical provides a description of the modes of flexibility prescription, explores factors that may influence flexibility and allows practice of prescription of flexibility exercises applied to case studies.

Anatomy

There are a number of anatomical structures and concepts that will assist in developing an understanding of how flexibility and joint range of motion are affected at different joints; these are described in Table 11.1.

TABLE 11.1	Description of Anatomical Structures and Concepts Related to Flexibility
Anatomical Features	**Description**
Musculotendinous unit (MTU)	Behaves as a contractile component (muscle fibres) in parallel with one elastic component (muscle membranes) and in series with another elastic component
Muscle spindles	Stretch receptors within a muscle that primarily detect changes in the length of a muscle
Golgi tendon organs	Proprioceptive sensory receptors that primarily detect changes in the tension of a muscle
Autogenic inhibition	Contraction of a target muscle activates Golgi tendon organs, resulting in reflexive inhibition of target muscles
Reciprocal inhibition	When a muscle spindle is stretched, the opposing muscle group is inhibited (reflexive antagonism)

Modes of Flexibility Exercise

Static

This form of flexibility exercise is frequently used by individuals and is generally considered to be one of the safest as the body is held in a static position during the stretch. The target muscle group should be lengthened and the position held for the recommended duration. The end position should be obtained slowly to avoid activating muscle spindles through high-velocity movement. The end position of a stretch can be obtained through applying individual force through the body or by utilising external aids to assist in achieving end range.

Ballistic

A ballistic stretch is characterised by repetitive, rapid bouncing movements to provide a stretch of a target muscle. It is less commonly prescribed, especially in untrained individuals, due to the high velocity component that is included in the stretch. It is important to distinguish between this and dynamic stretching which will be covered below. The distinguishing feature of a ballistic movement is that the bouncing movements mostly occur at end range of motion (ROM).

Dynamic

While previous literature has considered ballistic and dynamic flexibility to be similar, this practical distinguishes the two based on the ROM achieved in each. The primary focus of a dynamic flexibility exercise should be to take a joint through a full active ROM, under good motor control. Dynamic flexibility exercises are a key part of a good exercise warm-up as they assist in achieving muscle length. However, they also encourage muscle blood flow and a general increase in body and muscle temperature, which is important prior to exercise. Moving through the full available range may also improve the nerve conduction velocity and neural activation, prior to resistance and cardiorespiratory training.

Proprioceptive Neuromuscular Facilitation (PNF)

PNF stretching has grown in popularity in the last decade due to its successful application in improving muscle length. It is primarily comprised of combinations of concentric, isometric and eccentric muscle actions and passive stretching. The use of voluntary muscle actions is believed to affect the activation of neuromuscular mechanisms which contribute to muscle relaxation. These include autogenic and reciprocal inhibition. The application of PNF stretching varies in the literature with different combinations of contraction length (duration in seconds) and effort (% of maximum voluntary contraction) and the addition of the relaxation component.

Activity 11.1 Range of motion

There are many factors that may influence the ROM an individual is able to achieve at a given time. Age and gender are non-modifiable factors that influence flexibility but are not directly impacted through flexibility training. However, some factors can be remediated through the application of flexibility exercises (such as reduced muscle length from immobilisation) and will therefore improve over time with effective prescription.

AIM:
- To understand how flexibility training may or may not be able to improve flexibility

TASK:
- From the list below, identify which may change with flexibility training over time and which may not. Some have been completed for you.

Worksheet 11.1 Prescribing Core Exercises	
Factor	Influences Flexibility Exercise?
Bony configuration	No influence on flexibility exercise; usually congenital or the result of trauma or injury (e.g. ROM at the ankle is restricted because of a bony abnormality at the ankle)
Muscle bulk	No influence on flexibility exercise if the bulk is causing soft tissue approximation at end of range (e.g. large biceps may limit elbow flexion, making it difficult to stretch triceps)
Recreational overuse	Yes, flexibility exercises can improve this; due to repetitive sports movements or leisure activities, some muscles may tighten over time but flexibility exercise can have a positive impact

Worksheet 11.1 Prescribing Core Exercises (continued)	
Factor	Influences Flexibility Exercise?
Immobilisation/contracture	Yes and no—if the origin of contracture is from immobilisation (e.g. broken arm placed in a cast) then flexibility exercises will restore MTU length; however, if the contracture is neurological in origin (e.g. high muscle tone from cerebral palsy) then flexibility exercises are unlikely to change joint range
Connective tissue/fascia	
Pain	
Swelling/oedema	
Reduced neural (nerve) length	
Short muscle length	
Psychological/apprehension	
Adiposity	

Instructing Flexibility Exercises

Often, the instruction of flexibility exercises is not as rigorous as resistance exercises. However, it is important that effective cues are given, feedback is sought from the individual and modifications are made based on performance and capacity.

The key features of effective instruction are as follows.

- Positioning the client precisely to ensure the correct muscle groups are targeted and giving accurate feedback to correct their position.
- Considering characteristics such as the balance and strength required to move the body/limb into a position for a stretch and to ensure they are appropriate for an individual, modifying as required (e.g. an older adult may be better suited to perform a seated hamstring stretch from a chair with one leg outstretched, rather than getting onto the floor or performing it standing with the leg on a chair).
- Asking clients 'what they feel' and 'where they feel it' to ensure the muscle is effectively targeted (e.g. they should not feel lower back pain during a hamstring stretch).
- Describing to a client what they should feel at the end ROM is important. To achieve this, you can use phrases such as 'stretch to the point of discomfort, not pain' or a rating scale (e.g. 0–10, where 0 is 'I can't feel anything' and 10 is 'unbearable pain' may be useful).
- Breathing through the stretch may facilitate greater comfort and ROM. If instructing PNF stretching techniques for individuals to perform on their own, care needs to be taken to ensure both the passive stretch-assisted and the contract-relax sequence are appropriate in terms of force and comfort.

In order to maximise the effectiveness of flexibility prescription, it is important to approach the prescription as systematically as you would resistance training and cardiorespiratory training. This means:

- understanding the anatomy that underlies the position of the exercise; this is particularly important for multi-joint muscles which have opposing actions across their joints (e.g. rectus femoris which flexes at the hip, extends at the knee)
- having a strong rationale for the mode (static, ballistic, dynamic, PNF) you select, based on the current evidence and purpose of the flexibility prescription, and
- being aware of the key considerations related to the individual (age, gender), their history (previous exercise history, injuries and so on) and their capacity.

Flexibility by Body Region

The following section details flexibility by body region. That is, the anatomy that will optimise the position of the stretch, examples of different modes for that specific joint and some tips and considerations for prescription.

A suggested learning approach for this section is to encourage students to divide into pairs and select one stretch from each body region to demonstrate to the class with effective instructions and cues. Students should focus on justifying why they would select one variation of a stretch over another and demonstrate their reasoning. For example, a student may discuss that a ballistic pectoralis major stretch is not suitable for someone who has had previous shoulder pathology such as an anterior shoulder dislocation or subluxation of the glenohumeral joint.

Exercise 11a: Chest

Target muscles: Pectoralis major and minor, coracobrachialis, anterior deltoid

Primary action of target muscles: Horizontal flexion of the glenohumeral joint

Primary position of opposition: Horizontal extension of the glenohumeral joint as seen in Figure 11.1.

Useful cues:

- If the pectoralis major is the primary focus, ensure the shoulder is externally rotated.
- Think about opening through the front of your shoulder.
- Keep your shoulder blades depressed and set to focus on the chest.

Alternative positions can be seen in Table 11.2.

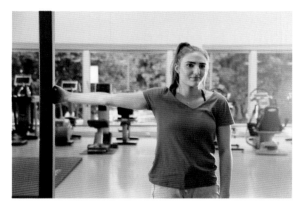

Figure 11.1 Basic chest stretch

TABLE 11.2	Variations of the Chest Stretch			
Variation	**Rationale**			**Considerations**
Bent elbow	The elbow is often flexed in this stretch to take elbow flexor length out of the stretch			Doorway stretches, especially if performed bilaterally may be increasing pressure through the anterior shoulder capsule

TABLE 11.2	Variations of the Chest Stretch (continued)		
Variation	**Rationale**		**Considerations**
Dynamic swimmer arm swing	Warm-up activity performed through full range		This exercise also impacts opposing muscle structure length concurrently
PNF floor stretch	Supported, less impact version of the lower limb position; the client can also widen their arms to target the chest if they experience stretch in their latissimus dorsi		Not suitable for older participants who have difficulty getting to the ground

Exercise 11b: Back

Target muscles: Rhomboids, serratus, posterior deltoid, latissimus dorsi, teres major, quadratus lumborum, erector spinae, trapezius

Primary action of target muscles: Glenohumeral adduction, shoulder extension, humeral external rotation and scapula retraction

Primary position of opposition: Glenohumeral abduction, shoulder flexion, humeral internal rotation, scapula protraction

Useful cues:

- If the latissimus dorsi is the primary focus, ensure the shoulder is externally rotated and the shoulder is in a flexed position with less emphasis on scapular protraction; the unilateral variation should also be encouraged to have lateral flexion to the contralateral side and trunk flexion as shown in Figure 11.2. Alternative positions for stretching back muscles can be seen in Table 11.3.
- Think about lengthening through your side.
- Think about pulling your shoulder blades apart.
- Focus on reaching through your arms.

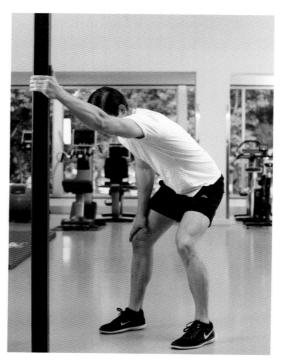

Figure 11.2 Lateral flexion to the contralateral side and trunk flexion

TABLE 11.3	Variations of the Back Stretch		
Variation	**Rationale**		**Considerations**
Mid-back focus	Concentrate on protracting the scapulae to target scapular retractors		Can be done bilaterally or unilaterally; if a person is feeling it more in the posterior deltoid in the unilateral version, try the alternative variation
PNF child's pose	More passive variation of stretch for latissimus dorsi		This variation allows you to easily internally or externally rotate the shoulder

TABLE 11.3   Variations of the Back Stretch (continued)

Variation	Rationale		Considerations
Leaning lateral flexion	The primary focus is quadratus lumborum and erector spinae		Able to be performed in kneeling or standing position, unilaterally
Cat/camel	Mobilises through the length of the spine		Able to perform standing or kneeling, unilaterally
Dynamic arm circles	Targets a number of different actions around a rotational plane which may be more specific prior to shoulder-dominant exercise or activities		This should be done initially at slower velocities and limited ROM and gradually increase in speed and range as the individual gets warmer

TABLE 11.3	Variations of the Back Stretch (continued)			
Variation	Rationale			Considerations
Seated quadratus lumborum stretch	Securing the pelvis allows people with challenges to balance to get a strong stretch through the quadratus lumborum			Hip adductor length can significantly impact on the seated position in this stretch and participants who may have trouble getting onto the ground (i.e. elderly client)

Exercise 11c: Arms Anterior

Target muscles: Anterior deltoid, biceps brachii, brachioradialis, brachialis, flexor carpi radialis, ulnaris, palmaris longus

Primary action of target muscles: Shoulder flexion, elbow flexion and wrist flexion

Primary position of opposition: shoulder extension, elbow extension and wrist extension as seen in Figure 11.3. Alternative positions for stretching anterior arm muscles can be seen in Table 11.4.

Useful cues:

- To maximally address biceps brachii, you need to add pronation.
- Adding lateral flexion or rotation of the cervical spine to these exercises may enhance the stretch of the scapular elevators as well.

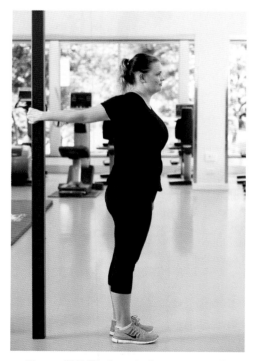

Figure 11.3 Basic anterior arm stretch

TABLE 11.4	Variations of the Anterior Arms Stretch		
Variation	**Rationale**		**Considerations**
Wrist extension	Stretch may be included in activities with high demands on grip strength		May be done with the elbow flexed or extended
Seated passive bodyweight	Using gravity and bodyweight to push into shoulder and elbow extension		Also consider length of anterior deltoid

Exercise 11d: Arms Posterior

Target muscles: Triceps (lateral, long and medial), anconeus, extensor carpi radialis longus and brevis, extensor carpi ulnaris

Primary action of target muscles: Elbow extension, shoulder extension, wrist extension

Primary position of opposition: Elbow flexion, shoulder flexion and wrist flexion as seen in Figure 11.4. Alternative positions for stretching posterior arm muscles can be seen in Table 11.5.

Useful cues:

- Ensure the chin is in a neutral position; some clients may find the cue 'slightly tuck your chin' useful to assist in alignment of the cervical spine and maintain neutral thoracic spine to maximise the stretch.
- Stay upright and tall and eyes should be looking straight ahead (if the neck flexes, the shoulder may also change position and lessen the stretch).
- A towel could be used for assistance in the other hand rather than pushing on the elbow.

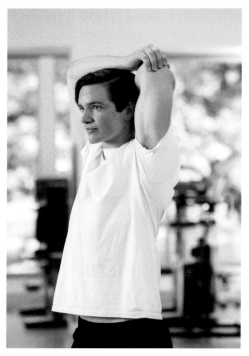

Figure 11.4 Basic triceps stretch

TABLE 11.5	Variations of the Posterior Arms Stretch		
Variation	**Rationale**		**Considerations**
Wrist flexion stretch	The forearm muscles may feel tight in individuals who participate in sports with high grip-related demands or occupations with considerable amounts of typing		End ROM for this stretch is not usually restricted by muscle length, so clients might not 'feel' the stretch as much as others of the upper limb

TABLE 11.5　Variations of the Posterior Arms Stretch (continued)			
Variation	**Rationale**		**Considerations**
Table-assisted prayer position	Using external forces may be more useful in intensifying the stretch compared with others		Consider latissimus dorsi length as well

Exercise 11e: Legs Anterior

Target muscles: Rectus femoris, vastus intermedius, vastus lateralis, vastus medius, iliopsoas, gracilis, adductor magnus, adductor longus, adductor brevis, pectineus

Primary action of target muscles: Hip flexion, knee extension

Primary position of opposition: Hip extension, knee flexion, as seen in Figure 11.5. Alternative positions for stretching anterior leg muscles can be seen in Table 11.6.

Useful cues:

- If no partner is available, this can be done with a towel.
- Make sure the hips stay square.
- Think about pushing your hips forwards and straightening your body rather than pulling on your foot.

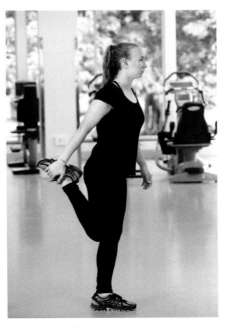

Figure 11.5　Basic quadriceps stretch

TABLE 11.6   Variations of the Anterior Legs Stretch

Variation	Rationale		Considerations
Kneeling hip flexors	As the iliopsoas attaches onto the lumbar spine, being in a position of posterior pelvic tilt will lengthen the iliopsoas		The position is important here as lunging too far forwards will place a significant amount of pressure on the anterior hip capsule
Bench assisted	For clients who cannot easily get onto the floor, this variation is a suitable alternative; for people with balance issues, provide an additional chair or pole for support		Make sure the bench is stable and fixed
PNF Thomas stretch	This stretch can be useful for clients who are unable to get onto the ground		Ideally needs a partner to make this effective
Side lying	This stretch allows the body to be supported when balance is an issue		Ensure the individual has no issues getting up and down from the floor; alternatively, use a plinth if available and stable

TABLE 11.6	Variations of the Anterior Legs Stretch (continued)		
Variation	**Rationale**		**Considerations**
Prone knee flexion	Useful to cue people to push their hip into the ground for this stretch		Watch for excessive anterior pelvic tilt; needs either a partner or band to assist; can prop up the knee to extend the hip passively
Dynamic leg swings	Targets the muscles through greater range as momentum will be used		Avoid twisting through the supporting knee and ankle joints when moving through the ROM

Exercise 11f: Legs Posterior

Target muscles: Semitendinosus, semimembranosus, biceps femoris, gluteus maximus, gluteus minimus, gluteus medius, piriformis, gemelli, obturators, quadriceps femoris, gastrocnemius, soleus

Primary action of target muscles: Hip extension, hip external rotation, knee flexion

Primary position of opposition: Hip flexion, hip internal rotation, knee extension as seen in Figure 11.6. Alternative positions for stretching posterior leg muscles can be seen in Table 11.7.

Useful cues:

- Keep the target leg straight to maximise the stretch.
- When the knee is extended, add dorsiflexion to intensify the stretch.
- Relax the neck or tuck the chin slightly to avoid hyperextension.

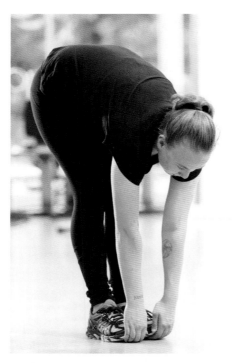

Figure 11.6 Basic posterior leg stretch

TABLE 11.7	Variations of the Posterior Leg Stretch			
Variation	**Rationale**			**Considerations**
Sit and reach	Effective stretch for the whole posterior chain in a seated, symmetrical position			Once the individual moves into a seated position and the pelvis is fixed, the range restrictions may be more evident than in standing
Seated toe touch (modified sit and reach)	This is a safe variation if balance, range and mobility are compromised			Keep a close eye on where the range is coming from as it may be thoracic and lumbar flexion rather than hip flexion

TABLE 11.7   Variations of the Posterior Leg Stretch (continued)

Variation	Rationale		Considerations
Glute max seated crossover or pretzel	Individuals with significant adipose tissue may find this stretch difficult to achieve		Use the arms for leverage and stretch modulation
Piriformis stretch seated	This stretch will target piriformis when the hip is in greater than 90° of flexion; if the hip is too open, this stretch will not target piriformis		Can be done in supine or standing position
Standing straight leg heel drop	Targets gastrocnemius as the knee is straight		If using bodyweight is not enough, the individual may want to hold extra weight or do this in a Smith machine

TABLE 11.7	Variations of the Posterior Leg Stretch (continued)		
Variation	**Rationale**		**Considerations**
Knee to wall	Targets soleus as the knee is bent		If ankle dorsiflexion range is restricted by bone, the individual may not feel this stretch in the soleus muscle
Lying torso knee rock	Targets gluteus maximus		Controlled movement of the lower limbs with back remaining in place; avoid this movement for those who can't easily transfer to the ground or who have existing lower back pain or disc problems

Exercise 11g: Legs Medial and Lateral

Target muscles: Medial—adductor longus, magnus, brevis, gracilis, pectineus; lateral—tensor fascia latae (TFL)

Primary action of target muscles: Hip adduction, and hip flexion, abduction and external rotation

Primary position of opposition: Medial—hip abduction, as seen in Figure 11.7; lateral—hip extension, adduction, lateral rotation; alternative positions to stretch medial and lateral leg muscles are shown in Table 11.8

Useful cues:

- You can add hip extension as most adductors also flex the thigh; however, you may also consider adding some slight hip flexion to target adductor magnus as it also contributes to extension of the hip.

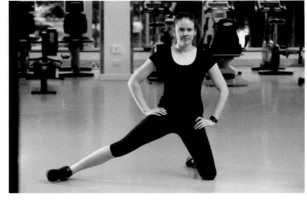

Figure 11.7 Medial hip stretch

TABLE 11.8   Variations of the Medial and Lateral Legs Stretch

Variation	Rationale		Considerations
Butterfly	Focuses on hip external rotation and abduction		In individuals with tight hips, it may be difficult to sit in this position effectively and a variation may be required
Semi-straddle	This stretch allows the individual to target the medial compartments more effectively		It may be useful to have something for the individual to hold in front of them to intensify the stretch
Happy baby	The individual can control the position of the lower limbs in this stretch and modulate the intensity, so it is a useful variation for less-trained individuals		This can be done prone if more resistance is required

TABLE 11.8 Variations of the Medial and Lateral Legs Stretch (continued)			
Variation	**Rationale**		**Considerations**
Standing TFL stretch	TFL tightness is a common issue in regular runners; this muscle inserts into the iliotibial band so it may require lengthening		This position can be challenging to feel the stretch in the same way the other stretches are felt; individuals should be made aware that they may not feel it in a muscle belly and that there are a lot of fascial connections in that region

Prescribing Flexibility Exercises

When instructing a flexibility program, a number of factors should be considered in order to ensure the prescription is optimal.

- What is the goal ROM? And why?
- Which joints are the target of the program and why?
- What is the current evidence supporting inclusion and prescription of this type of flexibility training?
- What is the current capacity of the individual? What is their initial range? What is their level of training?
- Which mode will be most affective to achieve the goal?
- How will improvements/changes be determined?
- What current injuries/conditions might impact on the performance of the exercise?

Worked Case Study for Flexibility Exercises

A 16-year-old male plays field hockey for his school and local club and has recently been selected in a state-based talent development squad. As a result of this, his training levels have increased and he is feeling 'tight', so he would like to incorporate more flexibility training into his program. Prior to implementation, what types of issues might you consider? A number of considerations and their implications are detailed for you in Table 11.9.

Critical thinking

As hockey is a highly explosive sport, this individual appears to require a full body stretch post training to maximise important muscle lengths and reduce the risk of injury, if possible.

Given we want to make this session a regular inclusion, static stretches are only ever performed after training, with pre-training inclusions relying on progressive dynamic flexibility to aid warm-up of all important joints used in hockey. The individual will be encouraged to perform the sessions as per exercise guidelines.[2]

A pre-hockey training session example flexibility program is shown in Table 11.10.

A post-resistance training and hockey training example flexibility program is shown in Table 11.11.

TABLE 11.9	Considerations for Flexibility Training and Some Example Implications
Consideration	**Implication**
Age	As a 16 year old, the client may have experienced a growth spurt. Sometimes, especially in males, this results in tight muscles of long bones like hamstrings. This may make hamstrings a key focus of the program, dependent on results from a test such as a sit and reach.
Sport	Hockey requires the development of speed and power from both the upper and lower limbs. The legs will require full flexion and extension ROM of the hip for running and when adopting a lunge position to strike the ball. The upper body will require good trunk, shoulder and scapular range; for example, when striking the ball the player will adopt a lunge combined with trunk flexion and scapular protraction to maximise force development for the ball.
Current injuries or conditions	The athlete hasn't reported any current issues that would impact on the positioning or equipment used; however, tight hamstrings may mean that certain long-seated positions are not ideal. It is also possible that restricted trunk rotation may impede performance and could be something to consider.
Goal of flexibility programming	The goal is to encourage full active ROM for resistance, aerobic and on-field training sessions and to lengthen and then maintain full static joint range over time.

TABLE 11.10	Example of a Pre-exercise Flexibility Program for Sport Specificity in Hockey	
Exercise	**Rationale**	
Shoulder crossovers	Arm range is important in hockey, especially in taking shots; crossovers are selected over arm circles because overhead movements are less important in hockey	

TABLE 11.10   Example of a Pre-exercise Flexibility Program for Sport Specificity in Hockey (continued)

Exercise	Rationale	
Trunk rotation	Key factor in developing rotational force through the trunk; this could be done standing or on the knees to ensure ROM is targeting the trunk and not the lower limbs	
Walking lunges	Hockey is a running-dominant sport, with alternating foot positions; therefore, lunging is more sport specific than squats, where a unilateral activity is more sports specific compared to a bilateral activity	
Side lunges	Multiple planes of lunges (e.g. front and side) included given the need to develop lateral leg force in hockey, and ensure warm-up for agility and change of direction	

TABLE 11.10   Example of a Pre-exercise Flexibility Program for Sport Specificity in Hockey (continued)

Exercise	Rationale	
Ankle circles and pumps	In such a dynamic sport, the need for ankle range and stability is important; while this exercise focuses on ankle range, it will also activate neural and neuromuscular structures	

TABLE 11.11   Example of a Post-exercise Flexibility Program for Sport Specificity in Hockey

Exercise	Rationale	
Calf stretches	Sprinting is dependent on ankle range and power and maintaining this in straight-leg and bent-leg positions will be important	
Hamstring seated	If a pre-assessment showed tight hamstrings, this would be a key flexibility exercise; prescribe in a seated position to stabilise the pelvis and ensure pure hip flexion	
Kneeling adductors	With constant change of direction, it will be important to keep the adductors long	
Pretzel	The glutes are a primary force generator in speed sports; therefore, they need stretching post training	

TABLE 11.11   Example of a Post-exercise Flexibility Program for Sport Specificity in Hockey (continued)

Exercise	Rationale	
Anterior cross-arm stretch	The back and posterior shoulder muscles will contribute to striking movements in hockey; therefore, maintaining the length of these muscles will be important	
Pec stretch	The chest and anterior shoulder muscles will contribute to striking movements in hockey; therefore, maintaining the length of these muscles will be important	

Activity 11.2 Prescribing flexibility exercises

AIM:
- to provide specificity in programming flexibility exercises

TASKS:
- Using the Worked case study for flexibility exercises, fill in the template below, selecting one of the following cases to develop an individualised flexibility program.
    1. A masters runner competing in the Gold Coast 10 km fun run who has previously had calf strains
    2. A 30-year-old body builder who has never done flexibility before despite regular gym use
    3. An older adult who has a sedentary job and spends large portions of their day doing computer work has some difficulty getting from the floor to standing positions.
    4. A ballerina who travels regularly for a Queensland ballet show and is working towards the summer schedule of at least two shows a day

Worksheet 11.2 Integrate Your Knowledge	
Case (1–4)	
Consideration	Implication

Critical thinking: Include here your overall thoughts regarding this client and sets/reps/prescription based on recommended guidelines and individual needs.

_____

_____

_____

_____

_____

_____

Flexibility Program		
Exercise	**Rationale**	**Picture**

Activity 11.3 Static stretching and maximal performance

Background

Implications of acute static stretching (SS) on maximal performance

A meta-analysis conducted in 2013 explored the impact of pre-exercise SS on maximal performance, determined by muscle strength (e.g. 1RM, maximal torque), muscle power (e.g. mean, peak power) and explosive muscle performance (e.g. rate of force development, jumping performance, sprint performance and throw performance).[1] The outcomes suggest that SS has a negative impact on maximum muscle strength performance (−5.4%), isometric strength (−6.5%) and dynamic strength tests (−3.9%). The effect of SS held for < 45, 45–90 and > 90 seconds per muscle group on muscle power were 0.4%, −1.7% and −3.3%, respectively, suggesting fewer clear outcomes, while the effect of SS on muscle power was negative (−2.2%).

Overall, the authors concluded that regardless of age, gender or training status, pre-exercise SS had a negative impact on muscle strength and explosive muscular performance, with the impact of SS on muscle power less clear.

Implications

This research suggests that SS should be avoided during warm-up regimens when maximal muscular performance is required.

- Avoid prescription of SS pre-exercise directly prior to performance of activities that require maximal muscular power, speed and strength, such as throwing and sprinting.
- Alternatively, prescribe sports-specific dynamic stretches prior to performance, such as those outlined in the Worked case study for flexibility exercises.
- As part of effective evidence-based flexibility prescription, SS would still be included in athletes' programs where increasing or maintaining ROM is important for the requirements of the sport and general ROM and joint health.

AIM:
- To read, interpret and critique evidence and apply it to flexibility exercise

TASK:
- Split into small groups. Review one of the following articles briefly and complete Worksheet 11.3. Present your findings to the class.
    1. McHugh MP, Cosgrave CH. 2010. To stretch or not to stretch: the role of stretching in injury prevention and performance. *Scand J Med Sci Sport.* 20:169–181.
    2. Loughrana M, Glasgowa P, Bleakley C, McVeigh J. 2017. The effects of a combined static-dynamic stretching protocol on athletic performance in elite Gaelic footballers: A randomised controlled crossover trial. *Phys Ther Sport.* 25:47–54.
    3. Sá MA, Matta TT, Carneiro SP, et al. 2016. Acute effects of different methods of stretching and specific warm-ups on muscle architecture and strength performance. *J Strength Cond Res.* 30(8):2324–2329.

Worksheet 11.3 Integrate Your Knowledge

Question 1: Identify the key outcomes from this research
a. _____
b. _____
c. _____

Question 2: List the implications of this research on your professional practice. That is, how does this inform your practice? How will you prescribe flexibility exercises in your practice, in general terms?

_____

_____

Question 3: Apply this knowledge to the following cases:
a. Middle-aged male, weight lifter who completes three sessions per week of resistance-strength training

_____

_____

_____

b. Javelin thrower, 23 years old, with previous history of hip tightness in the right leg

_____

_____

c. A 16-year-old female dancer, who predominantly does ballet

_____

_____

References

1   Simic L, Sarabon N, Markovic G. 2013. Does pre-exercise static stretching inhibit maximal muscular performance? A meta-analytical review. *Scand J Med Sci Sport.* 23(2):131–148.
2   Garber CE, Blissmer B, Deschenes MR, et al. 2011. American College of Sports Medicine position stand. Quantity and quality of exercise for developing and maintaining cardiorespiratory, musculoskeletal, and neuromotor fitness in apparently healthy adults. *Medicine & Science in Sports & Exercise*, July, 43(7):1334–1359. doi: 10.1249/MSS.0b013e318213fefb

PRACTICAL 12
EXERCISE IN WATER

Emma M. Beckman and Rosalind Beavers

Introduction

Water is an excellent yet underutilised medium for exercise that provides an alternative environment for exercise scientists to achieve positive outcomes in areas such as general fitness, training load modification and control, recovery, relaxation and rehabilitation.

This practical will provide the theoretical background on the physiological responses to immersion and the hydrodynamics of the aquatic environment. Practical group activities to be used in a water medium are also provided.

While exercise in water does include swimming, this area is well documented in other texts so the focus of this practical is on upright immersion exercise such as 'aqua aerobics' and deep-water running. The unique properties of water provide an excellent environment for exercise. Water is an effective conductor of heat. Additionally, buoyancy decreases load on the joints and the density of water (800 times that of air) allows for considerable energy expenditure.

The activities and worked case study in this practical provide a great opportunity for students to attempt water exercises, with the activities designed to ensure that students will develop knowledge resulting in the realistic and effective prescription of exercise in water.

Water and The Effects of Immersion

The physiological effects of water immersion were investigated in the late 1960s and early 1970s as the aquatic environment provided an ideal medium to study the effects of reduced gravity—an area of importance at the time of early space expeditions. We now know that physiological responses are depth and temperature dependent and that immersion has effects on cardiovascular, respiratory, hormonal and renal function.

The properties of the water environment; including hydrostatic pressure, buoyancy, turbulence and drag can be employed to create resistance during exercise, and as water is also a good conductor of thermal energy,[1] these properties then can combine to provide a unique and effective environment for exercise.

The capacity of a person to float in water is determined by their relative density. The relative density of water is greater than that of most humans, with the exception of the extremely lean and/or heavily muscled; therefore, most people tend to float when the lungs are inflated.

The effects of immersion are influenced by the temperature of the water in which a body is immersed therefore warmer water would elicit vasodilation and cooler water vasoconstriction, at rest. Water used for rehabilitation and swimming pools ranges from above thermoneutral (35°C), to that dictated by the ambient temperature for outdoor pools, and is generally around 27°C for climate-controlled indoor facilities. This is a temperature that is easily tolerated while still being comfortable for exercise.

Immersion has effects on blood volume distribution, and subsequently blood pressure and heart rate. During immersion in thermoneutral water (34.5°C), the temperature most commonly used in immersion studies, the hydrostatic pressure gradient causes an immediate shift in peripheral venous volume towards the thoracic area.[2,3]

The impacts of immersion on cardiac output can be viewed by considering that cardiac output (Q) is the product of heart rate (HR) and stroke volume (SV); that is, $Q = HR \times SV$. During immersion, the increase in central blood volume creates an increased preload (the volume of blood returning to the heart) that results in an increase in stroke volume through the Frank–Starling Law.[4] Therefore, during immersion in resting conditions adequate cardiac output can be maintained at a lower heart rate. The shift of the blood during upright immersion also results in reduced lung compliance.[5]

It is important to recognise that the physiological impacts of immersion mean that exercise in water is not suitable for all populations. A brief list of contraindications and precautions for exercise in water is presented in Table 12.1. For further information please consult Becker's article 'Aquatic therapy: scientific foundations and clinical rehabilitation applications'.[6]

TABLE 12.1 Contraindications and Precautions for Exercise in Water	
Conditions that May Contraindicate Water Exercise	Conditions Requiring Precaution in Water Exercise
• Uncontrolled medical conditions (epilepsy) • Central nervous system concerns (seizures, headaches, hypertonicity/flaccidity) • High-risk obstetric patients (uterine bleeding, fetal distress) • Alcohol consumption • Infections/open wounds • Gastrointestinal tract disorders (incontinence/diarrhoea) • Skin problems (rashes, tinea, ringworm, varicose veins, generalised eczema, active psoriasis)	• Frail or advanced debility • Renal insufficiency • Respiratory problems • Vital capacity < 1500 mL • Blood pressure issues, peripheral vascular disease • Radiotherapy (within 3 months) • Severe intellectual impairment • Gross involuntary movements (athetosis) • Heart conditions

Practical Application

In the water, target heart rates for exercise need to be adjusted as reports have shown heart rates to be 7–20 beats per minute (BPM) lower during water exercise than those during land exercise of a similar intensity.[7,8]

Equipment for Use in Water

A variety of equipment is available that is either specifically designed to facilitate water exercise or is able to be used in a way that enhances exercise prescription in water.

Examples of potential equipment and their use is presented in Table 12.2. Use range of motion (ROM), change of direction and change of body position to keep water exercise interesting and challenging.

TABLE 12.2 Equipment for Water-based Exercise	
Equipment	Sample Exercise
Noodle: inexpensive, accessible and buoyant 	Balance exercise: in deep water stand tall on the noodle (with it directly under you) and bring the noodle up and down slowly by bending your knees; try to touch the middle of the noodle. Resistance exercise: hold the noodle in front of you with both hands and move the noodle in a large circle under the water, first moving the noodle away from the body then down through the water.

TABLE 12.2 Equipment for Water-based Exercise (continued)	
Equipment	**Sample Exercise**
Buoyancy belt	In deeper water, the buoyancy belt allows for the body to be suspended upright in a neutral position in the water where only the head is out of the water. From here, a number of activities are possible. Deep-water running: using a running-type motion to move through the water in an upright position. Try exercises that you could do in the shallow water but increase the difficulty as there is no pool floor to push off.
Water weights	Water weights float: the force is in an upward direction meaning that the participant must apply force in a downward direction, so use these for working on the triceps using a push-down movement. Hold one weight in each hand, extend your arms to the side then bring them down through the water and clap the weights together in front of the thighs. Change the position of the body to lie prone on the surface then use the pectoral muscles to bring the weights down through the water and clap under the chest. These are an excellent addition to provide resistance, challenge stability and increase intensity.

Instructing Exercise in Water

Working in or near the water presents some challenges that are traditionally not relevant to many land-based exercise training sessions. Table 12.3 lists important factors to consider and presents some strategies that may be useful.

TABLE 12.3 Considerations and Strategies for Instructing Water-based Exercise	
Considerations for Session (Indoor or Outdoor Pool)	**Strategies**
Temperature (outdoor)	• If it is cool or windy, encourage clients to keep their hair dry where possible to reduce heat loss. • Adjust the duration of warm-ups and cool-downs; for example, if outdoor temperature is low, a longer warm-up might be necessary.
Temperature (indoor)	• Many indoor facilities present instructors with the challenge of working in very high humidity in warm conditions. Be prepared, pace yourself and wear cool clothing.

TABLE 12.3   Considerations and Strategies for Instructing Water-based Exercise (continued)

Considerations for Session (Indoor or Outdoor Pool)	Strategies
Temperature (in water)	• Intensity and duration might need adjustment when the water is too cold or too warm. Personal comfort often varies between participants so observe for signs of cold (shivering, blue lips) and heat stress (red faces).
Positioning of instructor	• Make sure you demonstrate exercises in a way that translates into easily understood instructions. Take care that clients do not need to spend long periods of time looking upwards if you are demonstrating by the side of the pool and they are already in the water. • If instructing in an outdoor environment, ensure the sun is not directly behind you. • Remember that movements are slower underwater so adjust your demonstrations to reflect this.
Can they hear me?	• In public places with additional noise, ensure that participants are within hearing distance when you deliver instructions. Do not give instructions until all the clients' heads are above water. Preserving your voice becomes extremely important if you spend large amounts of time in the water environment. Use a headset microphone when possible. • Use large, exaggerated movements to demonstrate exercises so clients can follow your lead even if it is hard for you to be heard.
Sun safety	• This issue pertains to both the practitioner and the clients. Always ensure you are modelling good sun safety behaviour in exercise sessions. Encourage participants to consider the impact of the sun and include messages related to sun safety on any material (printed or electronic) that is sent to clients prior to any session.
Jumping on hard surfaces to demonstrate exercises	• This consideration is predominantly for the practitioner. While many exercises will be low impact once performed in the water, the practitioner will often have to demonstrate exercises at the side of the pool, increasing their risk of injury. Consider the load when this is necessary and adjust intensity where necessary.
Attire	• This may be highly variable depending on the population group and the environment within which the sessions are conducted. Always aim for conservative, swimming-appropriate clothing if guidelines are not determined by your employer.
Session planning	• Traditional materials are water sensitive (e.g. electronic devices), so either laminate exercise cards or memorise the session. Laminated templates are useful to allow for recording information at the time that may then be transferred to electronic format for more secure and long-term record keeping. There should be some capacity for recording notes at the session to ensure nothing important is forgotten.
Pool access	• Access to the pool can be difficult for people with impairments to mobility. This should be something that is covered in an initial screening or asked prior to sessions commencing.
Hydration	• Water immersion may lead to dehydration and reduced fluid consumption as water bottles are often less available. Ensure you have a hydration strategy for yourself and the individuals in the pool.

Activity 12.1 Instructor positioning

As mentioned in the considerations, many new practitioners will have to decide how they will conduct a session: outside the water or in it? There are often many factors that should be considered. The pictures in Worksheet 12.2 show two possible perspectives for a practitioner: one looking down and one from within the water.

AIM:

- Consider the advantages and disadvantages of instructing inside (in water) versus outside the pool (pool deck)

TASK:

- In small groups, discuss each perspective and write down some advantages and disadvantages of each. Also count the number of individuals you can easily see in each photo.

Worksheet 12.2 Where Do I Stand?			
Perspective	Advantages	Disadvantages	Count
Instruct from the side of the pool			
Instruct from in the water			

Exercise in Water: Activity-based Examples

Individuals will undertake exercise in water to achieve a broad range or a variety of fitness or rehabilitation goals. The use of equipment and positioning provides almost endless options for exercises. This next section provides a case study that is worked through to include special considerations, pre-session preparations, a session plan and notes on the exercises and their rationale. It is recommended that students undertake this or a similar session to get a stronger understanding of the level of difficulty of various types of exercise in water!

Worked Case Study for Running a Water-exercise Session for Older Adults

You have been contracted to deliver a 30-minute water-exercise class for a group of older adults between the ages of 60 and 85 years (males and females) with varying levels of fitness and mobility at the local city council pool. The class is run in an outdoor pool during mid-morning.

Before the session, you have:

- contacted the pool, confirmed the session, asked if other groups have booked for the same time (Is it loud? Is it school holidays? Are there children's programs running?)
- confirmed your session plan (your template is on laminated card to make notes that you will transfer to your electronic device and electronic filing system straight after the session)
- reviewed the initial screening forms and noticed three participants who are likely to need the ramp access, so you have confirmed with the pool that this is available
- ensured the advertisement regarding the class included instructions to bring a hat, sunscreen and drinking water and you have confirmed that there is a drink fountain close by
- used the five minutes before to identify those who are attending, give them a location to gather and provided some safety instructions.

During the session you:

- start the class by giving a brief overview of the session to ensure they are aware of what is required
- check for recent injuries
- 'set the tone' for the class (more fun for this population than boot camp style) and you provide them with information related to the facilities and also what to do if they feel dizzy or tired.

After entering the water, the participants stand with the water up to around shoulder height (where possible). Aqua exercises are generally performed with the arms below the surface to use the resistance of the water. Instruct them to stand tall in the water—they should engage their abdominal muscles and try to have their heels on the pool floor during walking. Give instructions to them to work at their own pace.

An example of possible session activities is provided in Table 12.4.

Post-session Follow Up

After the session finishes, you talk to as many clients as possible and get an overall session rating of perceived exertion (RPE) from each to give you a sense of where the session was pitched for the majority of the clients. Transfer your notes to electronic format as quickly as possible to limit memory bias.

TABLE 12.4 Activities for An Exercise Session in Water			
Exercise	**Options for Progress and Regress**	**Components of Fitness Focused On by Exercise**	**Comments**
Circle walks: walk around in the shallow end in a circle	(Faster versus slower)	Aerobic, strength	During this time, each person passes by the trainer, giving the opportunity to develop rapport and create a friendly environment

TABLE 12.4   Activities for An Exercise Session in Water (continued)

Exercise	Options for Progress and Regress	Components of Fitness Focused On by Exercise	Comments
Side walking: line up and walk up and down the shallow end by side stepping	(Faster versus slower) use a high knee lift as if stepping over a fence or use a straight leg to step sideways against the resistance of the water	Balance and strength	The water environment provides a medium for the instructor to safely challenge balance and for people to perform movements they could not or would not feel comfortable and safe performing on land; consider counterintuitive exercises where the arms may move side to side and the legs in a front to back skiing motion to challenge the mind and body
Cross crawl: move hands backwards and forwards across the body, like you are clearing a path; create resistance using a flat hand to push against the water as it moves	In front of and behind the body	Strength endurance	
Aqua jacks: these are performed starting with the hands together in a clap position in front of the legs and the legs apart (so a little different to standard jumping jacks); the legs jump and the feet move together to meet under the body while the arms move out and up with a flat hand to stop just below the surface	Change speed; fingers open and closed	Strength, aerobic and power	
Arm work: this may include any exercises for the upper body; use movements in different directions to strengthen shoulders and arms (try underwater boxing with uppercuts!)	Fingers open and closed and ROM	Strength	
Noodle time: ride noodle ponies (noodle between legs); use travel here, considering turns and reversing using the arms	The noodle can be positioned under the foot and moved slowly up and down	Strength and aerobic	Strength, endurance and stability can all be challenged, with the noodle adding both buoyancy during supported floating-type work or resistance

TABLE 12.4	Activities for An Exercise Session in Water (continued)			
Exercise	Options for Progress and Regress	Components of Fitness Focused On by Exercise	Comments
Cool-down and stretch	Gentle slow movements should be used	Recovery	This is the same as land-based exercise but be mindful that in cool water people get cold quickly

Activity 12.2 Water exercise prescription for an individual

Background

You are an accredited exercise scientist (AES) with a new client who is a 35-year-old woman (BMI of 29) who does not like exercise due to her aversion to sweat and heat. A friend told her she might like aqua-based classes. She isn't ready to join a group (she has expressed some concerns and anxiety around wearing swimwear in public) but wants some one-on-one training.

AIM:
- Design a water-based exercise session for an individual

TASK:
- Complete Worksheet 12.3 by describing some considerations prior to the session (an example is provided for you), the content of the first session and some post-session considerations.

Worksheet 12.3 Improving General Health			
Pre-session considerations			
1. Consider the possible psychosocial considerations around body image given her reluctance to exercise as part of a group. This does not need explicit attention but your interactions with clients and your empathy for their individual considerations improve client outcomes. 2. _____ _____ _____ 3. _____ _____ _____			
Exercise	Progressions and regressions	Components of fitness	Rationale

Worksheet 12.3 Improving General Health (continued)
Post-session considerations
_____
_____
_____
_____

Activity 12.3 Water exercise for specific muscle groups

AIM:

- Design a water-based exercise strength endurance program

TASK:

- Using either the equipment listed earlier in the practical, or without equipment, design an exercise to use in the water to improve the strength endurance of the listed muscle groups. The first two are provided.

Worksheet 12.4 What and How		
Muscle group	**Description**	**Progressions and regressions**
Shoulder abductor (middle deltoid)	Standing in water up to armpits, start with arms next to sides, quickly push arms away from sides, then gently return arms to starting position	Close and open fingers for increased (decreased) resistance; slow movement down to make the exercise easier
Hip abductors	Standing in water up to waist height holding on to the side of the pool, from a feet-together position lift one leg away from the pool side	
Hip extensors		
Knee extensors		
Abdominals		
Shoulder flexors		

Activity 12.4 Deep-water running

Background

With the popularity of water running emerging in the industry and in research literature, it is important for practitioners to have a strong grounding in the theory surrounding its use, contraindications and special considerations for instruction.

Deep-water running is distinguished from regular running in a water environment by its location in the deep end of a swimming pool, where a flotation device is required. Clients may perform a running action where their feet touch the bottom of the pool as part of a water-exercise session; however, this would not be categorised as deep-water running.

The key reasons for performing deep-water running sessions are to reduce impact in those training for locomotor sports and maintain aerobic fitness when recovering from injury.[9]

Given these are the main reasons why it is included in exercise programs, research determining the effectiveness of deep-water running has concentrated on two main questions.

1. Can trained, competitive runners maintain their running performance by engaging in deep-water running, without supplemented on-land training?

2. Can the cardiorespiratory fitness of untrained individuals be improved through deep-water running?

The majority of research studies have shown maintenance of trained running performance with deep-water running only. Bushman and colleagues determined that running performance did not experience a significant decline after a period of 4 weeks of deep-water running 5 to 6 times a week.[10] Wilber and colleagues showed no significant declines in running performance after 6 weeks.[11]

With respect to untrained individuals, the improvement in $\dot{V}O_2$max of either a road or a deep-water running training program was evaluated. Similar improvements in $\dot{V}O_2$max occurred in both groups.[12] Other studies have found a greater improvement in those who trained on a treadmill when compared to a deep-water running group, although both improved significantly.[13]

It is easy to discern the benefits of deep-water running with respect to using buoyancy to decrease the physical load on the joints of the body, while achieving improvements in cardiorespiratory fitness. In addition, advocates also espouse the benefits of decreasing the compressive forces on the spine[14] and potentially aiding the recovery of land-based exercise by improving leg strength more rapidly and decreasing perceived soreness.[13] However, it is important for practitioners to consider the use of deep-water running when impact loading might be important, such as in those with low bone density. It has been suggested there is some transfer of capacity from water to land-based activity, with a deep-water running training program in elderly women showing an increase in power on a cycle ergometer test.[15] However, in this study (and others), no measures of functional activity were shown and it is important to consider exercises that will reduce the risk of falls in this particular population. Therefore, it is important to ensure appropriate land-based training in this population and utilise water as an adjunct medium, rather than as the sole training environment.

Moderating intensity can be a challenge in the water environment. With reduced resistive forces, achieving high intensity in deep-water running can often be more difficult for people. It is easy to shorten the stride length while keeping the stride frequency high, which decreases the effort required. The upper body is considered to contribute more significantly to deep-water running than on land, so it is important that cues are directed to the upper and lower body to make sure the intensity is maintained.

AIM:

- Understand how to program deep-water running for different intensities (through RPE)

TASKS:

- In small groups, complete 3 × 1-minute blocks of deep-water running. Have at least one practitioner instructing the bouts to allow groups to practise using effective cues during the activity. Record RPE following each bout and at the end.

- Now aim to prescribe a work set at an RPE of 6, 12 and 18. With the difficulties in moderating speed during water running, this might be challenging and good cues will be essential. Describe in depth how this will be achieved and what cues work most effectively.

Worksheet 12.4 Deep-water Running	
Block	**RPE**
1	
2	
3	
Part 1 reflections: _____	
_____	
_____	
_____	
_____	

Worksheet 12.4 Deep-water Running (continued)	
Block	RPE
1	6
2	12
3	18
Part 2 reflections: _____ _____ _____ _____ _____	

Activity 12.5 The power of music

Background

The power of music to motivate is well established, with reductions in RPE and increased work output during exercise with music shown consistently.[16] One of the unique challenges of aqua fitness instruction from the pool deck is that the movements of the participants are generally slower than the movements of the instructor due to the resistance of the water, making it difficult for the instructor to set the pace. Music can be used here to set the tone or mood of the session and to increase the tempo and pace of movement even if movements are not actually in time with the music. Different groups will respond to different types of music; therefore, music selection will inevitably be a part of the role of an exercise scientist.

AIM:
- Understand how music type can affect the elements of an exercise program

TASK:
- Think about the age group: is it older, mixed or young? Choose some all-time favourites for mixed age/ability groups to get everyone involved.
- Young groups will respond well to the use of music that is currently popular to get them into aqua.
- Pick one 3-minute activity for your class to undertake in the water and select three different songs with different tempos (some fast and some slow). You may also pick different styles of music or songs from different decades.
- Get the class to repeat the exercise three times with the different music playing each time. Reflect on whether the music complemented the activity and how it changed elements like RPE and enjoyment.

Worksheet 12.5 The Power of Music
Songs chosen:
1. _____
2. _____
3. _____
Reflections: _____ _____ _____ _____ _____

References

1   Haymes EM, Well CL. 1986. *Environment and Human Performance.* Champaign, IL: Human Kinetics.

2   Arborelius M Jr, Ballidin Ul, Lilja B, Lundgren CE. 1972. Hemodynamic changes in man during immersion with the head above water. *Aerosp Med.* 43(6):592–598.

3   Risch WD, Koubenec HJ, Beckmann U, et al. 1978. The effect of graded immersion on heart volume, central venous pressure, pulmonary blood distribution, and heart rate in man. *Pflügers Archiv: Eur J Appl Physiol.* 374(2):115–118.

4   Brooks GA, Fahey TD, White TP, Baldwin KM. 2000. *Exercise Physiology, Human Bioenergetics and its Applications.* (3d ed.). Mountainview: Mayfield Publishing Company.

5   Taylor NAS, Morrison JB. 1993. Static and dynamic pulmonary compliance during upright immersion. *Acta Physiologica Scandinavica.* 149(4):413–417.

6   Becker, BE. 2009. Aquatic therapy: scientific foundations and clinical rehabilitation applications. *PM&R.* 1(9):859–872.

7   Avellini BA, Shapiro Y, Pandolf KB. 1983. Cardio-respiratory physical training in water and on land. *Eur J Appl Physiol.* 50(2): 55–263.

8   Darby LA, Yaekle BC. 2000. Physiological responses during two types of exercise performed on land and in the water. *J Sports Med Phys Fitnes.* 40(4):303–311.

9   Reilly T, Dowzer CN, Cable NT. 2003. The physiology of deep water running. *J Sports Sci.* 21(12):959–972.

10 Bushman BA, Flynn MG, Andres FF, et al. 1997. Effect of 4 weeks of deep water run training on running performance. *Med Sci Sports Exerc.* 29:694–699.

11 Wilber RL, Moffatt RJ, Scott BE, et al. 1996. Influence of water in training on the maintenance of aerobic performance. *Med Sci Sports Exerc.* 28:1056–1062.

12 Davidson K, McNaughton L. 2000. Deep water running and road running training improve $\dot{V}O_2$max in untrained women. *J Strength Cond Res.* 14:191–195.

13 Reilly T, Cable NT, Dowzer CN. 2002. The effect of a 6-week land- and water-running training programme on aerobic, anaerobic and muscle strength measures. *J Sports Sci.* 21:333–334.

14 Dowzer CN, Reilly T, Cable NT. 1998. Effects of deep and shallow water running on spinal shrinkage. *Br J Sports Med.* 32:44–48.

15 Broman G, Quintana M, Lindberg T, et al. 2006. High intensity deep water training can improve aerobic power in elderly women. *Eur J Appl Physiol.* 98:117–123.

16 Karageorghis, CI, Priest DL. 2012. Music in the exercise domain: a review and synthesis (Part II). *Int Rev Sport Exerc Psychol.* 5(1):67–84.

PRACTICAL 13
GROUP TRAINING EXERCISE

Emma M. Beckman and Justin J. Holland

Introduction

Group exercise training is a popular training option for many reasons, largely related to the cost effectiveness of including groups of people together with one instructor (or multiple instructors) when compared to one-on-one instruction. The benefits of group exercise training are not only related to the health outcomes that are known to result from exercise in general but also include additional benefits due to the social aspects of the environment, and the potential improvements in adherence related to the social contract that is often formed between group members (Figure 13.1).

Group training must adhere to the general principles of exercise prescription; however, there are certain additional concerns and considerations that must be accounted for in the group setting. This practical will cover the safety, instruction, delivery and adjustments that must be made to run an effective group session.

The prevalence of group training in the health and fitness industry extends to the training of similar populations together. This might include participants with Parkinson's disease, postpartum women and older individuals. In addition to groups that are formed by condition or population, there are also countless examples of group training by particular activities, such as Pilates, yoga, dance, sports and established commercial fitness paradigms. Many of the characteristics relevant to instructing group sessions should be consistent across group training as a whole; however, due to the significant scope that this entails, the focus of this practical is small group sessions of between 2 and 15 people, with session goals related to strength and cardiorespiratory fitness.

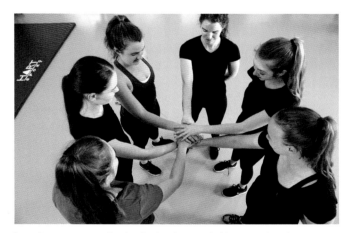

Figure 13.1 Benefits of group exercise include the social interaction between group members

Pre-session Preparation

The successful completion of a group session will largely reflect the preparation that an instructor puts into the session beforehand. Prior to running the session, you should develop a program that is relevant to your target population, the number of participants involved, equipment/facilities available and the surrounding environment. It is important to ensure that setting up a group session can be done efficiently and does not require elaborate attention and time. There are a number of tools that you can use to make sure your session runs smoothly and minimises the time spent off-task. Many factors must be considered in a group session, largely due to environmental, organisational and medical considerations that must be accounted for prior to conducting a session. There are also some legal considerations. It is important to ensure, prior to the delivery of a session, that you are working within the confines of your insurance coverage and scope of practice. This will relate to the number of people you can supervise at any one time, the environment that you can work within and the characteristics of the people that you can work with (including their medical conditions).

Activity 13.1 Environmental considerations

Background

Group sessions are often held in outdoor locations given the amount of space that is often required to run groups. Outdoor exercise has also been shown to increase mood in some individuals and it is often a cheaper option rather than hiring large indoor spaces. Should a session be planned for an outdoor location, the most pressing issue to consider is likely to be inclement weather such as rain or extreme temperatures (both hot and cold). Therefore, it is useful to have alternative session location plans to account for these issues. In addition to weather, the considerations related to outdoor locations are likely to be factors such as ground condition, the presence of animals and council or government regulations.

AIM:
- Develop strategies to address potential environmental issues

TASK:
- Complete Worksheet 13.1 by considering the potential issues and then developing strategies that may be useful to overcome them. The first one is completed for you.

Worksheet 13.1 Environmental Considerations	
Potential issue	**Strategies**
The local park where you run group sessions is only mowed by the city council in 12-week cycles and for the last 3 weeks before it is mowed the grass gets extremely long.	The council may be able to give you the mowing schedule for a particular area in advance, which will allow you to plan for times when areas are likely to experience greater overgrowth. Then you may either reschedule sessions for another location or record and/or document that the grass is overlong and contact the council requesting the mowing schedule be moved forwards.
It is spring and swooping magpies frequent the area where you generally run a group session.	
A local school has run a golf day on the oval that you use for group sessions and when you turn up for a session there are divots scattered throughout the area that are a risk for ankle sprains for group session participants.	
A notice has been distributed via social media that your local city council is requiring permits for group training at a number of locations in your city.	

Worksheet 13.1 Environmental Considerations (continued)	
Potential issue	**Strategies**
Hot temperatures (> 35°C) are expected for the next two days with the lowest temperature of the day (24°C) expected at 7 pm. Your sessions normally run at 4 pm.	
Your session includes exercises lying on the ground; however, you notice an extensive network of ant nests where you plan to run your session.	
There is extensive dew on the ground, making it slippery and dangerous for running and plyometrics.	

Activity 13.2 Organisational and medical considerations

Background

In group sessions, a number of organisational issues can arise related to groups of people, venues and medical conditions. If these issues are not planned for in advance, they can have serious consequences for both the instructor of a group session and the individuals participating. Other considerations may be less serious but will affect the enjoyment and engagement of participants and possibly influence their likelihood to continue attending sessions.

AIM:
- Develop strategies to address potential organisational and medical issues

TASK:
- Complete Worksheet 13.2 by considering the potential issues and then developing strategies that may be useful to overcome them. The first one is completed for you.

Worksheet 13.2 Organisational and Medical Considerations	
Potential issue	**Strategies**
Participants may have different medical conditions.	All instructors should have current first aid and CPR qualifications and a working, well-stocked first-aid kit. In addition, you should plan for conditions such as a person with diabetes having a hypoglycaemic event by having sugar-containing lollies or something similar on hand during group sessions. For participants with medical conditions, it is important that you are aware of signs and symptoms that may be a precursor to medical emergencies so you can observe and plan in advance. Easy phone access for instructors is crucial.
You are running sessions back-to-back and need to document observations from the sessions.	
Participants need a place to leave personal belongings such as keys, phones and wallets.	

| Worksheet 13.2 Organisational and Medical Considerations (continued) ||
Potential issue	Strategies
You are unable to take a group session (e.g. due to illness). What are some considerations you will need to put into place?	
Eight participants cancel 2 hours prior to the session being run, leaving you with only two participants. What policies and considerations should you put in place to avoid late cancellations?	
You run a bootcamp out of a local gymnasium and have a verbal contract that you will pay $100 per hour of usage; however, they now want to increase this to $150 per hour. This unexpected fee increase will lead to higher prices for your participants. How could you have prevented this from happening?	

Activity 13.3 Group communication

Background

Effective communication is an important component of a successful group exercise session. There are challenges in instructing exercise to any individual and the importance of good cues, giving strong effective feedback and maintaining enjoyment and motivation are no less important in a group setting than in individual instruction (Figure 13.2). Indeed, there are much greater challenges in ensuring these important aspects of exercise are maintained in the group setting. A group instructor should continually reflect on their communication. A common occurrence is to overuse phrases such as 'great work, guys' and 'that's good, that's good', so a variety of feedback phrases should be used with avoidance of gender-specific language such as 'guys' and words such as 'like'. Instructions should be kept succinct to avoid participants cooling down while waiting for you to explain something. If the sessions require substantial instruction or demonstration, it is best to do this prior to the warm-up or before the next exercise. Alternatively, you can use laminated cards and tablets with exercise names and pictures/videos where required. Depending on your group size, you should be positioned where you can be easily seen and heard. This may require the use of a microphone, megaphone or speaker system to project your voice over a longer distance.

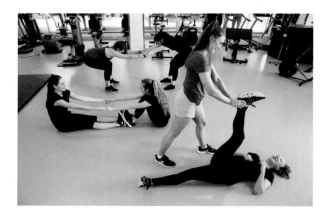

Figure 13.2 Effective communication is just as important in a group setting as in individual instruction

AIM:

- Develop strategies to address group communication issues

TASK:

- Complete Worksheet 13.3 by considering the potential issues and then developing strategies that may be useful to overcome them. The first one is completed for you.

Worksheet 13.3 Group Communication	
Potential issue	**Strategies**
Different people respond to or prefer different styles of instruction, ranging from bright and upbeat to a boot camp style of strict and demanding instructions.	Building rapport with multiple people at the same time is challenging, so it is often better to take a middle-of-the-road approach and set the tone of the group to be welcoming but motivating. When people start to repeat sessions and return, you can engage more on an individual level and gauge whether people respond to or comment on instances where you vary your style slightly. Group sessions require high amounts of energy from the instructor and it is important you can maintain your set tone for the duration of the session (and sessions that may run directly after).
You notice some of your group participants on some occasions will be less talkative or slightly less engaged, or you yourself might have a particularly challenging day and be required to run a group session in the evening.	
Many people may not realise it but they have a distinct style of language and often this is accompanied by repetitive phrases to fall back on in instruction. How can you avoid this?	.
Not everyone will come to a session with expertise in every exercise. How can you ensure safe and accurate prescription of exercises without lengthy periods of instruction and demonstration?	
You have been asked to run a conditioning session at the local football club. The session is for 60 players all at the same time. How will you communicate to ensure the players remain on task during the 30-minute conditioning task?	

Delivering group exercise sessions

Positioning

When you are demonstrating or instructing an exercise, try to remove any external distractions to the participants. This may include facing the sun when you address the group so that the sun is in your eyes—not theirs, facing the road to avoid the distraction from passing vehicles and avoiding running sessions at the same time as other groups.

Equipment

There is a range of equipment on the market that may help you deliver a group exercise session. Table 13.1 provides examples of common equipment used in group sessions, reasons for their inclusion and some sample exercises. New equipment and training devices are always evolving with different trends in training. Despite new equipment being developed, there are a number of standard pieces that can be utilised in a group exercise session.

Considerations when including equipment in sessions relate to the following.

- How heavy is it? Do you have to transport it to multiple places?
- How expensive is it? Will it be safe in a public place?
- What sort of surface will the session be conducted on? Does this change the equipment requirements?

TABLE 13.1   Equipment Used for Group Exercise Training

Equipment	Rationale	Examples	Considerations
Skipping ropes	• Aerobic-based activity that can be undertaken in a single spot	• Single/double skips • Side-to-side skips • High-knee skips	• Joint loading, arthritis, osteoporosis with fracture history, floor surface (e.g. grass, concrete)
Medicine balls (MB)	• Versatile and small piece of equipment that can target different areas of strength development	• MB throws • Side squat with MB press • MB woodchop squat • Russian twist	• One size won't fit all participants, may require hand-eye coordination, limitations in ball mass may restrict strength adaptations
Barbells	• Highly adaptable to suit individual clients • Enables the participant to undertake primary lifts	• Straight leg deadlift • Barbell row • Rollouts	• Storage/transport of plates and bars • Individual technique in association with adaptable load
Dumbbells	• Small and transportable pieces of equipment • Can target both upper and lower body movements • Increases degrees of freedom relative to barbells	• Renegade row • Squat press • Floor press	• The required size of the dumbbell will vary for each specific movement • Consider increased range of motion in relation to potential injury risk
Car tyres	• Allows participants to undertake an activity that they would not normally do in a gym or at home	• Tyre flips • Tyre jumps • Tyre chest press	• Transport and storage of large bulky tyres • Technique and safety in lifting and jumping

TABLE 13.1	Equipment Used for Group Exercise Training (continued)		
Equipment	**Rationale**	**Examples**	**Considerations**
Kettlebells	• Easily accessible, compact and portable • Handle and flat bottom kettlebells improve safety in stabilising positions compared to dumbbells	• Squat with upright row • Kettlebell swings • Turkish get-up	• Loss of control or grip (particularly during swings) may create an unsafe area • Improper technique during swings may lead to lower back pain • Given the degrees of freedom a kettlebell has, a participant should have appropriate shoulder stability before undertaking this form of training
Steps	• Can be used for both aerobic and muscular development depending on the client's goals • Easily portable and typically already found in parks, making them low-cost and highly functional	• Decline push-ups • Step-ups (aerobic and muscular development) • Single-leg skiers • Bulgarian squats	• Fatigue and poor body kinetics/awareness may result in the client falling or tripping over on the step
Ropes	• Versatile and easily transportable piece of equipment that is primarily used to target anaerobic and power adaptations	• Waves • Alternating waves • Power slams • Russian twist	• May be limited by client coordination (particularly in alternating movements) • Long ropes may require operating in larger areas to operate
Sleds	• Develops both muscular power and strength • Improves sprinting acceleration when compared to traditional bodyweight sprinting drills	• High/low sled push • Sled drag and row • Sled running	• Sufficient warm-up should be provided before undertaking sled training • Develop proper sprinting technique prior to working on sled drills

TABLE 13.1   Equipment Used for Group Exercise Training (continued)

Equipment	Rationale	Examples	Considerations
Logs (wooden and plastic)	• Versatile and unique piece of equipment that can develop strength and power	• Log toss • Log carry • Log press	• Splinters and cuts are a risk if using wooden logs
Unstable surface (e.g. Swiss ball, BOSU ball, Dura Disc)	• Easily portable pieces of equipment that promote the development of proprioception, stability and balance	• Single-leg balance on DuraDisc • Swiss ball squat • BOSU ball lunges	• Increased falls risk when undertaking exercise on unstable surfaces
Sporting equipment (e.g. tennis racquet, soccer ball, tennis balls)	• Provide the opportunity for games	• Small games • Soccer game • Catch and pass	• May isolate some clients who are uncomfortable in game/team-based sports • The size of the area, time of task and intensity need to be considered in accordance with the participants' goals

Bodyweight Exercises

Bodyweight exercises can be used in a variety of indoor and outdoor settings and in a range of populations from the young to the elderly. Group exercise instructors should include bodyweight exercises as part of their session. Among the many benefits of bodyweight training is the opportunity for participants to understand that resistance training can be performed without equipment. A limitation of bodyweight exercises is that the inability to increase external loading may require more repetitions to promote muscular adaptation. Increasing repetitions may not suit the client's goals or appropriate training status (e.g. a bodyweight squat will not develop strength for a well-trained football player). Table 13.2 provides common bodyweight exercises; a number of these have already been covered in detail in previous practicals.

Plyometric Exercises

Plyometric exercises help develop power, speed and rate of force development, and were discussed in detail in Practical 10. They can be undertaken with limited or no equipment and performed in a variety of different settings. They are well suited to a group exercise environment. Plyometrics are associated with a higher risk of injury and therefore should be used with cautioned in untrained or injured clients. They should be implemented after an appropriate warm-up.

Exercise Names

The use of only a small amount of equipment in group-based exercise training has led to the development of new exercises using little to no equipment and modifications to more common exercises. The names of some of these exercises can reflect the movement (e.g. side squat with medicine ball press), whereas others may be more difficult to understand (e.g. Turkish get-up). Tables 13.1 and 13.2 contain some exercises not previously mentioned in this manual. There are many more in addition to these, with new names popping up regularly. It is outside the scope of this manual to attempt to provide a comprehensive list of exercises and their variations, so it is suggested that when a new exercise name is encountered, you use online resources to obtain the necessary information about it.

TABLE 13.2	Bodyweight Exercises
Body Region	**Exercises**
Upper body	• Push-up (Exercise 6b) • Wall press • Chin up/pull up (Exercise 8f) • Triceps dips
Lower body	• Squat (Exercise 9a) • Lunge (Exercise 9b) • Hip extension—supine bridge (Exercise 9e) • Calf raise (Exercise 9h)
Abdominals	• Prone bridge (Exercise 5a) • Side bridge (Exercise 5b) • Bird dog (Exercise 5c) • Abdominal crunch (Exercise 5e) • Oblique crunch (Exercise 5f) • Leg lowers
Combined upper and lower body	• Burpees • Tiger crawls • Inchworm

Designing a Group Exercise Session

The exercise options presented above make it clear there are many choices to make when designing a group exercise session. The use of these and/or other exercises and where they are placed in a program will require consideration of the following questions.

- What are appropriate exercises for a warm-up?
- Do you have a good balance of upper and lower body exercises and are they performed in an alternating fashion?
- Do any of these exercises require high levels of skills, making it necessary to consider fatigue? Should they be done early in the session?
- Do you cover all body parts? Often when minimal equipment is used it is more challenging to include exercises that train the back muscles and sessions may emphasise the chest muscles as there are more variations that are easy to implement.

Worked Case Study for Designing a Group Exercise Session

You are asked to design a 60-minute group exercise session for 10 people aged between 22 and 47 years of age. Their goals are to improve cardiorespiratory fitness and strength and there are no medical contraindications to exercise.

The session you design includes 45 minutes of activity and 15 minutes for instruction and breaks. A focus is on high intensity with all major muscle groups targeted. The general parameters are:

- warm-up 10 minutes
- circuit approximately 20 minutes
  - each circuit has 10 exercises

- each exercise is for 20 seconds using the 'as many reps as possible' (AMRAP) approach
- 10 seconds rest/move to next station
- 3 times through each circuit with 2 minutes rest between circuits
- cool-down 15 minutes.

An example of a session is provided in Table 13.3. Feel free to refer to it, but try and be creative when creating your session.

TABLE 13.3 Designing a Group Exercise Session

Session Timing	Exercise	
Warm-up (10 minutes) 3 of each × 20 seconds	High knees Butt kicks Hip openers Jog Grapevine Leg swings Arm circles Cossack squats	
Circuit exercises (20 minutes)	1. Bodyweight squats	
	2. Decline push-ups	

TABLE 13.3 Designing a Group Exercise Session (continued)		
Session Timing	**Exercise**	
	3. Bulgarian squats	
	4. Renegade row with dumbbells	
	5. Double skips	

TABLE 13.3 Designing a Group Exercise Session (continued)		
Session Timing	**Exercise**	
	6. Log press	
	7. Prone bridge	
	8. Hip extension—supine bridge	
	9. Leg lowers	

TABLE 13.3   Designing a Group Exercise Session (continued)

TABLE 13.3 Designing a Group Exercise Session (continued)		
Session Timing	**Exercise**	
	10. Russian twist	
Cool-down (15 minutes)	Slow jog (5 minutes) Stretches for upper and lower body	

Activity 13.4 Modifying exercises in a group session for a specific population

Background

It is extremely rare that a trainer would get through a whole group training session without making adjustments to technique or modifying exercises. This challenge is magnified with increasing numbers of participants in a session. The most common elements requiring adjustment will be because of: population characteristics; musculoskeletal limitations/injuries and medical conditions; and poor technique. Factors associated with each of these that need to be considered are as follows.

- Population factors:
  - age
  - cardiorespiratory fitness and strength (athlete's vs sedentary population)
  - body mass and anthropometrics (e.g. height).
- Musculoskeletal limitations/injuries and medical conditions:
  - low back pain
  - shoulder pain or instability
  - knee pain
  - general soreness and tightness (particularly when people start training more than once a week).
- Technique:
  - poor body position
  - compensations to carrying heavy objects (e.g. water bottles, sandbags).

AIM:
- Modify exercises in a group session for a specific population

TASKS:

- In groups of three, select a population based on their age and fitness levels (e.g. 18 to 30 year olds with moderate cardiorespiratory fitness and strength).
- Complete Worksheet 13.4 by providing a modification to each of the exercises below to suit this population.
- Deliver one circuit of this modified session to the rest of the class.

Worksheet 13.4 Modifying Exercises in A Group Session for A Specific Population	
Population (age range, fitness level): _____	
Exercise	Modification
Bodyweight squats	
Decline push-ups	
Bulgarian squats	
Renegade row with dumbbells	
Double skips	
Log press	
Prone bridge	
Hip extension—supine bridge	
Leg lowers	
Russian twist	

Activity 13.5 Modifying exercises in a group session for various participants

AIM:

- Modify exercises in a group session for various participants

TASKS:

- The participants in your group exercise session have various issues that require you to modify the exercise during the class.
- Complete Worksheet 13.5 by providing a modification to the exercise for each issue.
- The modifications to the first exercise are provided (in *italics*).

Worksheet 13.5 Modifying Exercises in A Group Session for Various Participants			
Exercise	Issue 1	Issue 2	Issue 3
Bodyweight squats	Client has pain in the knees at 90° flexion	Poor ankle range of motion	Experienced athlete
	Change depth of squat	*Put the heels on a slight rise*	*Add weight with kettlebell*

Worksheet 13.5 Modifying Exercises in A Group Session for Various Participants (continued)			
Exercise	Issue 1	Issue 2	Issue 3
Decline push-ups	Previous history of shoulder subluxations; this position makes him nervous	A 69-year-old man	Scapular winging throughout movement
Bulgarian squats	Chronic lower back pain	Vestibular disorder	A 60-year-old female with osteoporosis
Renegade row with dumbbells	Very poor posture (exaggerated thoracic kyphosis)	Carpal tunnel	Fractured big toe 6 weeks ago
Double skips	Woman with pelvic floor issues	Double knee replacement	Person with type 2 diabetes
Log press	Mild hypertension	Locks out elbows at top of movement	Pain when reaching overhead
Plank	Goes into lumbar lordosis	Tight hip flexors with reduction in hip extension range	BMI of 34 kg/m^2
Hip extension—supine bridge	Older man who has difficulty getting onto the ground	Feels the exercise in her hamstrings	Athlete doesn't feel this anywhere (too easy)
Leg lowers	Lumbar curve increases after 2 reps	Feels this in hip flexors	Older man that has difficulty getting onto the ground
Russian twist	Feels this in hip flexor and unable to cue them out of it	Unable to coordinate the movement	Pregnant

Activity 13.6 Risk management

Given the nature of group exercise training, with usually one trainer supervising multiple people exercising concurrently, the risks of a participant experiencing an adverse event are increased compared to typical one-on-one training. Mitigating risk by providing a safe environment should be the trainer's major aim. If safety concerns cannot be addressed to an acceptable level then the session should not commence. Identifying risks is an important skill.

In the indoor and outdoor environments risks may include poor flooring/ground surfaces, faulty/damaged equipment or hazards (e.g. broken glass). When outdoors, extreme weather (e.g. lightning) can provide an additional risk. The type of exercise may also increase risk. More difficult exercises that require close monitoring of technique may not be suitable for larger groups. Exercises that use equipment in a confined area may also increase the risk of someone getting injured (e.g. throwing medicine balls).

There are usually four approaches that need to be considered in a risk-management plan.

1. Accept the risk; for example, you have identified and recorded the risk but no action is required.
2. Avoid the risk; for example, change plans to avoid the risk.
3. Transfer the risk; for example, use 'waivers' to transfer the risk to the participant by making them aware of the risk. It is important to understand that obtaining a waiver from a participant does not preclude your duty of care towards the individual.
4. Mitigate the risk; for example, limit the impact of a risk so that if it does occur, the problem it creates is small and easy to fix. This is the most common approach to risk management.

Risk management is an ongoing activity, so you should continue to identify and record new risks as they arise.

AIM:

- Recognise risks when conducting group exercise training and adapt a situation to minimise the risks

TASKS:

- Identify three risk factors in the picture below.
- Outline your management plan for this scenario.

Worksheet 13.6 Risk Management

Risk factors:
1. _____
2. _____
3. _____

Management plan

_____
_____
_____
_____

Activity 13.7 Group exercise training goals

There is a difference between group training as a concept and individual training that occurs with a number of people together in the same place at the same time. For example, if the purpose of a group session is to enhance social connectedness (often the goal of group training), is this goal achieved by individuals working their way around circuit stations?

In group-based training it is important to consider activities that can get people working together during a session. For example, play-based games, partner stretching and using body weight between people may all be effective ways to allow stronger group cohesion during an exercise session.

AIM:
- Design exercises to meet group exercise training session goals

TASKS:
- You are a group training instructor who has been asked to take an exercise class for 10 employees of a company. You are told that this should be designed to improve the workers' cardiorespiratory fitness and strength and it should be as social as possible.
- Worksheet 13.7 contains exercises for a session presented in previous activities. Complete it by adding games/exercises that can be used in the session. Some have been provided (in *italics*). Figures 13.3 and 13.4 show examples of games and social exercises.

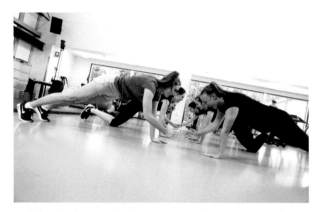

Figure 13.3 Paper, scissors, rock in plank position is one example of a game that can be used in a group session

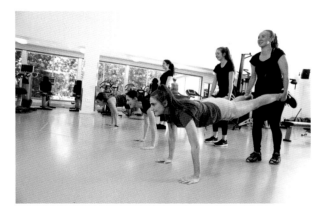

Figure 13.4 Wheelbarrow races is an example of a social exercise that can be used in group sessions

Worksheet 13.7 Group Exercise Training Goals		
Session timing	**Exercise**	**Group session exercise**
Warm-up (10 minutes)	High knees	*Games*
3 of each × 20 seconds	Butt kicks Hip openers Jog Grapevine Leg swings Arm circles Cossack squats	*1. Ship to shore* *2. Deck of cards* *3. Offside touch football*
Stations (20 minutes)	Bodyweight squats	*Squat and high-five your partner*
	Decline push-ups	
	Bulgarian squats on park bench	
	Renegade row with dumbbells	
	Double skips	
	Log press	
	Prone bridge	*Partner taps: Two people plank face to face and have to try and touch each other's elbows (to make it more difficult, they aren't allowed to touch your elbow if one of your feet is lifted off the ground—use this for more advanced groups)*
	Hip extension—supine bridge	
	Leg lowers	
	Russian twist with rope	
Cool-down (15 minutes)	Slow jog (5 minutes) Stretches for upper and lower body	*Partner-assisted stretching*

Activity 13.8 Design and deliver a group exercise session

AIM:
- Design and deliver a group exercise session

TASKS:
- The activity is completed in groups of around six people.
- One student will be required to design and deliver a segment of a group exercise session for the remaining group members.
- The segment should run for approximately 10 minutes and can be a warm-up, a part of the conditioning section or a cool-down.

- The student should pick a focus or goal for the session and explain this to the group prior to delivery of the session, including any contextual factors (e.g. what population it is aimed at).
- At the end of the 10-minute segment each member of the group completes a peer assessment tool (Worksheet 13.8) on various characteristics of the session.
- As a group, come to a consensus about how the student performed on the items in the peer assessment tool. One member of the group provides the student with this feedback.

Worksheet 13.8 Design and Deliver a Group Exercise Session—Peer Assessment Tool		
Characteristic	Circle (rating out of 10) (1 = easiest/least appropriate, 10 = the best/most effective)	Comments
How appropriate was the segment for the goal stated at the start of the session?	1 2 3 4 5 6 7 8 9 10	
How would you rate the complexity and variety of exercises provided?	1 2 3 4 5 6 7 8 9 10	
How enjoyable was the segment?	1 2 3 4 5 6 7 8 9 10	
How effective was the instruction of the segment (e.g. cues and demonstration)?	1 2 3 4 5 6 7 8 9 10	
How optimal was the organisation of the session in terms of equipment, timing, structure and transitions?	1 2 3 4 5 6 7 8 9 10	
How effective was the student's adherence to the principles of exercise prescription (e.g. rest, sets and repetitions)?	1 2 3 4 5 6 7 8 9 10	
To what degree was the instructor engaging, positive and had a professional attitude throughout the session?	1 2 3 4 5 6 7 8 9 10	
List two items the student did well.	1.\n2.	
List two items the student could have improved on.	1.\n2.	

PRACTICAL 14
NEUROMOTOR AND FUNCTIONAL FITNESS TRAINING

Emma M. Beckman and Kelly M. Clanchy

Introduction

The aim of neuromotor exercise training is to ensure that motor responses are optimal when balance, coordination, agility or gait is challenged.[1] This will ensure that an individual's capacity meets their requirements for activities of daily living, occupation and leisure. This practical will detail the principles behind exercise prescription designed to train the components of the neuromotor system and provide direction regarding how to tailor prescription to an individual's requirements and task demands.

When investigating literature in this field, it is important to recognise the variations in terminology that are commonly used. Terms including 'neuromotor exercise' and 'proprioceptive and functional training' are often used interchangeably to describe similar prescription practices. Conceptual clarity related to the underlying needs and requirements of an individual is necessary to ensure optimal outcomes from exercise prescription. That is, there is a need to identify which component(s) of neuromotor functioning is impairing an individual's ability to perform a task (e.g. balance, coordination and agility) and tailor your prescription to address the deficit.

In this practical, each of the components of neuromotor exercise are addressed individually; however, this is done with the important caveat that there is significant crossover between each component. The practical concludes with a short section on functional exercise to encourage students to practise their skills in creating exercises that replicate important activities. Important considerations for training and example exercises are provided. It is recommended that students form small groups when working through this practical and not only try each suggested activity but also practise the instruction of each and determine the most important cues that will allow optimisation of the prescription.

Anatomy: Neuromuscular and Sensory Systems

Neuromotor exercises target structures of the neuromuscular and sensory systems to allow information to be processed regarding joint position and movement (referred to collectively as 'proprioception'). This is largely mediated by mechanoreceptors (both articular and tenomuscular) that send afferent feedback to be processed by the central nervous system (CNS) and subsequently produce motor responses. This process whereby sensory information results in motor responses is most often termed neuromuscular control.

Articular mechanoreceptors such as Pacinian corpuscles, Meissner's corpuscles and free nerve endings provide information regarding joint position by responding to mechanical deformation that is then processed to provide enhanced joint stiffness, coordinated motor patterns or reflex activity—all undertaken to enhance the stability of the joint.

Tenomuscular mechanoreceptors (muscle spindles and Golgi tendon organs) have been shown to play a similar role in optimising joint stability by sending information to the CNS related to joint rotations and muscle length. This is then processed to optimise joint stability, coordination and control.

The role that these structures play in moderating motor responses means that neuromotor training becomes of great importance. This can occur when there is damage to afferent pathways due to injury or pathology, or simply when greater capacity is required of a joint or a number of joints than has previously been required. Therefore, training to gradually progress the capacity of the body to cope with the new demands is necessary (e.g. training a new skill, beginning a new sport or performing a new activity at work or in the home).

Generally, the neural input that is processed in the CNS from the mechanoreceptors results in one of three levels of motor control response: spinal reflexes, brainstem control or cortical pathways. Given that all three of these pathways contribute to optimising neuromuscular control, they should each be incorporated into exercise prescription. An example of this is in Table 14.1.

TABLE 14.1 Motor Control, Neuromuscular Control and Implications for Exercise Prescription		
Motor Control Level	**Role in Neuromuscular Control**	**Implications for Exercise Prescription**
Spinal reflexes	Provides reflex joint stabilisation during positional change	Consider exercises and activities that include sudden alterations in joint position which will necessitate reflex control; this response may be optimal when utilising closed-chain activities (e.g. coordination)
Brainstem control	Integrates mechanoreceptor input with visual input to maintain posture and balance	Exercise prescription should aim to challenge the centre of gravity in relation to the base of support and may be done by also altering the contribution of the visual system (e.g. closed eyes during balance exercises)
Cortical pathways	Cognitive awareness of body position and movement and incorporates voluntary movements	When considering exercises, there may be indications for repetitive actions that require joint positioning preferably at the end ROMs with the intended result to be improvements in unconscious motor programming (e.g. agility)

Balance Training

Balance is defined as a task-specific multi-joint skill that requires the effective performance and interaction of the neuromusculoskeletal, visual, vestibular and somatosensory systems. Balance relates to the position of the centre of gravity over the base of support (defined as the area within an outline of all ground contact points) and is challenged through alterations to a person's stability and mobility.[2] The response to these challenges is undertaken for the purposes of maintaining the body's equilibrium, which relates to an equal balance between two opposing forces or processes.

Balance is an important component of all voluntary movements; the postural adjustments that are required before, during and after movements are numerous and are task and context specific.

Balance is essential for optimising performance. Force production and agility is optimised when the body is in a stable position.

Important Considerations for Balance Training

The design of specific and functional balance training programs requires: 1. an understanding of the systems that interact to produce voluntary and involuntary movements (e.g. neuromusculoskeletal and visual systems); and 2. a progressive overload of these systems specific to the function or outcome of the movement (e.g. understanding the role that balance has in allowing the person to complete the movement successfully). There are two types of balance training programs:

- static balance, which includes drills designed to improve an individual's ability to stand in place
- dynamic balance, which improves an individual's ability to maintain equilibrium during motion.

In order to improve the components of balance, progressions that increase the difficulty of executing the exercise are needed. These modifications are targeted primarily at the postural control systems that contribute to executing the movement. There are many factors that can be used to modify the demands of an activity or to add a balance component into an exercise. Table 14.2 presents common balance exercises.

There are a number of ways to modify balance exercises, including:

- altering the base of support (e.g. sitting versus standing, one versus two legs)
- altering stance width
- increasing the range of motion (ROM) that the exercise is completed in (e.g. lifting a leg higher in a single leg stance)
- performing exercises unilaterally in preference to bilaterally
- alternating between having eyes open and closed
- increasing the movement speed
- completing the task on an unstable surface (e.g. foam)
- introducing an additional task to complete during the completion of the task (e.g. a cognitive element such as counting backwards from 100 in threes) or a physical element (e.g. standing on one leg while bouncing a ball)
- performing combination exercises in unstable positions (e.g. squat with a simultaneous shoulder press).

Different individuals will find various aspects of balance more challenging, depending on their skills and prior experience. The next activity will allow you to practise these balance exercises and modifications.

TABLE 14.2   Balance Exercises with Their Rationale and Considerations

Exercise	Rationale and Considerations
Sitting and standing exercises with external support (e.g. use of a bar) progressed to sitting and standing exercises with no external support	These exercises require the translation of the centre of mass from a low position to a higher position with a focus on strength in specific muscles. Inclusion of the bar allows for the movement to be completed safely; progressively reducing the reliance on the external bar increases the stabilisation required from key muscle groups which increases the balance component required to complete the movement.
Progressive standing exercises (listed in order of increased difficulty): • normal stance • split stance • tandem stance • standing on one leg with eyes open • standing on one leg with eyes closed	These exercises allow for the training of postural responses related to standing upright including proprioception (maintain the body's position in space); vestibular function (maintain the head's position in space); and vision (maintain and adjust for changes in body position). Changing the stance from a comfortable stance to split and/or tandem stance challenges the maintenance of the centre of mass with a reduced and/or altered base of support. Standing on one leg challenges the maintenance of the centre of mass that is displaced towards the stance leg with half of the required base of support. Closing the eyes removes the visual system as a source of monitoring and adjusting for changes in body position. This creates an increased reliance on neuromusculoskeletal, vestibular and somatosensory balance systems.

TABLE 14.2 Balance Exercises with Their Rationale and Considerations (continued)	
Exercise	**Rationale and Considerations**
Hopping (eyes open) Hopping (eyes closed)	Hopping progresses the standing on one leg exercise by adding an increased need for a neuromuscular and somatosensory responses, particularly when landing on the stance leg. Closing eyes increases the reliance on the vestibular system to monitor and adjust for changes in body position as a replacement for input from the visual system.
Spinning in a circle five times and then standing on one leg with eyes open, progressing to spinning in a circle five times and standing on one leg with eyes closed	Spinning in a circle disorientates the vestibular balance system which increases the demands on the visual, somatosensory and neuromuscular systems in order to maintain a balanced posture on one leg. Closing the eyes eliminates input from the visual system, which in turn increases the reliance on input from the somatosensory system and responses from the neuromuscular system to maintain a balanced posture.
Standing on one leg while bouncing a ball	Standing on one leg bouncing a ball increases the difficulty of standing on one leg by adding an additional task to divert conscious attention away from maintaining balance (i.e. maintenance of balance becomes secondary to the bouncing of the ball).

Activity 14.1 Balance exercises

AIM:
- To complete balance exercises and understand how modifications may increase the difficulty

TASK:
- Complete the balance exercises in Worksheet 14.1 and rate each for level of difficulty by placing an X on the scale.
- Provide a modification to each exercise and rate this exercise for level of difficulty.

Worksheet 14.1 Balance Exercises	
Balance exercise	**Difficulty rating**
Normal stance Modification: _____ _____	Very easy Easy Difficult Very difficult ⌊___⌊___⌊___⌊___⌊ Very easy Easy Difficult Very difficult ⌊___⌊___⌊___⌊___⌊

Worksheet 14.1 Balance Exercises (continued)

Balance exercise	Difficulty rating
Split stance Modification: _____ _____	Very easy — Easy — Difficult — Very difficult Very easy — Easy — Difficult — Very difficult
Tandem stance Modification: _____ _____	Very easy — Easy — Difficult — Very difficult Very easy — Easy — Difficult — Very difficult
Standing on one leg with eyes open Modification: _____ _____	Very easy — Easy — Difficult — Very difficult Very easy — Easy — Difficult — Very difficult
Standing on one leg with eyes closed Modification: _____ _____	Very easy — Easy — Difficult — Very difficult Very easy — Easy — Difficult — Very difficult
Hopping with eyes open Modification: _____ _____	Very easy — Easy — Difficult — Very difficult Very easy — Easy — Difficult — Very difficult
Hopping with eyes closed Modification: _____ _____	Very easy — Easy — Difficult — Very difficult Very easy — Easy — Difficult — Very difficult
Spinning in a circle five times and then standing on one leg with eyes open Modification: _____ _____	Very easy — Easy — Difficult — Very difficult Very easy — Easy — Difficult — Very difficult

Worksheet 14.1 Balance Exercises (continued)	
Balance exercise	**Difficulty rating**
Spinning in a circle five times and then standing on one leg with eyes closed Modification: _____ _____	Very easy Easy Difficult Very difficult Very easy Easy Difficult Very difficult
Standing on one leg while bouncing a ball Modification: _____ _____	Very easy Easy Difficult Very difficult Very easy Easy Difficult Very difficult

Activity 14.2 Exercise prescription for balance

AIM:

- To prescribe balance exercises

Case study 14.1
A 75-year-old man complains of poor balance and concerns getting around on his own without falling. His primary goal is to walk up his 10 steps at home independently. During your assessment, you measure his tandem stance at 3 seconds.

TASKS:

- Based on the information provided in Case study 14.1, complete Worksheet 14.2 by prescribing three balance exercises you would use to progress the client towards his goal.
- Provide a brief justification for your choices.

Worksheet 14.2 Balance Case Study
Exercises: 1. _____ 2. _____ 3. _____ **Brief justification:** _____ _____ _____

Coordination Training

Coordination is defined as the ability to voluntarily execute fluid, accurate and controlled movements at a desired velocity. This definition is relevant from an exercise delivery perspective as it relates to a number of tasks including the ability to perform both repetitive and discrete movements with the limbs at various speed (i.e. throwing a ball at a target, or performing repetitive split jumps) as well as the ability to achieve optimal segmental control for performing whole body movements such as a maximal jumping, throwing or running.

Coordination is a key component when attempting to maximise performance efficiency of a movement.[4,5] While the coordination of slow movements might be important in some tasks, the demands of many activities are for a coordinated and accurate movement performed at a high velocity. This is of importance to athletes who need to perform optimally in both competition and practice, and for people who are required to perform fast and accurate movements as part of their occupation or leisure activities.

Considerable research has focused on the impact of fatigue on the coordination of movement and has shown significant reductions in movement speed and precision when muscular fatigue is induced. This has significant implications for training. Two considerations should be made relating to training coordination as a neuromotor component.

1. If learning a new skill, the coordination of this skill should be practised with as little local and systemic fatigue as possible to maximise the opportunity for learning, ensure optimal movement timing and reduce timing errors.
2. Training coordination under fatigued conditions may be necessary to improve coordinated performance of repetitive movements in a task that requires endurance.

Important Considerations for Training

In order to train coordination through neuromotor exercise, the first step is to identify the task demands and prescribe exercises that replicate these demands within the individual's current capacity. These exercises are progressed gradually in order to allow the person to complete the task in conditions that replicate the required context.

Worked Case Study for Exercise Prescription for Coordination Training

Aafia is a 17-year-old javelin thrower who has recently won the event at her school's athletics competition. Her parents approach you and ask for advice on how she can improve her throwing distance. After watching her throw, you believe it is important to focus on improving her coordination. You develop the exercise plan in Table 14.3 identifying the aspects of coordination that are important for a javelin thrower and including one exercise to address the components of coordination required for improved performance.

TABLE 14.3 Exercises to Address Aspects of Coordination for A Javelin Thrower		
Aspect of Coordination	**Exercise**	**Rationale**
Joint dynamic stability at end range (muscles firing)	TheraBand shoulder extension at 180° of flexion	The javelin is released at the top of the throwing position, requiring large forces at the end range. This exercise activates the stabilising muscles of the shoulder in a sport-specific position in order to allow for maximal force upon release.
	Wall ball throws	Catching a heavy ball mimics the high forces that are required to coordinate the stabilisers of the shoulder at the end ROM.
Sequencing of proximal to distal muscles (legs to torso to arms)	Cross-body flexion wood chops with cable	This requires the coordination of muscles from the legs to the torso in the same sequence as the required activity with a decreased load.

Activity 14.3 Exercise prescription for coordination

AIM:

- To prescribe coordination exercises

You own a strength and conditioning business that focuses on providing support to underage athletes. Your business has been employed to work with the state's under-17 basketball team that is preparing for the national championships. Your new client is 16 years old and the tallest player on the team. The coach has told you that he will be competing at the starting tip-offs and wants you to provide some exercises to improve his ability to win tip-offs.

TASK:

- Complete Worksheet 14.3 in reference to the basketball tip-off movement for Case study 14.2. Provide exercises and their rationale to improve performance for the two aspects of coordination (from Table 14.3).

Worksheet 14.3 Coordination Case Study

Aspect of coordination	Exercise	Rationale

Functional Exercise Training

Functional training relates to the application of the exercise prescription principle of specificity to design exercises that replicate the demands of activities required for an individual's occupation, sport or leisure activities. For functional training to be effective, the overload principle needs to be applied in order to promote adaptation to the exercises performed. This section uses a worked case study to demonstrate how the individual components of neuromotor exercise may be combined into a sequential, functional training program.

Worked Case Study for Exercise Prescription for Functional Training

Belinda is a 35-year-old female who wishes to take up social tennis to meet new people. Previously she was a runner and had limited experience completing resistance training. She asks for your advice regarding the new sport-specific demands that require consideration in her training program. You develop Table 14.4 that identifies the new demands and one exercise for each of these.

TABLE 14.4   Exercises to Address Demands of Tennis

Demand	Exercise	Notes
Ability to internally rotate and flex the shoulder of her dominant arm in an overhead position (required to serve a ball)	TheraBand internal rotations with the arm at 90° abduction and the TheraBand attached behind	Progressions include a ball being thrown repetitively at a rebounding surface. This will allow force to be generated while the arm is in internal rotation and flexion.

TABLE 14.4 Exercises to Address Demands of Tennis (continued)		
Demand	**Exercise**	**Notes**
Ability to change direction in both the frontal and sagittal planes will mimic moving between the sides of the court and also between the net and the baseline	Multi-directional lunges	This exercise replicates the movement required to take off and change direction. Progressions include increasing speed, with a dumbbell in hand and completing a push-to-press movement and transitioning the lunges to split squats.
Ability to perform trunk rotation and shoulder horizontal flexion/extension simultaneously	Single-arm wood chop	This exercise replicates the movements required to hit a tennis ball. Progressions include continuous repetitions with increased speed, inclusion of a ball and inclusion of a forward step or lunge.
Reaction time for volley pass	As per the exercise for the first demand with addition of a light stimulus that signals when to start and stop the exercise	The exercise described in the first demand will also allow the eccentric absorption of force when catching, which may replicate the requirements of preparing for a fast overhead volley. Progression of the first exercise described to incorporate a reaction time challenge better develops this demand.

Activity 14.5 Exercise prescription for functional fitness

AIM:
- To prescribe exercises for functional fitness

TASKS:
- Using the principles described above, form small groups and choose one of the following three case studies:
  1. an older adult who has an increased risk of falling and is struggling in their community to cross the road
  2. a physical education teacher returning to full-time work teaching athletics, after having twins 6 months ago
  3. a retired gentleman (60 years old) who has spent many years in an office-based job and was predominantly sedentary but would like to climb Mt Kilimanjaro with his wife in 12 months.
- Complete the table with demands that the goal or activity places on the individual, what exercises might be appropriate to meet these demands and your rationale for selecting these exercises.

Worksheet 14.5 Functional Fitness		
Case study: _____		
Demand	**Exercises**	**Rationale**

References

1   Bushman B. 2012. Neuromotor exercise training. *ACSM's Health Fit J.* 16(6):4–7.
2   Woollacott MH, Shumway-Cook A. 1996. Concepts and methods for assessing postural instability. *J Aging Phys Act.* 4:214–33.
3   Samaan MA, Hoch MC, Ringleb SI, Bawab S, Weinhandl JT. 2015. Isolate hamstrings fatigue alters hip and knee joint coordiantion during a cutting maneuver. *J Appl Biomech.* 31(2):102–10.
4   Apriantono T, Nunome H, Ikegami Y, Sano S. 2006. The effect of muscle fatigue on instep kicking kinetics and kinematics in association football. *J Sports Sci.* 24(9):951–60. DOI: 10.1080/02640410500386050

SECTION 3
EXERCISE ADHERENCE

Nicola W. Burton

PROFESSIONAL STANDARDS AND LEARNING OBJECTIVES

Practical 15: Understanding exercise non-adherence

This practical aims to address professional standards related to the following:

- demonstrate practice consistent with client-centred care
- analyse and understand behaviour and behavioural constructs in the health, exercise and sport contexts from an ecological perspective
- identify behaviours non-conducive to exercise participation and/or progression
- identify clients in need of additional strategies for behaviour modification
- examine barriers and their implication for exercise participation and/or progression.

By the end of this practical, it is anticipated that students will be able to:

- identify the key components of assessing exercise non-adherence and calculate a basic rate of exercise non-adherence
- discuss the relative advantages and disadvantages of self-report and objective methods of collecting data related to exercise adherence
- identify and discuss common individual, social and contextual factors that can contribute to exercise non-adherence including personal meaning, instrumental and affective attitudes, knowledge, exercise attributes, exercise experiences, competing demands, social support, cultural norms and exercise settings
- describe the difference between intentional and non-intentional non-adherence
- describe the fundamental attribution error and the implications for understanding exercise non-adherence.

Practical 16: Promoting exercise adherence

This practical aims to address professional standards related to the following:

- strategies for behaviour modification to increase adherence of clients to exercise and manage negative influencing factors
- help clients to work through behaviour change and develop self-management strategies to engage with exercise
- design exercise plans that consider individual factors beyond referral and risk factors to include the client's goals, perspectives, preferences, opportunities, barriers, facilitators, exercise settings and other influencing factors
- understand and demonstrate fundamental behaviour change principles and their application to improving engagement with exercise
- employ motivational techniques to deliver exercise programs and promote engagement in a manner that is sensitive to the specific needs and abilities of clients.

By the end of this practical, it is anticipated that students will be able to:

- discuss and demonstrate a range of strategies that can be used to promote exercise adherence including action planning, competing demand and coping plans, empathic responses, motivational interviewing, optimising support, preference matching, self-regulatory strategies, self-monitoring and values exploration
- discuss the different types of social support, and how practitioners might contribute to each of these to promote exercise adherence
- describe the transtheoretical model and the applied implications of this for exercise adherence
- discuss the potential role of context in exercise adherence
- define exercise efficacy and identify examples of strategies that may impact efficacy
- discuss intrinsic and extrinsic satisfaction in relation to exercise adherence.

Practical 17: Behavioural counselling for exercise

This practical aims to address professional standards related to the following:

- recognise, interpret and demonstrate practice consistent with client-centred care

- design and deliver exercise plans that consider individual factors beyond referral and risk factors to include the client's goals, perspectives, preferences, opportunities, barriers, facilitators, exercise settings and other influencing factors
- illustrate fundamental behaviour change principles and strategies and their application to improving client adherence and lifestyle choices including exercise
- employ behavioural change strategies and revise communication to facilitate mitigation of cognitive, behavioural and other influencing factors on exercise participation/progression
- employ motivational techniques to deliver exercise programs in a manner that is sensitive to the specific needs of clients
- basic counselling, support and communication skills for best practice in delivery of health and exercise advice and to help clients work through behaviour change and develop self-management strategies.

By the end of this practical, it is anticipated that students will be able to:

- describe the key components of person-centred communication and demonstrate client-centred communication (e.g. reflective listening, shared decision-making)
- describe the primary components of the 5A framework for behavioural counselling
- identify key assessment information for exercise behaviour counselling
- describe and demonstrate how to respond to exercise ambivalence using a client-centred approach
- describe and demonstrate the key principles of behavioural counselling for exercise, including client-centred problem-solving.

DEFINITIONS

5As counselling: A specific client-centred framework for behaviour counselling. It identifies five key communication tasks: assess, advise, agree, arrange and assist.

Action planning: A behaviour change technique that involves detailed consideration of the context, frequency, duration and intensity of behaviour to be done. The context can be environmental (physical or social) or intrapersonal (emotions or thoughts).

Adherence: Accordance with an agreed-on, expected, desired or pre-determined standard.

Adherence criterion: A specified level or standard used to define concordance (e.g. 80% of sessions).

Ambivalence: Having mixed feelings or contradictory thoughts.

Appraisal support: Also known as esteem support. The provision of information that contributes to self-evaluation.

Attitude: Thoughts, feelings and actions regarding an entity, with some degree of favour or disfavour.

Attributes of exercise: Characteristics of exercise such as intensity, duration, frequency, complexity and so on.

Behavioural counselling: A conversation-based approach to assist people to adopt, change or maintain behaviour.

Behavioural review: An analysis of the extent to which the desired behaviour was achieved.

Client-centred communication/counselling: An approach that *prioritises* responsiveness to the client's needs and values, and *actively* includes the client in shared decision-making.

Competing demands: Multiple requirements, interests or activities that require a common resource (e.g. time, money).

Context: The circumstances and setting: this can refer to physical, social or other attributes.

Coping plans: A process of identifying and analysing situations when desirable behaviour may lapse *and* generating and selecting strategies to manage this.

Decisional balance: Evaluation of 'pros' (advantages) and 'cons' (disadvantages) of a choice.

Demonstration/modelling: Observable sample of performance to aspire to. This may be done directly (i.e. in person) or indirectly (e.g. via picture).

Efficacy: An individual's belief of their ability to organise and do the behaviour required for the desired outcomes.

Emotional support: An interpersonal process of assistance and caring that targets feelings (e.g. sympathy).

Empathy: The ability to understand and share the feelings of others from their position/context.

Environmental factors: Factors that are physically external to the person, such as availability of resources, accessibility of facilities and climate. This may include the physical built and/or natural context.

Exercise readiness: A process of motivation for, willingness to do and performance of, behaviour.

Experiential attitudes: The affective response (i.e. feelings) about the evaluation of an entity.

Extrinsic satisfaction: Positive reaction associated with external factors of the experience (e.g. rewards/returns).

Feedback: Monitoring and providing information on performance.

Fundamental attribution error: The tendency to explain behaviour based on intrapersonal factors, such as personality or disposition, and to underestimate the influence of external factors, such as social and environmental support.

Informational support: The provision of advice, guidance, suggestions or data that contributes to knowledge.

Instruction: Information on how to perform.

Instrumental attitude: The evaluation of an entity's favourable and unfavourable outcomes.

Instrumental support: The provision of assistance via tangible, material, physical or service means (e.g. providing resources).

Intentional non-adherence: When the person is aware of the discrepancy between the actual and prescribed behaviour.

Intrapersonal factors: Aspects of psychological being that originate from within people, such as attitudes, confidence and motivation.

Intrinsic satisfaction: Positive reaction associated with the intrapersonal experience (e.g. enjoyment).

Motivation: A theoretical construct to explain behaviour, reflecting a desire, need, want or drive, that stimulates action.

Motivational interviewing: A client-centred conversational process to elicit clients' expectations (pros *and* cons), minimise resistance and resolve ambivalence.

Network support: Connections with, and the presence of, others to engage in shared activities/interests and providing a sense of belonging.

Non-adherence: A lack of concordance with an agreed-on, expected, desired or pre-determined standard.

Non-compliant: Used interchangeably with 'nonadherent'. The term is out of favour because of implying a paternalistic and passive process without shared responsibility.

Objective assessment: Information based on observable data or physical measures (e.g. attendance records, heart rate).

Outcome review: An analysis of the extent to which desired outcomes were achieved.

Partial adherence: Performance that is in part, but not wholly, in accordance with an agreed-on, expected, desired or pre-determined standard.

Problem-solving: A process of identifying and analysing behavioural influences *and* generating and selecting strategies to overcome barriers and increase enablers.

Reward: Experience or event occurring after performance that promotes repeat performance. Rewards may be verbal, non-verbal, material or social.

Satisfaction: Fulfilment of desires, expectations or needs.

Self-monitoring: A method by which someone tracks their own action and performance. This can focus on thoughts, feelings, behaviour, or outcomes or related processes.

Self-regulation: Processes by which people manage their own behaviour (e.g. goal setting, planning, scheduling, problem-solving, rewards, prompts).

Social connections: The experience of belonging, feeling close to others or being part of a network of people.

Social desirability: A potential source of bias where someone responds in a manner which they think will be viewed favourably (e.g. over-reporting 'good' behaviour or underreporting 'bad' behaviour).

Social/relational factors: Processes that occur between and among people, such as support, discouragement and norms.

Social support: An interpersonal process of assistance and caring; this can include emotional, material, informational and network components.

Subjective assessment: Information based on self-report (e.g. data from questionnaires, practitioner opinions).

Transtheoretical model: A framework to understand motivational readiness. It includes five stages: precontemplation (not considering action); contemplation (considering action); preparation (intention to take action); action (initiation) and maintenance (sustained action over time).

Unintentional non-adherence: When the person is not aware of the discrepancy between the actual and prescribed behaviour.

Value: A principle or standard of what is important, meaningful and of worth.

Values exploration: A process to identify the principles or standard of what is important, meaningful and of worth.

Walkability: the extent to which an area enables walking; this is determined by factors such as traffic, aesthetics, destinations and safety.

PRACTICAL 15
UNDERSTANDING EXERCISE NON-ADHERENCE

Nicola W. Burton

Introduction

Behavioural adherence is the extent to which a person acts in accordance with an agreed on, expected, desired or pre-determined standard (such as professional advice). Exercise non-adherence is, therefore, exercise behaviour that is inconsistent with exercise advice, recommendations or prescriptions.

Although typically interpreted as *under* performance (i.e. not doing enough), exercise non-adherence also includes *over* performance (i.e. doing too much) which can also be undesirable in some contexts (e.g. exceeding exercise rehabilitation recommendations can increase risk of injury, over training can increase risk of exhaustion).

Although the terms can be used interchangeably, contemporary practice is to use '*non-adherent*' rather than '*non-compliant*'. 'Compliance' is interpreted as indicating a paternalistic and passive process, with the non-compliant person seen as deviant or incapable. Many behavioural practitioners, therefore, prefer to use 'adherence' or 'concordance' to imply a shared responsibility for behaviour, and that non-adherence reflects a complex interplay of multi-level factors.

This practical will discuss how to collect information on and quantify exercise non-adherence. It will also highlight key exercise, personal, social and environmental factors that may contribute to exercise non-adherence.

Implications of Assessing Exercise Non-adherence

Non-adherence is typically assessed for a specific group of people, site, type of behaviour or context. The following are some statements from research about exercise nonadherence.

- In older adults with diabetes, 55% to 75% were not meeting physical activity guidelines.[1]
- Of older adults attending community-based exercise programs, 14% to 35% did not complete the program, and the proportion of available sessions not attended ranged from 23% to 64%.[2]
- Non-adherence for exercise interventions targeting bone mineral density in adults was 24%, with dropout rates averaging 21% in the exercise groups and 16% in the control groups.[3]
- The proportion of people with depression not meeting activity guidelines was higher in studies using objective versus self-report measures (86% versus 62%).[4] The overall dropout rate across exercise interventions was 17%.[5]
- Non-uptake of exercise referral schemes ranged from 19% to 34% and non-adherence was 51% to 57%, with women more likely to begin, but less likely to adhere, than men.[6]
- Although the uptake of exercise programs varied markedly, non-adherence rates were low, ranging from 2% to 32% for supervised programs, 6% to 30% for home-based programs and 19% for programs with both supervised and home-based components.[7] Low adherence with established physical activity and cancer prevention guidelines was associated with increases in cancer incidence and mortality overall.[8]
- Non-adherence was 18% for people doing moderate-intensity aerobic and resistance training, and 25% for those doing high-intensity interval functional training (HIFT), with HIFT dropouts reporting lower baseline exercise enjoyment than participants.[9]
- Approximately 60% of heart failure patients did weekly training sessions below the recommended 90 minutes per week; this is likely to have contributed to the considerably smaller than expected increments in peak oxygen uptake (peak $\dot{V}O_2$) and 6-minute walking distance. Adherence to larger exercise volumes resulted in significantly greater benefits in peak $\dot{V}O_2$.[10]

Such information on exercise non-adherence can be used to, for example:

- identify who is less likely to engage with exercise, and therefore priority groups to target
- determine or compare acceptability and feasibility of exercise interventions and components
- justify and inform resources/interventions to support exercise engagement
- provide a rationale for/against a specific approach to exercise programming
- understand the relationships between exercise and outcomes
- inform the development of a business case (e.g. likely uptake/completion of exercise training programs and required resources).

Assessing Non-adherence Rates

There are four stages in determining exercise non-adherence rates.

1. Define the behaviour.
2. Collect related information.
3. Calculate rates.
4. Define criteria for non-adherence.

Define the Behaviour

The previous statements about exercise non-adherence refer to different types of behaviour; for example, not commencing, not attending sessions, not completing an exercise program or not meeting exercise specifications. An important aspect of measuring exercise non-adherence is, therefore, to specify *what* behaviour is being considered.

As exercise behaviour can be described in terms of frequency, intensity, interval, type and duration (see Table 15.1), exercise non-adherence can also be assessed across these dimensions. Non-adherence may also refer to other qualitative aspects of exercise (e.g. technique, equipment used). These components of exercise behaviour may be considered separately or in combination; the more elements involved in defining adherence, the more likely it is that people will be identified as non-adherent.

TABLE 15.1	**Components of Exercise Behaviour That Can Be Used to Define Non-adherence**	
Component	**Definition**	**Examples**
Frequency	The number of times the exercise is done in a specified frame of reference	• 3 sessions per week • 10 repetitions per set
Intensity	The physiological effort required to perform the exercise	• $> 50\%$ of maximum heart rate • Light, moderate, vigorous, high • Rating of perceived exertion $\geq 7/10$
Intervals	The ratio of exercises done in a specified frame of reference	• Alternating high-intensity bouts of exercise with moderate-intensity bouts during the session • Alternating chest and leg exercises during the week • Continuous exercise (no intervals) during the session
Type	The style of exercise	• Resistance, aerobic, anaerobic • Yoga, walking, cycling, swimming, weights • Low impact, high impact • Leg extension, chest press

TABLE 15.1 Components of Exercise Behaviour That Can Be Used to Define Non-adherence (continued)		
Component	**Definition**	**Examples**
Duration	The period of time for exercise	• 30-minute sessions • ≥ 150 mins/week
Technique	Style parameters	• Sitting • Slowly • With small increments
Setting	Location and characteristics of physical and social context	• Home based, facility based • Supervised, unsupervised • Group, individual

Collect Related Information

Once the behaviour of interest is defined, data on adherence and non-adherence can be collected using a range of methods.

Subjective methods involve client self-report and include behaviour logs, visual analogue scales, interviews, questionnaires and ratings. Clients can be asked to provide information on various dimensions of exercise (i.e. frequency, duration, weights used, perceived exertion). Additional descriptive information can also be obtained to understand non-adherence, such as affective state and associated cognitions (i.e. feelings and thoughts).

Objective methods are based on observation or physical measures and include attendance records, observer recordings, behaviour monitoring and physiological monitoring. Records of attendance can be maintained manually or derived from other sources (e.g. electronic records from secure access to exercise facilities). Observers can record specific components of exercise behaviour. Behavioural monitors such as pedometers provide information on steps/day and accelerometers measure acceleration during movement. Physiological monitors can be used to record heart rate and other indicators of performance.

Objective and subjective methods of collecting data on exercise adherence and non-adherence have relative advantages and disadvantages in terms of client/practitioner burden, acceptability, cost, intrusiveness, precision/accuracy, vulnerability to bias (e.g. recall, social desirability), type of data provided and appropriateness for exercise type.

Activity 15.1 Self-report and objective measures of collecting exercise non-adherence data

For each of the following methods to assess exercise non-adherence, consider the potential advantages and disadvantages in terms of client/practitioner burden, cost, intrusiveness, precision/accuracy and vulnerability to bias (e.g. recall, social desirability).

Also consider the type of data provided and (in)appropriateness for specific types of exercise data.

An example response is provided for the first method.

Method	Advantages	Disadvantages
Telephone interview	• Low equipment cost versus physiological monitoring • Vulnerable to social and recall bias • Good for descriptive information (can use clarification and follow-up probes) • Means participant does not have to come in to facility	• Time burden for practitioner • Could be intrusive for client • High cost compared to questionnaires • Poor precision

Method	Advantages	Disadvantages
Participant diary		
Recall questionnaire		
Perceived exertion rating by client		
Perceived exertion rating by practitioner		
Observer recording of exercise attendance		
Observer recording of exercise performance		
Pedometer data on steps/day		
Accelerometer data on time spent in moderate to vigorous intensity activity		
Heart rate monitoring		

Calculate Rates

Exercise non-adherence is often evaluated in a defined period (e.g. a session or week), or for the program duration. A common unit of measurement for adherence is the amount of behaviour done per defined time period as a proportion of prescribed exercise for the same period. For example:

- (number of sessions done in past week ÷ number of sessions prescribed for the week) $\times$ 100%
- (number of sessions attended during the exercise program ÷ number of sessions prescribed for the exercise program) $\times$ 100%
- (total amount of time spent in exercise during past month ÷ total amount of time exercise prescribed for a month) $\times$ 100%
- (number of sessions target heart rate met during exercise sessions ÷ total number of exercise sessions during the training) $\times$ 100%
- (number of people actioning an exercise referral during a year ÷ number of exercise referrals made during the year) $\times$ 100%.

Define Criteria

What level of behaviour constitutes adherence and non-adherence is often arbitrarily defined, and **good practice is to report these criteria**. Adherence criteria can be based on different requirements such as the minimal 'dose' required to achieve benefits, formal recommendations of exercise dose, the number of training sessions considered necessary to observe clinically meaningful changes, and so on. Adherence criteria could represent a logistic minimum (e.g. the number of people attending an exercise training program to make it a financially viable proposition over time, or the number of sessions to be completed to receive an award/prize).

Some measures of adherence and non-adherence involve a simple dichotomy (e.g. meeting/not meeting recommendations to do $\geq$ 150 minutes per week of exercise). For other types of data, a common criterion for *adherence* is $\geq$ 80%. This could be operationalised as, for example:

- attending $\geq$ 80% of training sessions during a 12-week exercise program
- completing $\geq$ 80% of the total time recommended for exercise during the week
- achieving $\geq$ 80% of the target heart rate during exercise training sessions.

Activity 15.2 Calculating exercise non-adherence rates

You are implementing a group training program for 10 people. The program involves two training sessions a week for 10 weeks and attendance records were kept for each session.

Session Attendance

Id	1	2	3	4	5	6	7	8	9	10	11	12	13	14	15	16	17	18	19	20
1	Y	Y	Y	Y	Y	Y	Y	Y	Y	Y	Y	Y	Y	N	Y	Y	Y	Y	Y	Y
2	Y	N	Y	Y	Y	Y	Y	N	Y	Y	Y	Y	N	N	Y	Y	Y	Y	Y	Y
3	N	Y	Y	Y	Y	Y	Y	Y	N	Y	Y	Y	Y	Y	N	N	Y	Y	Y	Y
4	Y	Y	Y	Y	Y	Y	N	Y	N	Y	N	Y	Y	Y	Y	Y	Y	Y	Y	Y
5	Y	Y	N	N	N	N	N	N	N	N	N	N	N	N	N	N	N	N	N	N
6	Y	Y	Y	Y	Y	Y	Y	Y	Y	Y	Y	Y	Y	Y	Y	Y	N	N	N	N
7	N	Y	Y	Y	Y	Y	Y	Y	Y	Y	Y	Y	N	Y	N	Y	N	Y	N	Y
8	Y	Y	Y	Y	Y	Y	Y	Y	Y	Y	Y	Y	Y	Y	N	Y	N	Y	Y	Y
9	Y	Y	Y	Y	Y	N	Y	Y	Y	Y	N	Y	Y	Y	Y	Y	Y	N	Y	Y
10	Y	Y	N	Y	Y	Y	Y	Y	Y	Y	Y	Y	N	N	Y	Y	N	Y	Y	Y

1. What is the overall rate of non-adherence for session attendance across the program?

_____

2. How would you describe non-adherence for session attendance during the first versus second half of the program?

_____

3. Using the criterion of 75% session attendance to indicate program adherence, what proportion of clients were non-adherent?

_____

4. Using the criterion of 80% session attendance to indicate program adherence, what proportion of clients were non-adherent?

_____

5. Using the criterion of 85% session attendance to indicate program adherence, what proportion of clients were non-adherent?

_____

6. Given your answers to Questions 4, 5 and 6, what do you conclude about the potential impact of different criteria on non-adherence?

_____

_____

The simple corollary to this is a criterion of $<$ 80% for *non-adherence*; for example:

- attending $<$ 80% of training sessions during a 12-week exercise program
- completing $<$ 80% of the total time recommended for exercise during the week
- achieving $<$ 80% of the target heart rate during exercise training sessions.

To increase sensitivity, additional criteria may be used to indicate *partial* adherence; for example:

- non-adherence was defined as attending $<$ 50% of available training sessions, partial adherence was defined as attending 51% to 79% of available sessions, and adherence was defined as attending $\geq$ 80% of available sessions during the 12-week program
- non-adherence was defined as completing $<$ 30% of the total time recommended for exercise during the week, low adherence was defined as 30% to 50%, moderate adherence as 51% to 85%, and high adherence as $\geq$ 85%
- achieving 75% to 99% of the target heart rate during training sessions was categorised as partial adherence and achieving $<$ 75% was categorised as non-adherence.

Partial adherence can be used to describe behaviour that reflects, but is not completely consistent with, the prescription. Partial adherence reflects the multidimensional aspect of exercise prescription. It can also reflect that benefits can still be obtained from exercise different from that prescribed, or that clients are making some progress. Partial adherence can enable examination of dose response relationships. It can also facilitate critical reflection of the exercise prescription to inform strategies to promote adherence. If someone adheres to one component of the exercise prescription and not another, considering how these components differ may indicate how the program could be modified to optimise engagement. For example, someone may engage more with exercise of high frequency and short duration than exercise of low frequency and long duration.

MAKE-UPP: a Framework for Understanding Factors Contributing to Exercise Non-adherence

An understanding of the factors associated with exercise non-adherence can come from client conversations, questionnaires or telephone interviews; from observation; and from information from significant others and external sources or theories of behaviour. This understanding can inform the development of strategies to promote exercise adherence.

Exercise non-adherence has been associated with a range of modifiable and non-modifiable factors including:

- *sociodemographics*; for example, age, gender, socioeconomic status (education, income), occupation and employment status
- *health and wellbeing*; for example, general health, health conditions, condition-related symptoms, medication effects, physical limitations, comorbidities, injury, mood, stress and fatigue
- *exercise attributes*; for example, type, intensity, duration, resources required, complexity, perceived burden, competence/skill required, consistency with preferences/interests and associated pain/ discomfort
- *intrapersonal factors*; for example, confidence, enjoyment, exercise beliefs/attitudes (e.g. personal salience, outcome expectations, perceived value, perceived effort/risks), knowledge and motivation
- *social/relational factors*; for example, support, stigma, social cohesion, caring responsibilities, practitioner advice, practitioner–client relationship, life events, sociocultural norms
- *environmental factors*; for example, accessibility and availability, costs, safety, climate, aesthetics, convenience and policy.

The MAKE-UPP acronym is a way to think about key factors potentially contributing to non-adherence, and can be used by practitioners in exercise and sport contexts.

Motivation/meaning

Attitudes

Knowledge

Exercise experiences and attributes

Understand competing demands

People

Place

Motivation/meaning

Lack of motivation is a common explanation for exercise non-adherence. Motivation is a theoretical construct to explain behaviour, and reflects a desire, need, want or drive that stimulates individuals to action. The salience of exercise motives differs by age, gender, health, personality, physical activity level, stage of exercise (initiation, maintenance) and other personal circumstances.

Activity 15.3 Differences in exercise motives by age, gender, activity level, personality and socioeconomic status

The following statements are from research on exercise motives. For each sentence, select one answer from the options within the curly brackets to identify which group you think matches the information provided.

1. Motivators for {young/middle-aged/older} adults participating in resistance training included preventing disability, reducing risk of falls, building muscles (toning), feeling alert and better concentration.[11]

2. Social contact with other participants was a primary reason for {men's/women's} adherence during the program, and a desire to maintain wellness benefits derived during the program was the reason for continuing exercise after the program.[12]

3. Motives of mastery, fitness, social aspects, enjoyment and appearance were more important to {inactive/active people} and conforming to others' expectations was higher for {inactive/active} people.[13]

4. {Men/Women} endorsed mood improvement more as a motive for exercise.[14]

5. During {young/middle-aged} adulthood, {men/women} reported greater weight control motivation and during {young/middle-aged} adulthood, {men/women} reported greater weight control motivation.[14]

6. {Introverts/Extroverts} were more likely to endorse exercise motivations of general appearance and enjoyment.[14]

7. Rehabilitation from health conditions, and seeing similarly aged people exercising, were described as motivators among the {low/high} socioeconomic status group.[15]

8. {Men/Women} reported higher motivation for appearance and physical condition, and {men/women} were more motivated by competition and mastery.[16]

9. {Young/Middle-aged} adults reported higher mastery and enjoyment exercise motives, and {young/middle-aged} adults reported others' expectations as important exercise motives.[16]

10. Extrinsic motives {e.g. appearance, weight management} were more dominant during {early/maintenance} stages of exercise. Intrinsic motives {enjoyment and revitalisation} were more dominant during {early/maintenance} stages.[17]

11. Social benefits and life balance were more salient exercise motives to {low/high} socioeconomic status participants.[18]

12. {Introversion/Extroversion} was more likely to correlate with exercise motives of socialisation and meeting people, and {introversion/extroversion} was more likely to correlate with motives of stress relief.[19]

13. {Middle-aged/older} women reported greater health commitment than {middle-aged/older} women.[20]

Motivation is low when behaviour has a low personal value, or a personal meaning that conflicts with other needs/values. For example, exercise to 'stay healthy' may have little value to someone who sees themself as already healthy and unlikely to become ill.[18] Exercise may have a personal meaning of hard work (which could conflict with a value of relaxation), being seen as non-competitive (which could conflict with a value of achievement or competence) or less free time to spend with friends (which could conflict with a value of being social).[18] People can act on the same value in different ways; for example, 'being a good mother' may motivate one woman to exercise so as to be a role model for her children, but motivate another woman not to exercise so as to spend more time with her children.[21]

Activity 15.4 Exercise meaning and values

Collect exercise meaning statements from three different people. Ask 'What does that exercise mean to you?' If possible, ask the person about an exercise they do not do, or is not motivated to do; for example, if someone does swimming and not weights training, then ask about weights training.

What values are suggested by these meaning statements? Check your values interpretation with the person who provided the meaning statement. Is this right or not? Is it in conflict with a core value? For example, a personal meaning of exercise as 'hard work' could be consistent with a value of pushing oneself to the limits, or in conflict with a value of taking things easy. Does the value have high or low personal salience?

Exercise and meaning statement	Suggested value	Value check
Cycling: Cycling around here means being on busy roads, as I live in a busy area and there are no off-road cycle paths. That would worry me.	Safety	Highly salient
Exercise class: Doing an exercise class means having to watch the clock to be sure I get away from work on time, and that means I can't always finish the task I am working on.	Flexibility, task completion	Conflict
Walking: To me walking means getting outdoors and being close to nature and that's important to clear my head.	Being in nature	Highly salient
1.		
2.		
3.		

Attitudes

Attitudes refer to thoughts, feelings and actions regarding an entity, with some degree of favour or disfavour. Instrumental attitudes are the evaluation of the behaviour's outcomes (i.e. consequences) and experiential attitudes are the affective response (i.e. feelings) about the behaviour itself.

Instrumental attitudes involve an evaluation of both positive *and* negative outcomes. Behaviour theories with a decisional balance process purport that potential benefits are weighed up against perceived costs ('pros' vs 'cons'). Costs refer to what must be given up or an unfavourable impact. Financial costs are commonly identified as a barrier to organised exercise and sport,[22,23] and may be highly salient among those who are socioeconomically disadvantaged,[24] culturally diverse or disabled,[23] or older and with chronic conditions.[25] Non-financial costs of exercise include time, energy, pain, etc. Exercise non-adherence is likely when the perceived costs outweigh the potential benefits.[1,26,27]

Affective attitudes predict exercise intentions and behaviour, and may be a better predictor than instrumental attitudes.[28–33] Positive affective responses include pleasure, energy, pride and so on; and negative responses include dislike, frustration, fear, anger, distress, anxiety, embarrassment and so on. Affective attitudes are influenced by perceptions of competence,[34] and poor fitness is a predictor of dropout.[35] People often expect exercise to be less pleasant than the actual experience,[36] and anticipated negative affect is a strong predictor of (low) physical activity intentions among inactive people.[37] Low active people experience less positive affect during exercise than active people.[38] Affective responses can be influenced by exercise intensity, with reductions in pleasure mainly above the ventilatory or lactate threshold or the onset of blood lactate accumulation.[39]

Activity 15.5 Exercise attitudes and costs
. . . .

Identify five examples of specific behaviour that could indicate that a client has a negative attitude to an exercise or exercise program. Consider both verbal and non-verbal actions.

1. _____
2. _____
3. _____
4. _____
5. _____

Identify five potential costs/cons of exercise and sport that could contribute to non-adherence.

1. _____
2. _____
3. _____
4. _____
5. _____

Knowledge

The majority of people know that exercise is beneficial; however, there can be misunderstandings about condition-specific benefits and inherent risks. For example, the benefits of exercise for cancer and neurological conditions are less understood than for cardiovascular conditions.[40] The benefits for serious mental illness, such as schizophrenia, are less understood by patients[41] or mental health professionals[42] than for other conditions such as depression. Intermittent claudication is a symptom where the person experiences pain (often in the leg) which begins during exercise and is relieved by rest. People with intermittent claudication can be unaware of the role of exercise in improving symptoms and reducing risk of mortality, and believe that pain experienced during walking is harmful.[43] Older adults may think that resistance training increases the risk of a heart attack or stroke,[11] or that exercise will exacerbate preexisting health problems or result in physical harm.[44,45] People may consider themselves too old or unwell to derive benefits from exercise.[18,46]

Clients may have a limited understanding of exercise requirements. Some people think they are already sufficiently active[47-51] (e.g. from other exercise, occupational activities or general life busyness). Clients may not understand what to do[48] or how to exercise safely.[45] Lack of confidence in operating gym equipment is a barrier to adherence.[22] Clients may exceed the prescribed dose of exercise because of a misbelief that this will speed up recovery. Similarly, the belief of 'no pain, no gain' may precipitate clients to persist with exercise beyond a safe level.

Exercise Experiences and Attributes

Personal experiences of exercise are a major source of both affective and instrumental attitudes. Exercise experiences can also be vicarious; that is, learned from others such as friends, family or online information. It is a key principle of behaviour theory that negative consequences—either the presence of an aversive event (positive punishment) or the absence/removal of a pleasant experience (negative punishment)—decrease the likelihood of the behaviour being repeated. Therefore, clients with aversive past exercise experiences, who lack positive experiences or who know others with aversive exercise experiences, are at risk of non-adherence.

Past behaviour is a predictor of future behaviour. Physical activity or sports participation in adolescence, early adulthood or mid-adulthood is positively associated with participation in later stages of life.[52-56] This association is stronger for a high number of types of activity[57] and for people with an athletic self-concept.[58] Therefore, clients with a limited experience of exercise or who have a poor self-concept related to physical activity are at risk of non-adherence. Clients with a history of poor adherence are likely to be non-adherent.[59]

Activity 15.6 Exercise experiences contributing to negative attitudes

Describe five exercise experiences that could contribute to a negative attitude about exercise.

1. _____
   _____
   _____

2. _____
   _____
   _____

3. _____
   _____
   _____

4. _____
   _____
   _____

5. _____
   _____
   _____

Exercise attributes can also impact on adherence. Exercise programs perceived as low variety, complex, inflexible or overly restrictive can have poor adherence.[60-62] Increased pain during exercise is associated with poor adherence in rehabilitation clients;[59] this may also apply to experiences of discomfort, nausea, weakness, dizziness, physiological instability and so on. Exercise considered to be unsafe can discourage people who are worried about falling, or who have comorbidities or a critical illness.[45,63] Some types of exercise may not appeal because of being perceived as more suited for the opposite gender[64,65] or embarrassing (e.g. water-based activities that require overweight people to be seen in swimwear).[66]

Understand Competing Demands

'Competing demands' or 'lack of time' is a commonly identified barrier to exercise.[24,45,48,51,67-70] The nature and source of this differs among people; for example, work demands, irregular hours (such as shift work), family and/or child care responsibilities, other caring activities, study, travel requirements. Poor health or wellbeing can create competing demands of stress, fatigue, pain, low energy, weakness and low/negative mood.[1,25,41,50,59,63,71-74] Competing demands may also come from more appealing activities (e.g. socialising, screen use, sedentary leisure).[75] Some competing demands may be episodic (e.g. holidays).[76] People with low confidence to overcome exercise barriers are more likely to drop out of exercise.[77]

Activity 15.7 Exercise competing demands

Ask three people about major competing demands against exercise; for example, 'What are the main activities or interests in your life that can make it difficult for you to exercise?'

Ask each person to rate their confidence in managing these competing demands (e.g. on a scale of 1 to 10, where 1 is low and 10 is high confidence).

1. _____
2. _____
3. _____

People

Group or public settings can create social barriers to exercise adherence. Clients in group-based activities may have unsatisfactory interactions with, or not relate to, other participants. Overweight people can feel embarrassed and intimidated about exercising around young, fit and healthy-weight people.[78,79] Perceived stigma or an expectation of discrimination is an exercise barrier among people with obesity[80] and people with mental illness.[81] Inactive or older people are concerned about slowing others down.[45,82] Older adults may feel a social awkwardness about groups that involve people of different ages or physical capabilities.[45] Perceived pressure to keep up and complete exercises can lead to a sense of incompetence and disconnection from others.[45] Unfavourable upward social comparisons (i.e. seeing others doing better) can be aversive for women.[83] A male-oriented exercise culture may discourage participation by women,[83] and programs perceived as for women can discourage men.[64] Sociocultural issues can be a barrier[23,46] and some cultures may have specific social requirements (e.g. gender segregation).[84] Privacy concerns may discourage employees from participating in workplace programs.[85] Employers/managers may be perceived as not supporting movement breaks in the workplace because of concerns for productivity.[86] Low social cohesion in neighbourhoods reduces the likelihood of older adults walking for exercise.[87]

Lack of social support contributes to exercise non-adherence. Isolated or vulnerable people such as some older adults,[46] those with mental illness[88] or the culturally diverse[23] may lack support and companionship for exercise. Lack of company may be an issue for middle-aged and older adults,[48] and those concerned about safety when exercising.[1] Divorce/separation or having a weak social network is associated with low physical activity in men.[89] Carers can overestimate the difficulty of activities[63] and actively discourage exercise in others because of overprotective concerns.[45,63] Adolescents from socioeconomically disadvantaged backgrounds can lack exercise role models.[90] Women commonly report having children as a constraint against exercise,[91] and can lack support to overcome barriers associated with child care and housework.[84] People who are frail may be reliant on others to assist with transportation.[45] Perceptions of a lack of management support can discourage employees from attending workplace programs.[92] Media images may have a negative impact on exercise engagement.[93]

Activity 15.8 Social influences on exercise non-adherence

Describe a social interaction in an exercise or sport context that impacted negatively on your/someone else's participation.

_____

_____

_____

_____

_____

_____

_____

_____

_____

Exercise non-adherence may be a consequence of clients' negative reactions to exercise practitioners. Overweight people feel more embarrassed and intimidated about health club salespeople than non-overweight people.[78] Exercise supervision/leadership characterised by general instruction and technical feedback, low interaction and encouragement, lack of a personally meaningful rationale for exercise, lack of choice, non-individualised feedback and discouragement of questions can compromise participants' enjoyment, attendance, motivation and intentions to continue.[94–98] Clients who feel unsupported during exercise training programs are at risk of non-adherence.[99]

Activity 15.9 Social influences on exercise non-adherence

Identify five potential indicators of an unsatisfactory relationship between an exercise practitioner and client. Consider verbal and non-verbal indicators, as well as inter- and intrapersonal indicators.

1. _____

   _____

2. _____

   _____

3. _____

   _____

4. _____

   _____

5. _____

   _____

Place

The physical setting of exercise can contribute to non-adherence. Accessibility may be constrained by inconvenient schedules[100] or transportation/travel difficulties, especially for those who are older, are disabled, are socioeconomically disadvantaged or have chronic conditions.[23,25,46,101] Fitness facilities can be intimidating[82,102] and poor-quality facilities discourage use.[103] A lack of showers, change rooms and lockers makes it difficult for employees to engage with exercise opportunities onsite or around work times (e.g. walking/cycling to work).[104]

Walking outdoors for exercise may be constrained by 'low walkability' areas; that is, few destinations (e.g. parks, services, shops), no or poor-quality footpaths and pedestrian infrastructure, poor aesthetics (e.g. little green space, unclean, litter, graffiti, pollution), poor traffic control, low residential density and limited street connectivity.[105–109] Safety fears can be salient for women and older adults,[84,110] and reflect concerns with poor street lighting, uncontrolled dogs, rowdy youth or crime. Parents may have safety concerns for children walking and cycling in the local area.[111] Unlevel floor surfaces, poor lighting, no rest areas/benches, and trip hazards can constrain walking in public spaces.[101,108]

Activity 15.10 Place factors related to exercise non-adherence
· ·

Identify five characteristics of an exercise setting that could discourage use. Consider a range of settings (e.g. indoors, outdoors, commercial facilities, residential facilities).

1. _____
   _____

2. _____
   _____

3. _____
   _____

4. _____
   _____

5. _____
   _____

The Fundamental Attribution Error

Exercise non-adherence can be categorised as intentional or non-intentional. Non-adherence is *intentional* when done deliberately by the person with awareness of the discrepancy between actual and desired behaviour. Intentional non-adherence may <u>not</u> be spiteful or malicious, and may instead be an informed choice reflecting for example, limited resources, perceptions of potential harm/risk, aversive exercise experiences etc. *Unintentional* non-adherence is when the person is not aware of the discrepancy between the actual and prescribed behaviour. This can reflect issues related to knowledge, such as an inaccurate or misunderstanding of the role of exercise and what or how exercise is to be done. Non-intentional non-adherence could be due to inaccurate or reduced capacity for monitoring of exercise, poor insight or conflicting information.

The *fundamental attribution error* is the tendency to explain behaviour based on intrapersonal factors, such as personality or disposition, and to underestimate the influence of external factors, such as social and environmental support. In the exercise context, this tendency would attribute clients' non-adherence as intentional because of, for example, laziness or a lack of motivation. While this may be true for some clients, it is a narrow and unhelpful explanation that does not acknowledge or prompt consideration of multilevel factors or proactive strategies to optimise adherence.

Summary

Understanding exercise non-adherence can help identify priority target groups, determine feasibility and acceptability, explain exercise outcomes, justify resource allocation and specific approaches and inform strategies to optimise exercise engagement. Assessing exercise non-adherence involves defining engagement criteria across specific dimensions of behaviour, and comparing actual and desired behaviour against an established criterion. Exercise non-adherence data can be collected using self-report or objective methods, which each have relative advantages and disadvantages. Criteria for adherence and non-adherence are often set arbitrarily, and so should be clearly specified.

The MAKE-UPP acronym provides a framework to identify key modifiable factors potentially contributing to exercise non-adherence and includes:

- motivation and personal meaning of behaviour
- attitudes: affective and instrumental
- knowledge
- exercise experiences and attributes
- understanding competing demands
- people: social barriers, lack of support and poor/unsatisfactory relationships with practitioners
- place: the physical setting of exercise including accessibility, aesthetics and characteristics.

Non-adherence can be intentional or unintentional. The fundamental attribution error refers to the tendency to attribute behaviour, such as exercise non-adherence, to dispositional factors and underestimate other situational factors. This constrains consideration of opportunities to promote adherence.

Activity Answers: Understanding Exercise Non-adherence

Activity 15.2

1. $48 \div 200 \times 100\% = 24\%$

2. Non-adherence almost doubled in second half of program: $(17 \div 100) \times 100\%$ versus $(31 \div 100) \times 100\%$

3. 75% adherence is 15/20 sessions: 10% were non-adherent

4. 80% adherence is 16/20 sessions: 20% were non-adherent

5. 85% adherence is 17/20 sessions: 70% were non-adherent

6. High criterion values increase rates of non-adherence. Impressions and results for non-adherence can be easily manipulated to be less or more favourable.

Activity 15.3

1. older

2. women's

3. active people; inactive people

4. Women

5. young; women; middle-aged; men

6. Extroverts

7. high

8. Women; men

9. Young; middle-aged

10. early; maintenance

11. high

12. Extroversion, extroversion

13. Older; middle-aged

References

1 Qiu S, Sun Z, Cai X, et al. 2012. Improving patients' adherence to physical activity in diabetes mellitus: A review. *Diabetes Metab J.* 36(1):1–5.

2 Picorelli A, Pereira L, Pereira D, et al. 2014. Adherence to exercise programs for older people is influenced by program characteristics and personal factors: a systematic review. *J Physiother.* 60(3):151–156.

3 Kelley G, Kelley K. 2013. Dropouts and compliance in exercise interventions targeting bone mineral density in adults: a metaanalysis of randomized controlled trials. *J Osteoporos.* 250423.

4 Schuch F, Vancampfort D, Firth J, et al. 2017. Physical activity and sedentary behavior in people with major depressive disorder: A systematic review and meta-analysis. *J Affect Disord.* 210:139–150.

5 Stubbs B, Vancampfort D, Rosenbaum S, et al. 2016. Dropout from exercise randomized controlled trials among people with depression: A meta-analysis and meta regression. *J Affect Disord.* 190:457–466.

6 Pavey T, Taylor A, Hillsdon M, et al. 2012. Levels and predictors of exercise referral scheme uptake and adherence: a systematic review. *J Epidemiol Community Health.* 66:737–744.

7 Szymlek-Gay E, Richards R, Egan R. 2011. Physical activity among cancer survivors: a literature review. *N Z Med J.* 124(1337):77–89.

8 Kohler L, Garcia D, Harris R, et al. 2016. Adherence to diet and physical activity cancer prevention guidelines and cancer outcomes: A systematic review. *Cancer Epidemiol Biomark Prev.* 25(7):1018–1028.

9 Heinrich K, Patel P, O'Neal J, Heinrich B. 2014. High-intensity compared to moderate-intensity training for exercise initiation, enjoyment, adherence, and intentions: an intervention study. *BMC Public Health.* 14:789.

10   Conraads VM, Deaton C, Piotrowicz E, et al. 2012. Adherence of heart failure patients to exercise: barriers and possible solutions. *Eur J Heart Fail.* 14(5):451–458.

11   Burton E, Farrier K, Lewin G, et al. 2017. Motivators and barriers for older people participating in resistance training: A systematic review. *J Aging Phys Act.* 25(2):311–324.

12   Viljoen J, Christie C. 2015. The change in motivating factors influencing commencement, adherence and retention to a supervised resistance training programme in previously sedentary post-menopausal women: a prospective cohort study. *BMC Public Health*, 15:236.

13   Aaltonen S, Rottensteiner M, Kaprio J, Kujala U. 2014. Motives for physical activity among active and inactive persons in their mid30s. *Scand J Med Sci Sports.* 24(4):727–735.

14   Davis C, Fox J, Brewer H, Ratusny D. 1995. Motivations to exercise as a function of personality characteristics, age, and gender. *Pers Indiv Diff.* 19(2):165–174.

15   Gray P, Murphy M, Gallagher A, Simpson E. 2016. Motives and barriers to physical activity among older adults of different socioeconomic status. *J Aging Phys Act.* 24(3):419–429.

16   Patel AS, Schofield GM, Kolt GS, Keogh JWL. 2013. Perceived barriers, benefits, and motives for physical activity: two primary-care physical activity prescription programs. *J Aging Phys Act.* 21(1):85–99.

17   Ingledew D, Markland D, Medley A. 1998. Exercise motives and stages of change. *J Health Psychol.* 3(4):477–489.

18   Burton NW, Turrell G, Oldenburg B. 2003. Participation in recreational physical activity: why do socioeconomic groups differ? *Health Educ Behav.* 30(2):225–244.

19   Courneya KS, Hellsten LAM. 1998. Personality correlates of exercise behavior, motive, barriers and preferences – an application of the five-factor model. *Pers Indiv Differ.* 24(5):625–633.

20   Holahan C, Holahan C, Li X, Chen Y. 2017. Association of health-related behaviors, attitudes, and appraisals to leisure-time physical activity in middle-aged and older women. *Women Health.* 57(2):121–136.

21   Miller Y, Brown W. 2005. Determinants of active leisure for women with young children – an 'ethic of care' prevails. *Leis Sci.* 16(27):405–420.

22   Morgan F, Battersby A, Weightman A, et al. 2016. Adherence to exercise referral schemes by participants – what do providers and commissioners need to know? A systematic review of barriers and facilitators. *BMC Public Health.* 16:227.

23   Smith B, Thomas M, Batras D. 2016. Overcoming disparities in organized physical activity: findings from Australian community strategies. *Health Promot Int.* 31(3):572–581.

24   Sequeira S, Cruz C, Pinto D. 2012. Prevalence of barriers for physical activity in adults according to gender and socioeconomic status. *Br J Sports Med.* 45:A18–A19.

25   Desveaux L, Goldstein R, Mathur S, Brooks D. 2016. Barriers to physical activity following rehabilitation: Perspectives of older adults with chronic disease. *J Aging Phys Act.* 24(2):223–233.

26   Karnes S, Meyer B, Berger L, Brondino M. 2015. Changes in physical activity and psychological variables following a web-based motivational interviewing intervention: pilot study. *JMIR Res Protoc.* 4(e129).

27   Lewis BA, Marcus BH, Pate RR, Dunn AL. 2002. Psychosocial mediators of physical activity behavior among adults and children. *Am J Prev Med.* 23(2S):26–35.

28   Rhodes RE, Fiala B, Conner M. 2010. A review and meta-analysis of affective judgments and physical activity in adult populations. *Ann Behav Med.* 38(3):180–204.

29   Conner M, Rhodes RE, Morris B, et al. 2011. Changing exercise through targeting affective or cognitive attitudes. *Psychol Health.* 26(2):133–149.

30   McEachan R, Taylor N, Harrison R, et al. 2016. Meta-Analysis of the Reasoned Action Approach (RAA) to understanding health behaviors. *Ann Behav Med.* 50(4):592–612.

31   Lowe R, Eves F, Carroll D. 2002. The influence of affective and instrumental beliefs on exercise intentions and behavior: a longitudinal analysis. *J Appl Psychol.* 32(6):1241–1252.

32   Rhodes R, Fiala B, Nasuti G. 2012. Action control of exercise behavior: evaluation of social cognition, cross-behavioral regulation, and automaticity. *Behav Med.* 38(4):121–128.

33   Liao Y, Intille S, Dunton G. 2015. Using ecological momentary assessment to understand where and with whom adults' physical and sedentary activity occur. *Int J Behav Med.* 22(1):51–61.

34   Sudeck G, Schmid J, Conzelmann A. 2016. Exercise experiences and changes in affective attitude: direct and indirect effects of in situ measurements of experiences. *Front Psychol.* 7:900.

35   Nam S, Dobrosielski D, Stewart K. 2012. Predictors of exercise intervention dropout in sedentary individuals with type 2 diabetes. *J Cardiopulm Rehabil Prev.* 32(6):370–378.

36   Kwan B, Stevens C, Bryan A. 2017. What to expect when you're exercising: an experimental test of the anticipated affect-exercise relationship. *Health Psychol Rev.* 36(4):309–319.

37   Wang X. 2011. The role of anticipated negative emotions and past behavior in individuals' physical activity intentions and behaviors. *Psychol Sport Exerc.* 12(3):300–305.

38   Magnan R, Kwan B, Bryan A. 2013. Effects of current physical activity on affective response to exercise: Physical and social-cognitive mechanisms. *Psychol Health.* 28(4):418–433.

39   Ekkekakis P, Parfitt G, Petruzzello SJ. 2011. The pleasure and displeasure people feel when they exercise at different intensities: Decennial update and progress towards a tripartite rationale for exercise intensity prescription. *Sports Medicine.* 41(8):641–671.

40   Loprinzi P, Darnell T, Hager K, Vidrine J. 2015. Physical activity related beliefs and discrepancies between beliefs and physical activity behavior for various chronic diseases. *Physiol Behav.* 151:577–582.

41   Fraser SJ, Chapman J, Brown WJ, et al. 2016. Physical activity attitudes and preferences among inpatient adults with mental illness. *Int J Ment Health Nurs.* 24:413–420.

42   Burton NW, Pakenham KI, Brown WJ. 2010. Are psychologists willing and able to promote physical activity as part of psychological treatment? *Int J Behav Med.* 17(4):287–297.

43   Cunningham M, Swanson V, Pappas E, et al. 2014. Illness beliefs and walking behavior after revascularization for intermittent claudication: a qualitative study. *J Cardiopulm Rehabil Prev.* 34(3):195–201.

44   Horne M, Skelton D, Speed S, Todd C. 2013. Perceived barriers to initiating and maintaining physical activity among South Asian and White British adults in their 60s living in the United Kingdom: a qualitative study. *Ethn Health.* 18(6):626–645.

45   Franco M, Tong A, Howard K, et al. 2015. Older people's perspectives on participation in physical activity: a systematic review and thematic synthesis of qualitative literature. *Br J Sports Med.* 49(19):70–78.

46   Liljas A, Walters K, Jovicic A, et al. 2017. Strategies to improve engagement of 'hard to reach' older people in research on health promotion: a systematic review. *BMC Public Health.* 17:349.

47   Chaudhury M, Shelton N. 2010. Physical activity among 60–69-year-olds in England: knowledge, perception, behaviour and risk factors. *Ageing Soc.* 30:1343–1355.

48   Justine M, Azizan A, Hassan V, et al. 2013. Barriers to participation in physical activity and exercise among middle-aged and elderly individuals. *Singapore Med J.* 54(10):581–586.

49   Rogers A, Harris T, Victor C, et al. 2014. Which older people decline participation in a primary care trial of physical activity and why: insights from a mixed methods approach. *BMC Geriatr.* 14:46.

50   Normansell R, Holmes R, Victor C, et al. 2016. Exploring non-participation in primary care physical activity interventions: PACE-UP trial interview findings. *Trials.* 17:178.

51   Yang D, Hausien O, Aqeel M, et al. 2017. Physical activity levels and barriers to exercise referral among patients with cancer. *Patient Educ Couns.* 100(7):1402–1407.

52   Smith L, Gardner B, Aggio D, Hamer M. 2015. Association between participation in outdoor play and sport at 10 years old with physical activity in adulthood. *Prev Med.* 74:31–35.

53   Bélanger M, Sabiston C, Barnett T, et al. 2015. Number of years of participation in some, but not all, types of physical activity during adolescence predicts level of physical activity in adulthood: Results from a 13-year study. *Int J Behav Nutr Phys Act.* 12:76.

54   Hamer M, Kivimaki M, Steptoe A. 2012. Longitudinal patterns in physical activity and sedentary behaviour from mid life to early old age: a substudy of the Whitehall II cohort. *J Epidemiology Community Health.* 66(12):1110–1115.

55   Morseth B, Jørgensen L, Emaus N, et al. 2011. Tracking of leisure time physical activity during 28 yr in adults: The Tromsø Study. *Med Sci Sport Exerc.* 43:1229–1234.

56   Bonn S, Alfredsson L, Saevarsdottir S, Schelin M. 2016. Correlates of leisure time physical inactivity in a Scandinavian population: a basis for interventions. *J Phys Act Health.* 13(11):1236–1242.

57   Borodulin K, Mäkinen TE, Leino-Arjas P, et al. 2012. Leisure time physical activity in a 22-year follow-up among Finnish adults. *Int J Behav Nutr Phys Act.* 9:121.

58   Wichstrom L, von Soest T, Kvalem I. 2013. Predictors of growth and decline in leisure time physical activity from adolescence to adulthood. *Health Psychol.* 32(7):775–784.

59   Jack K, McLean SM, Moffett JK, Gardiner E. 2012. Barriers to treatment adherence in physiotherapy outpatient clinics: A systematic review. *Man Ther.* 15(3):220–228.

60   Sylvester B, Standage M, McEwan D, et al. 2016. Variety support and exercise adherence behavior: experimental and mediating effects. *J Behav Med.* 39(2):214–224.

61   Palazzo C, Klinger E, Dorner V, et al. 2016. Barriers to home-based exercise program adherence with chronic low back pain: Patient expectations regarding new technologies. *Ann Phys Rehabil Med.* 59(2):107–113.

62   George ES, Kolt GS, Duncan MJ, et al. 2012. A review of the effectiveness of physical activity interventions for adult males. *Sports Med.* 42(4):281–300.

63   Parry S, Knight L, Connolly B, et al. 2017. Factors influencing physical activity and rehabilitation in survivors of critical illness: a systematic review of quantitative and qualitative studies. *Intensive Care Med.* 43(4):531–542.

64   Gavarkovs A, Burke S, Petrella R. 2016. Engaging men in chronic disease prevention and management programs: A scoping review. *Am J Men's Health.* 10(6):N145–N154.

65   Vrazel J, Saunders R, Wilcox S. 2008. An overview and proposed framework of social-environmental influences on the physical-activity behavior of women. *Am J Health Promot.* 23(1):2–12.

66   Evans A, Sleap M. 'You feel like people are looking at you and laughing': Older adults' perceptions of aquatic physical activity. *J Aging Stud.* 26(4):515–526.

67   Rodrigues I, Armstrong J, Adachi J, MacDermid J. 2017. Facilitators and barriers to exercise adherence in patients with osteopenia and osteoporosis: a systematic review. *Osteoporos Int.* 28(3):735–745.

68   Borodulin K, Sipila N, Rahkonen O, et al. 2016. Socio-demographic and behavioral variation in barriers to leisure-time physical activity. *Scand J Public Health.* 44(1):62–69.

69   Leijon ME, Faskunger J, Bendtsen P, et al. 2011. Who is not adhering to physical activity referrals, and why? *Scand J Prim Health Care.* 29(4):234–240.

70   Strazdins L, Welsh J, Korda R, et al. 2016. Not all hours are equal: could time be a social determinant of health? *Sociol Health Illn.* 38(1):21–42.

71   Stults-Kolehmainen M, Sinha R. 2013. The effects of stress on physical activity and exercise. *Sports Med.* 44:81–121.

72   Clark M, Jenkins S, Hagen P, et al. 2016. High stress and negative health behaviors: A five-year wellness center member cohort study. *J Occup Environ Med.* 58(9):868–873.

73   Malone L, Barfield J, Brasher J. 2012. Perceived benefits and barriers to exercise among persons with physical disabilities or chronic health conditions within action or maintenance stages of exercise. *Disabil Health J.* 5(4):254–260.

74   Baert V, Gorus E, Mets T, et al. 2011. Motivators and barriers for physical activity in the oldest old: A systematic review. *Ageing Res Rev.* 10(4):464–474.

75   Smith LN, Ng SW, Popkin BM. 2014. No time for the gym? Housework and other non-labor market time use patterns are associated with meeting physical activity recommendations among adults in full-time, sedentary jobs. *Soc Sci Med.* 120:126–134.

76   Venditti E, Wylie-Rosett J, Delahanty L, et al. 2014. Short and long-term lifestyle coaching approaches used to address diverse participant barriers to weight loss and physical activity adherence. *Int J Behav Nutr Phys Act.* 11:16.

77   Mullen SW, Wojecki TR, Mailey, EL, et al. 2013. A profile for predicting attrition from exercise in older adults. *Prev Sci.* 14(5): 489–496.

78   Miller WC, Miller TA. 2009. Attitudes of overweight and normal weight adults regarding exercise at a health club. *J Nutr Educ Behav.* 42(1):2–9.

79   Dunlop WL, Schmader T. 2014. For the overweight, is proximity to in-shape, normal-weight exercisers a deterrent or an attractor? An examination of contextual preferences. *Int J Behav Med.* 21(1):139–143.

80   Thomas SL, Lewis S, Hyde J, et al. 2010. 'The solution needs to be complex': Obese adults' attitudes about the effectiveness of individual and population based interventions for obesity. *BMC Public Health.* 10:420.

81   Alba A, Weich S, Griffiths FE. 2011. Service users' experiences of a physical activity and lifestyle intervention for people with severe mental illness: A longitudinal qualitative study. *J Epidemiol Community Health.* 65:A19.

82   Costello E, Kafchinski M, Vrazel J, Sullivan P. 2012. Motivators, barriers, and beliefs regarding physical activity in an older adult population. *J Geriatr Phys Ther.* 34(3):138–147.

83   Pridgeon L, Grogan S. 2012. Understanding exercise adherence and dropout: an interpretative phenomenological analysis of men and women's accounts of gym attendance and non-attendance. *Qual Res Sport Exerc Health.* 4(3):382–399.

84   Abbasi I. 2014. Socio-cultural barriers to attaining recommended levels of physical activity among females: a review of literature. *Quest.* 66(4):448–467.

85   Rongen A, Robroek S, van Ginkel W, et al. 2014. Barriers and facilitators for participation in health promotion programs among employees: a six-month follow-up study. *BMC Public Health.* 14:573.

86   Gilson N, Burton NW, van Uffelen JGZ, Brown W. 2011. Occupational sitting time: Employees' perceptions of health risks and intervention strategies. *Health Promot J Austr.* 22(1):38–43.

87   Ory M, Towne S, Won J, et al. 2016. Social and environmental predictors of walking among older adults. *BMC Geriatr.* 16:155.

88   Ussher M, Stanbury L, Cheeseman V, Faulkner G. 2007. Physical activity preferences and perceived barriers to activity among persons with severe mental illness in the United Kingdom. *Psychiatr Serv.* 58(3):405–408.

89   Hakola L, Hassinen M, Komulainen P, et al. 2015. Correlates of low physical activity levels in aging men and women: The DR's EXTRA study. *J Aging Phys Act.* 23(2):247–255.

90   De Cocker K, Artero E, De Henauw S, et al. 2012. Can differences in physical activity by socio-economic status in European adolescents be explained by differences in psychosocial correlates? A mediation analysis within the HELENA (Healthy Lifestyle in Europe by Nutrition in Adolescence) Study. *Public Health Nutr.* 15(11):2100–2109.

91   Prince S, Reed J, Martinello N, et al. 2016. Why are adult women physically active? A systematic review of prospective cohort studies to identify intrapersonal, social environmental and physical environmental determinants. *Obes Rev.* 17(10):919–944.

92   Kilpatrick M, Blizzard L, Sanderson K, et al. 2017. Barriers and facilitators to participation in workplace health promotion (WHP) activities: results from a cross-sectional survey of public-sector employees in Tasmania, Australia. *Health Promot J Austr.* 28(3):225–232.

93   Stahl T, Rutten A, Nutbeam D, et al. 2001. The importance of the social environment for physically active lifestyle – results from an international study. *Soc Sci Med.* 52(1):1–10.

94   Moustaka FC, Vlachopoulos SP, Kabitsis C, Theodorakis Y. 2012. Effects of an autonomy-supportive exercise instructing style on exercise motivation, psychological well-being, and exercise attendance in middle-age women. *J Phys Act Health.* 9(1):138–150.

95   Annesi J. 1999. Relationship between exercise professionals' behavioural styles and clients' adherence to exercise. *Percept Mot Skills.* 89:597–604.

96   Fox L, Rejeski W, Gauvin L. 2000. Effects of leadership style and group dynamics on enjoyment of physical activity. *Am J Health Promot.* 14(5):277–283.

97   Maher J, Gottschall J, Conroy D. 2015. Perceptions of the activity, the social climate, and the self during group exercise classes regulate intrinsic satisfaction. *Front Psychol.* 6:1236.

98   Izumi B, Schulz A, Mentz G, et al. 2015. Leader behaviors, group cohesion, and participation in a walking group program. *Am J Prev Med.* 49(1):41–49.

99   Burton E, Hill A, Pettigrew S, et al. 2017. Why do seniors leave resistance training programs? *Clin Interv Aging.* 12:585–592.

100   Blake HS, Stanulewicz N, Mcgill F. 2017. Predictors of physical activity and barriers to exercise in nursing and medical students. *J Adv Nurs.* 73(4):917–929.

101   King D, Allen P, Jones D, et al. 2016. Safe, affordable, convenient: environmental features of malls and other public spaces used by older adults for walking. *J Phys Act Health.* 13(3):289–295.

102   Hogg L, Grant A, Garrod R, Fiddler H. 2012. People with COPD perceive ongoing, structured and socially supportive exercise opportunities to be important for maintaining an active lifestyle following pulmonary rehabilitation: a qualitative study. *J Physiother.* 58(3):189–195.

103   Lee J, Kim Y. 2017. Application of the social ecological constructs to explain physical activity in middle aged adults. *Int J Sport Psychol.* 48(2):99–110.

104   Watts A, Masse L. 2013. Is access to workplace amenities associated with leisure-time physical activity among Canadian adults? *Can J Public Health.* 104(1):E87–E91.

105 Choi J, Lee M, Lee J-K, et al. 2017. Correlates associated with participation in physical activity among adults: a systematic review of reviews and update. *BMC Public Health*. 17:356.

106 Zapata-Diomedi B, Veerman J. 2016. The association between built environment features and physical activity in the Australian context: a synthesis of the literature. *BMC Public Health*. 16:484.

107 Sallis JC, Cerin E, Conway TL, et al. 2016. Physical activity in relation to urban environments in 14 cities worldwide: a cross-sectional study. *Lancet*. 387(10034):2207–2217.

108 Moran M, Van Cauwenberg J, Hercky-Linnewiel R, et al. 2014. Understanding the relationships between the physical environment and physical activity in older adults: a systematic review of qualitative studies. *Int J Behav Nutr Phys Act*. 11:79.

109 Adams M, Ding D, Sallis JF, et al. 2013. Patterns of neighborhood environment attributes related to physical activity across 11 countries: a latent class analysis. *Int J Behav Nutr Phys Act*. 10:34.

110 van Dyck D, Cerin E, De Bourdeaudhuij I, et al. 2015. Moderating effects of age, gender and education on the associations of perceived neighborhood environment attributes with accelerometer-based physical activity: The IPEN adult study. *Health Place*. 36:65–73.

111 Lorenc T, Brunton G, Oliver S, et al. 2008. Attitudes to walking and cycling among children, young people and parents: a systematic review. *J Epidemiol Community Health*. 62(10):852–857.

PRACTICAL 16
PROMOTING EXERCISE ADHERENCE

Nicola W. Burton

Introduction

There is substantial evidence and consensus regarding the benefits of exercise across the lifespan for people with or without clinical conditions. However, these benefits are only realised when the person actually engages with exercise over a period of time. Non-adherent clients don't have the opportunity to experience associated physical and psychological benefits—which can compromise quality of life and increase the burden of disease and healthcare costs. Non-adherence can frustrate exercise practitioners and contribute to a financial loss for service providers.

Exercise adherence is a dynamic process, and a shared responsibility between a practitioner and the client. It requires proactive planning. Just as the practitioner plans what and how exercises will be done to promote gains, planning is also required to consider what and how strategies will be used to promote adherence. This practical focuses on planning for exercise adherence, which is conceptualised as both participation in and maintenance of exercise.

A Framework for Planning for Exercise Adherence

The previous practical introduced the MAKE-UPP acronym as a framework to understand potential factors contributing to non-adherence. The A-SUCCESS acronym is a framework to help planning for behavioural adherence.

Action planning

Social support and connections

Understand exercise readiness and relevance

Context

Competing demands and coping plans

Efficacy

Self-regulation

Satisfaction

Action Planning

Action planning is a behaviour-change technique that involves detailed consideration of what will be done, *as well as* how, when and where.[1] Plans may also include details on who is involved, and other pre-action steps to be done, or resources required, to perform the behaviour.

Action planning is more than goal setting, which is a future-oriented resolution about a specific behaviour (e.g. do exercise training three times next week) or an outcome of a behaviour (e.g. lose 5 kg over next 6 months).[1] It can help habit formation,[2] and be useful for people with established (positive) intentions[3] or weak habits.[4]

Action planning has demonstrated efficacy for promoting physical activity and exercise among a range of people including university students,[3] the general population,[5-7] middle-aged and older adults,[6,8,9] older adults with multiple illnesses,[10] people at risk of or with diabetes,[11,12] people with intermittent claudication[13] or musculoskeletal conditions[14] and rehabilitation clients.[15]

Action planning complements exercise prescription. It involves considering the following.

- *When* the exercise will be done (e.g. on what days of the week, what time of day). 'When' may also reflect links with other events/behaviours (e.g. after work, before school, on shiftwork days, while on holidays, on presentation of specific signs or symptoms).
- *Where* the exercise will be done (i.e. the exercise location and physical setting). This may involve identifying convenient and accessible facilities, what outdoor areas are suitable, where walking can be done safely in the local area and so on.
- *How* the exercise will be done. This can include frequency and duration, and how to integrate exercise with other activities of daily life. It may also include information on how to respond to possible contraindications (e.g. pain).

Although detailed, action planning can be done at the expense of minimal time (e.g. 5 minutes).[16]

Activity 16.1 Action planning

In pairs, each develop an action plan to do a total of 2 hours of walking during the following week (assume there is agreement to do so). Ensure the action plan includes the following elements:

- how it will be done (e.g. in several bouts, as part of travel to and from places, on equipment, as part of other activities, alone/with others)
- when it will be done (i.e. time of day, what days)
- where it will be done (e.g. local neighbourhood, at gym, outdoors, specific walking route)
- back up plans if required (e.g. if adverse weather)
- any cues/prompts that can be used (e.g. when to increase/decrease).

Write your action plan:

_____
_____
_____
_____
_____
_____
_____
_____
_____
_____
_____
_____
_____
_____

Social Support and Connections

Social support and connections are strong determinants of exercise adoption, adherence and maintenance,[17–23] and potentially more important than intrapersonal factors.[24,25] Social support may be particularly relevant for clients with vulnerabilities such as obesity,[26,27] mental illness[28] or clinical conditions such as diabetes.[29]

Potential sources of social support for exercise include family, friends, peers, co-workers, employers, other exercise participants, staff, professionals, acquaintances and group/community links. Importantly, the preferred nature, source and degree of social support for exercise can vary by age, gender, personal style and life circumstances. Parents and teachers are salient sources of support for children and adolescents.[30,31] Partner support is important for people in a couple relationship.[32,33] Family support can be important for older adults,[19,34] and older adults are more likely than younger adults to want assistance from a health professional.[35] Younger adults are more likely than older adults to want support from group exercise.[35]

Practitioners can contribute to social support for exercise in different ways.

- As a *direct source* of support (e.g. providing information, education, encouragement, feedback). They can help clients overcome anxieties about the exercise environment and assist confidence and motivation.[36] Supervision is a common type of support for exercise, and adherence is higher for supervised than unsupervised exercise.[37]
- By collaborating with clients to *plan how to elicit support* for exercise. This can consist of discussions about increasing the give and take of social support from significant others, identifying and highlighting role-models, problem-solving social barriers, facilitating the integration of physical activity into social routines, linking in with community resources and identifying (friendly and non-threatening) social comparisons.[24]
- By *enabling and managing social connections* among exercise clients. This could involve, for example, linking exercise clients into buddy systems, moderating interpersonal dynamics in group-based activities or introducing clients to exercise networks.

There are also different types of social support.

- *Emotional* support targets affect and provides encouragement (e.g. empathy, caring).
- *Instrumental* support involves material assistance (e.g. transport, resources).
- *Informational* support contributes to knowledge (e.g. advice, suggestions).
- *Appraisal* support is a specific type of information support for self-evaluation purposes (e.g. constructive feedback and affirmation).
- *Network* support involves links with other people (e.g. companionship, group cohesion/identity).

Activity 16.2 Social support for exercise

Identify who in your social network contributes support for your exercise and how this is done. Do this for each type of support. If you are unable to identify a current source or type of support, think about past experiences or potential options.

1. Who provides *emotional* support and how is this done?

_____

_____

_____

2 What *instrumental* support have you received for exercise? How was it helpful?

_____

_____

_____

3 Who/what are your sources of exercise-related *information*?

_____

_____

4. Who provides *appraisals* of your exercise performance?

_____

_____

5. Who do you link with for *network* support? How do you do this? Are there exercise-related groups that you identify with?

_____

_____

_____

_____

Emotional Support

Emotional support is what is typically thought of when conceptualising social support. Emotional support promotes exercise adherence in part by enabling better self-regulation, in particular self-efficacy,[38] and assuring the person that they are valued.

Activity 16.3 Providing emotional support to exercise clients

In small groups, discuss how exercise practitioners and exercise facilities/businesses (e.g. fitness centre, rehabilitation centre, gym) could demonstrate to clients that they are valued. Write your answers below.

_____

_____

_____

_____

_____

_____

_____

_____

_____

_____

Sources of emotional support are usually close others (e.g. partner, parent, good friend, carer). Accordingly, exercise practitioners may involve significant others in exercise programming as exercise companions or champions. Individuals are more likely to increase their exercise if their partner does as well.[39,40] Significant others may be involved in client sessions, so that they understand exercise requirements and processes. Peer champions can provide direct encouragement and facilitate wider support in workplace programs.[41] Practitioners can also talk with clients to identify preferred/likely sources of emotional support among significant others and problem-solve social support barriers (e.g. how to respond to unhelpful comments or criticisms).

Exercise practitioners can also be a direct source of emotional support. The previous practical on understanding exercise non-adherence highlighted that people often have expectations of or experience exercise as unpleasant, particularly those who are inactive, unfit or who see themselves as not competent.[42–45] Clients can also have negative emotions that generalise to exercise from other contexts such as work, relationships or life events. Responding to emotions is a major component of practitioner good communication skills, which in turn are positively associated with adherence.[46] Exercise practitioners can provide empathic responses that acknowledge (versus deny, dismiss or contest) clients' negative emotional experiences and can highlight and celebrate positive affective experiences.

Some practitioners may have concerns about the level of emotional support that can be offered to clients without creating dependence.[36] This may be particularly salient for socially isolated clients or those with interpersonal difficulties (e.g. people with mental illness). This can be managed in part by limiting the duration, frequency and detail of emotional discussions and working with the client to identify alternative appropriate sources of support. The issue of dependence can also be discussed (sensitively) with clients.

Activity 16.4 Providing emotional support to exercise clients

Below are some examples of emotional statements about exercise. Develop an empathic response for each. This can be done by acknowledging the emotion (e.g. paraphrasing or reflecting the client's information) and offering assistance. Ensure your responses demonstrate acceptance of the expressed emotion.

To provide a contrast, also develop a low empathic response for each statement. This may deny, dismiss or contest the emotion; prioritise the practitioner's perspectives over the client's; or not include an offer of assistance.

I hate doing this part of the program.	Low empathy: This is a really important exercise for you. When you get better at it you'll like it more.
	High empathy: This is one of the exercises you dislike. Maybe we can find an alternative, or change the order of when you do it in the program.
I am just so overwhelmed at work right now I don't know if I have the time to exercise.	Low empathy: It's really important that you keep up with your exercises so that you don't lose the gains you've made.
	High empathy: It's hard to keep up with everything when work is so busy and stressful. I could help you develop a shorter program until things settle down.
I'm feeling so pleased with how I'm going.	Low empathy: Great! Now we can take your exercise up to the next level of difficulty.
	High empathy: It's wonderful that you are so happy with your progress. Congratulations!
I've been trying really hard with this exercise but I am not getting any better.	Low empathy:
	High empathy:
I get so bored.	Low empathy:
	High empathy:
I think I am finally getting better at this.	Low empathy:
	High empathy:
My kids make it difficult to get here, and I feel guilty leaving my partner to look after things at home.	Low empathy:
	High empathy:
I am worried about making things worse.	Low empathy:
	High empathy:
I'll never be able to do that.	Low empathy:
	High empathy:
I am so tired at the end of the day that it's hard to motivate myself to do anything.	Low empathy:
	High empathy:
You ask and expect too much of me.	Low empathy:
	High empathy:

Instrumental Support

Instrumental support relates to material assistance such as transport, resources, finances and related services. This type of support is an important enabler for exercise clients with accessibility difficulties such as those who are older or who have a disability or socioeconomic disadvantage.[34,47–49] Women may require instrumental support to overcome the commonly identified exercise barriers of child care and housework.[50–54] Change rooms and options to secure valuables can be useful for clients to attend exercise facilities. Clients with clinical conditions may require specific types of instrumental support for exercise adherence.

Activity 16.5 Providing instrumental support to exercise clients

In a group, brainstorm what instrumental support exercise practitioners or exercise facilities/businesses (e.g. fitness centre, rehabilitation centre, gym) could offer to clients to support adherence. Consider clients across a range of different needs and contexts: young people, working adults, parents, couples, singles, older adults, adolescents, people from culturally diverse backgrounds, people with specific conditions or limitations. Write your answers below.

_____

_____

_____

_____

_____

_____

_____

_____

_____

_____

_____

_____

_____

_____

Informational Support

Information giving is one of the most common behaviour-change techniques used in exercise interventions.[22,55] Information can be provided using a range of modalities (e.g. in person, written, using images, remotely using telephone or online facilities) and address a range of topics such as:

- benefits of exercise and risks of inactivity; this can be generalised or specific to the individual
- exercise recommendations (e.g. from clinical practice guidelines, position statements)
- specific exercise programming (i.e. how to exercise, use equipment)
- inherent risks and contraindications
- information about what/how other people are doing
- related resources.

Exercise practitioners are a key source of informational support for exercise. Information should be age-appropriate and not too scientific.[56] Information such as correct technique, intensity and equipment needed may be important for older adults[57] or those with condition-specific concerns.[58] Information on performance that contributes to self-appraisal and esteem is valued by young adult women.[59]

Clients may also access other sources of exercise information, such as friends, family and acquaintances; other professionals; written materials (e.g. books, brochures); media (e.g. magazines, television); and online resources. Women are more likely than men to share information about exercise.[56] Apps are a contemporary source of information for self-education and can have a role in maintaining exercise adherence.[60] Clients with clinical conditions may value some types of information from condition specialists, people with the same condition or exercise practitioners affiliated with a condition-specific facility.[61-63] Identifying reliable and accurate sources of information may, therefore, be useful to direct information gathering by clients.

Note that although potentially important, providing information is _not_ the most effective behaviour-change technique[22] and knowledge does not predict adherence.[64]

Network Support

Network support is about connecting with similar people and provides a sense of belonging and group identity. Exercise networks can occur as part of group activities (e.g. exercise classes, weight-loss meetings), interest forums (e.g. online communities) or informal connections (e.g. work colleagues with similar interests). Some social connections may be indirectly related to exercise (e.g. walking in the local area and seeing neighbours, cycling/jogging and seeing others doing likewise).

Demographic homogeneity is a key factor that contributes to a sense of social connectedness. This enables people to share the same language, feel more at ease and receive empathy for similar experiences and constraints.[65] Exercise with people of the same gender can help lower feelings of embarrassment.[65] Condition-specific exercise groups can support adherence by lowering potential stigma, and providing opportunities for vicarious learning and information sharing. Being around similar others can be a central motive for continued exercise participation.[66]

Exercise networks can provide pleasant social interactions that promote exercise adherence. Affiliation is an important exercise motive for young adults.[67] Studies of older adults' experiences in exercise programs have highlighted opportunities to meet and interact with new people, which contribute to positive affective attitudes and motivation and increases sources of instrumental and emotional support.[65,68,69] Once people are physically active, high levels of social interaction can promote retention.[70]

Networks can provide social norms, role models, social comparisons and companions to promote exercise adherence. People are more likely to be active if their friends are active[71,72] or if they perceive others in their neighbourhood are active.[73] Employees are more likely to engage in health promotion programs if they perceive participation is expected by colleagues and supervisors.[74] Social modelling from family members can promote physical activity in people with diabetes.[75] Peer involvement, co-leadership or leadership in exercise groups can promote adherence among people with chronic conditions and older adults.[76–78] Group/buddy exercise participants may develop a sense of accountability that is associated with ongoing engagement.[79] *Friendly* social comparisons can promote adherence[24,80] and can be a component of team-based or competitive events. Companionship during exercise is valued by young women[59] and people with safety concerns.[29] Men and women are five times more likely to become physically active if their partner does too.[40] Online social networks can connect people looking for exercise companions and network support,[81] and are a common function of many physical activity monitors, apps and online programs.

Understand Exercise Readiness and Relevance

Motivation is consistently identified as a predictor of exercise adherence. The transtheoretical (stage of change) model[82] is a framework to understand motivational readiness, and identifies five stages.

1. Precontemplation: no intention to take action.
2. Contemplation: considering action.
3. Preparation: intention to take action, may have done some behaviours towards this.
4. Action: action initiated.
5. Maintenance: action sustained over time (e.g. > 6 months).

Some representations of the model identify a sixth stage—termination when there is no temptation to relapse and 100% confidence.

Client needs may differ according to stage of readiness; for example, awareness-raising when inactive, addressing fears when considering exercise, advice and companionship for starting, reinforcement for action, or resources to sustain exercise outside of facility-based programs. Exercise stage of readiness can predict adherence in clients with clinical conditions.[83,84] Therefore, practitioners need to be sensitive to the client's stage of motivational readiness and not move to action precipitously.

Activity 16.6 Client readiness for exercise

Discuss how you might differentiate between an exercise client in precontemplation, contemplation and preparation. Write your answers below.

_____

_____

_____

_____

_____

_____

_____

_____

_____

_____

How could your interactions differ between the following?

1. a client in contemplation

_____
_____
_____
_____
_____
_____
_____
_____
_____
_____

2. a client in preparation

_____
_____
_____
_____
_____
_____
_____
_____
_____
_____

3. a client in action

_____
_____
_____
_____
_____
_____
_____
_____
_____
_____

People can move backwards and forwards through the stages. For example, someone may be in maintenance, have an injury and then move back to contemplation. Stage progression occurs in part as people perceive the pros of exercise to increase and cons to decrease.[85] Positive expectations (pros) are positively associated with exercise adherence[86] and need to be personally relevant. Motivational interviewing strategies can be used to elicit clients' expectations (pros *and* cons), minimise resistance and resolve ambivalence to promote adherence.[87] This involves asking questions to explore the pros and then the cons of the status quo, as well as the cons and then the pros of change. For example:

- What are the advantages of continuing to do what are you are doing now?
- What are the disadvantages of continuing to do what are you are doing now?

- What are the disadvantages of doing more exercise?
- What are the advantages of doing more exercise?

Values exploration is another strategy for evoking personal relevance and motivation. This is done by asking people to identify important life goals and values, and how the behaviour fits with these.[88] For example:

- What things are important to you?
- What do you want in life?
- How is exercise consistent with that?

Exercise may be consistent with values of, for example, looking good, having self-respect, being a good parent, independence, quality of life and so on. Focusing on a client's goals and values can foster motivation by decreasing defensiveness, moving the focus away from the 'undesirable' behaviours (i.e. not exercising) and highlighting personal relevance.[88]

Activity 16.7 Personal relevance of exercise

In pairs, do a values exploration and link this to exercise.

- What things are important to you?
- What do you want in life?
- How could exercise fit in with these priorities and values?

_____

_____

_____

_____

_____

_____

Context

Context refers to the circumstances and setting. Exercise contexts reflect attributes of how, when, where and with whom exercise is done. Examples of these attributes are provided in Table 16.1.

TABLE 16.1	Contextual Variables for Exercise
Context	**Examples**
How	- Competitive - Varied/repetitive routine - Skilled, unskilled activities - Supervised, unsupervised
Where	- Outdoors, indoors - Home - Facility based - In the local area - At a worksite
When	- Morning, afternoon, evening - Weekday, weekend - Fixed time, variable schedule

TABLE 16.1	Contextual Variables for Exercise (continued)
Context	**Examples**
With whom	• Alone/with one other/small group/large group • Team-based • With others of the same level of ability • With others of the same gender • With others of comparable age • With others with same condition

Clients will have different preferences for exercise contexts. Exercise that is supervised, with people of the same gender, and at a fixed time with scheduled sessions can appeal to people with psychological distress[89,90] or high body mass index (BMI).[91,92] Team-based activities may suit people with high BMI[91] or with socioeconomic disadvantage.[93] Age similarity is important for people with high BMI, and middle-aged and older adults.[91,94–96] Middle-aged men may also want exercise companions to be of the same gender.[94,95] People with a low income may prefer exercise that is supervised, skill-based and not outdoors.[93] Exercise that involves friendly competition and opportunities for mastery may appeal to men more than women.[21,67,95] Some clients may be interested in complementary activities that make it not just about exercise (e.g. social activities)[17,93,97] while others dislike music and television in exercise settings.[98] Exercise that matches diurnal preferences (morningness-eveningness) promotes adherence.[99]

People with clinical conditions may prefer condition-specific exercise programs/groups with professional supervision/support.[90,97,100–103] However, this is not always the case. People living in the community with mental illness can prefer not to exercise with others recovering from mental illness, which may reflect a desire for 'normalisation'.[104] People with some types of cancer prefer exercise that is done alone.[105,106] People with arthritis and/or osteoporosis prefer activities with a set routine or format.[93]

Activity 16.8 Exercise context preferences

Use the following questionnaire to assess your exercise context preferences.

I Prefer Exercise That: (Please Tick one Box for Each Item)	Strongly Disagree	Disagree	No Preference	Agree	Strongly Agree
Is done on my own	☐	☐	☐	☐	☐
Involves competition	☐	☐	☐	☐	☐
Is done with people around my age	☐	☐	☐	☐	☐
Is done in my neighbourhood/local area	☐	☐	☐	☐	☐
Is done outdoors	☐	☐	☐	☐	☐
Requires skill and practice	☐	☐	☐	☐	☐
Has a set routine or format	☐	☐	☐	☐	☐
Is done with people who have the same health concerns that I do	☐	☐	☐	☐	☐
Is supervised	☐	☐	☐	☐	☐
Is team-based	☐	☐	☐	☐	☐
Is done at a scheduled time	☐	☐	☐	☐	☐

I Prefer Exercise That: (Please Tick one Box for Each Item)	Strongly Disagree	Disagree	No Preference	Agree	Strongly Agree
Is done with people of my gender	☐	☐	☐	☐	☐
Includes a range of different types of activities	☐	☐	☐	☐	☐
Is vigorous	☐	☐	☐	☐	☐
Is done with an exercise partner/buddy	☐	☐	☐	☐	☐
Is done in a small group (e.g. 3–6 people)	☐	☐	☐	☐	☐
Can be done at home	☐	☐	☐	☐	☐
Is done with people at my level of ability	☐	☐	☐	☐	☐
Can be done at any time that suits me	☐	☐	☐	☐	☐
Includes a social aspect	☐	☐	☐	☐	☐
Lets me choose the level of difficulty	☐	☐	☐	☐	☐
Includes a fun element	☐	☐	☐	☐	☐
Is in a climate-controlled setting (e.g. with air-conditioning/heating)	☐	☐	☐	☐	☐

Source: © Nicola Burton 2020. Reproduced with permission.

Convenience and aesthetics are key contextual attributes for exercise adherence.[17,18,107–109] Quality facilities are important to encourage use[110] and include accessible parking and clean toilets.[48] Travel time/transportation requirements impact on adherence,[34,98] and may be more important than health benefits among older adults with mobility issues.[111] Work-based programs can be convenient for employees.[112] Level surfaces, sufficient lighting, footpaths, seating for rest breaks, aesthetics and quality recreational destinations (e.g. parks) enable older adults' walking for exercise in public spaces.[48, 113–115]

Competing Demands and Coping Plans

As competing demands and lack of time are commonly identified barriers to exercise,[69,116–122] adherence planning needs to consider strategies to manage these issues. Problem-solving and coping plans are behaviour-change techniques for initiating and maintaining adherence.[1] Problem-solving involves identifying potential barriers and competing demands in specified situations (as well as enablers of the behaviour), and coping planning identifies situations when the behaviour may not be maintained. Practitioners can collaborate with clients to identify factors that might or do constrain exercise adherence, and how these can be managed. People with a high level of coping planning are better able to implement exercise action plans,[123] and coping plans can improve confidence for and actual exercise participation and maintenance.[10,27,75,124]

Competing demands and coping plans may target issues relating to behavioural (e.g. program complexity), intrapersonal (e.g. unhelpful self-talk, low knowledge), interpersonal (e.g. criticism) or physical (e.g. accessibility) factors. Associated strategies include time management, environmental restructuring, cues/prompts, planning social support, contingent rewards and stress management. Flexible timing and content of exercise programming may help clients cope with competing time demands as well as poor health and wellbeing (e.g. fatigue, weakness, nausea, dizziness, fluctuating abilities, deterioration). Referral to other practitioners may be useful for specific coping needs (e.g. psychological issues, pain, nutritional support, footcare and footwear).

Efficacy

Efficacy refers to an individual's belief of his/her ability to organise and do the behaviour required for the desired outcomes.[125] It is consistently identified as one of the strongest predictors of exercise participation, adherence and maintenance.[18,29,50,107,126–131] General approaches for increasing efficacy (not specific to exercise) are:[125,132]

- mastery experiences—successful performance
- vicarious experiences/social modelling—learning from others' experiences or seeing similar people do the behaviour
- improving physical and emotional states (e.g. reducing tension or stress)
- expressions of encouragement or faith.

The effectiveness of various approaches to improve exercise efficacy can differ across clients. Among healthy adults aged < 60 years, feedback on past performance, feedback by comparing performance to others, vicarious experiences, action planning, instruction and praising/rewarding effort can improve efficacy for recreational physical activity (e.g. walking, aerobics, gym); but verbal persuasion, graded mastery (increasing difficulty of tasks), barrier identification and relapse prevention planning (identifying barriers to maintenance) may not.[6,133] Action planning, time management, prompting self-monitoring of *outcomes* and planning social support/change can improve physical activity efficacy in adults with obesity.[26] Setting goals, prompting self-monitoring of *behaviour*, relapse planning, providing normative information and providing performance feedback have been associated with *lower* levels of efficacy in older adults.[134] Therefore, exercise practitioners need to be flexible with, and confirm the impact of, strategies aiming to improve exercise confidence.

Activity 16.9 Exercise efficacy
. . . .

Discuss why/how the following behaviour-change techniques could *lower* a client's exercise efficacy (confidence).

1. verbal persuasion

_____

_____

_____

_____

_____

2. increasing difficulty of tasks

_____

_____

_____

_____

_____

3. barrier identification

_____

_____

_____

_____

_____

4. goal setting

_____
_____
_____
_____
_____

5. self-monitoring of behaviour

_____
_____
_____
_____
_____

6. providing normative information

_____
_____
_____
_____
_____

7. performance feedback

_____
_____
_____
_____
_____

Self-regulation

Self-regulatory strategies are the actual processes by which people manage their own behaviour, and include goal setting, planning, scheduling, problem-solving, rewards and prompts. Self-regulatory skills are associated with physical activity participation and improvement[23,86,135,136] and can influence maintenance.[129,137,138]

Exercise programs that are flexible and have adaptable content can promote adherence and maintenance.[17,139] This enables clients to self-regulate exercises to suit their needs and constraints (e.g. short duration, low impact, less demand). Flexibility in timing and location of exercises may enable self-regulation.

Exercise practitioners can assist clients to develop self-regulatory skills for exercise. This may be important for adolescents and for clients with a low level of education, who don't identify themselves as 'exercisers' or who have self-regulatory problems (e.g. people with depressive symptoms or mental illness).[140–143]

One of the major components of self-regulation is self-monitoring. This can focus on the behaviour itself or the expected outcome of the behaviour.[1] Self-monitoring is one of the most effective techniques to support behaviour change generally and physical activity interventions specifically.[1,22,26,144,145] Exercise practitioners can develop, provide and identify tools to assist clients with exercise self-monitoring.

Activity 16.10 Exercise self-monitoring

Discuss how clients could self-monitor exercise performance, progress and outcomes. Write your answers below.

_____

_____

_____

_____

_____

_____

_____

_____

_____

What do you think are some key characteristics of exercise self-monitoring tools that could encourage clients to use them?

_____

_____

_____

_____

_____

Satisfaction

Client satisfaction reflects client experiences; attitudes; emotions, feelings and perceptions of services; and congruency between expectations of and actual services received.[146] Satisfaction is different from enjoyment, which is primarily affective, in that it reflects fulfilment of a need or desire: someone can be satisfied with an experience that is not necessarily enjoyable. Satisfaction has both affective and cognitive elements, and so can contribute to both affective and instrumental attitudes. Satisfaction has been hypothesised as one of the main determinants of behaviour maintenance generally[147] and can predict exercise adherence and maintenance.[148-151]

Intrinsic satisfaction with exercise is based on positive affective experiences. Perceived competence is one of the major factors influencing emotions during exercise[152] and, in combination with practitioner encouragement, can promote intrinsic satisfaction.[153] Once people are active, high levels of interest and enjoyment are associated with improved levels of retention.[70] Client satisfaction tends to be higher with practitioners who use encouragement, positive reinforcement and individualised feedback; and who don't overly control the social environment or only use feedback on the technical nature of exercise.[154] In exercise groups, intrinsic satisfaction can be influenced by clients' perceptions of involvement, which could be facilitated by, for example, practitioners offering multiple options for a given exercise so that each person can participate regardless of ability.[153] Intrinsic satisfaction is dynamic, and fluctuates over time as attributes of the exercise experience changes.

However, not all clients intrinsically enjoy exercise. Extrinsic satisfaction reflects the realisation of external goals (e.g. weight loss, approval from significant others, symptom management). Extrinsic satisfaction may also come from congruency between expectations of and actual services received. Although intrinsic motivation is more strongly associated with adherence,[155] instrumental attitudes can promote adherence if they have personal value and utility.

Practitioner courtesy, respect and careful listening are strong drivers of client extrinsic satisfaction.[146] Personality, professionalism and a humanistic approach are key practitioner attributes; that is: demonstrating care and concern; being enthusiastic, lively and encouraging; trying to make exercise enjoyable; being approachable; being aware of individual clients' concerns; discretion; being non-judgmental; personalising information and activities; prioritising safety; and seeking client feedback.[17]

Activity 16.11 Client satisfaction

How can client satisfaction be assessed? Consider both formal and informal options. Write your answers below.

_____
_____
_____
_____
_____
_____
_____
_____
_____
_____

What could client satisfaction be assessed in relation to? That is, what specific topics are clients being asked about?

_____
_____
_____
_____
_____
_____
_____
_____
_____

When could this assessment be done?

_____
_____
_____
_____

Summary

The benefits of exercise are only realised when clients are adherent. Adherence is a dynamic process and a shared responsibility between practitioner and the client that requires proactive planning.

The A-SUCCESS acronym is a framework to help planning for adherence and involves the following.

- Action planning: considering when, where, how and with whom exercise is done, and relevant cues and preparatory action.
- Social support: providing and enhancing emotional, instrumental, informational and network support.
- Understanding: being sensitive to clients' motivational readiness and the personal relevance/value of exercise.
- Context: optimising exercise contexts to be convenient, aesthetic and consistent with client preferences.
- Competing demands and coping plans: developing plans to problem-solve barriers and cope with competing demands.
- Efficacy: enabling client perceptions of confidence and competence.
- Self-regulation: developing client management skills such as self-monitoring.
- Satisfaction: enabling intrinsic and extrinsic satisfaction.

References

1 Michie S, Ashford S, Sniehotta F, et al. 2011. A refined taxonomy of behaviour change techniques to help people change their physical activity and healthy eating behaviours: the CALO-RE taxonomy. *Psychol Health.* 26(11):1479–1498.

2 Fleig L, Pomp S, Parschau L, et al. 2013. From intentions via planning and behavior to physical exercise habits. *Psychol Sport Exerc.* 14(5).

3 Conner M, Sandberg T, Norman P. 2010. Using action planning to promote exercise behavior. *Ann Behav Med.* 40:65–76.

4 Maher J, Conroy D. 2015. Habit strength moderates the effects of daily action planning prompts on physical activity but not sedentary behavior. *J Sport Exerc Psychol.* 37(1):97–107.

5 Parschau L, Fleig L, Warner L, et al. 2014. Positive exercise experience facilitates behavior change via selfefficacy. *Health Educ Behav.* 41(4):414–422.

6 Williams SL, French DP. 2011. What are the most effective intervention techniques for changing physical activity self-efficacy and physical activity behaviour—and are they the same? *Health Educ Res.* 26(2):308–322.

7 Mistry C, Sweet S, Latimer-Cheung A, Rhodes R. 2015. Predicting changes in planning behaviour and physical activity among adults. *Psychol Sport Exerc.* 17:1–6.

8 Mesters I, Wahl S, Van Keulen H. 2014. Socio-demographic, medical and social-cognitive correlates of physical activity behavior among older adults (45–70 years): a cross-sectional study. *BMC Public Health.* 14:647.

9 Arbesman M, Mosley LJ. 2012. Systematic review of occupation- and activity-based health management and maintenance interventions for community-dwelling older adults. *Am J Occup Ther.* 66(3):277–283.

10 Schuz B, Wurm S, Ziegelmann J, et al. Contextual and individual predictors of physical activity: interactions between environmental factors and health cognitions. *Health Psychol.* 31(6):714–723.

11 Cradock K, O'Laighin G, Finucane F, et al. 2017. Behaviour change techniques targeting both diet and physical activity in type 2 diabetes: a systematic review and meta-analysis. *Int J Behav Nutr Phys Act.* 14:18.

12 Hankonen N, Absetz P, Ghisletta P, et al. 2010. Gender differences in social cognitive determinants of exercise adoption. *Psychol Health.* 25(1):55–69.

13 Cunningham M, Swanson V, Holdsworth R, O'Carroll R. 2013. Late effects of a brief psychological intervention with intermittent claudication in a randomized clinical trial. *Br J Surg.* 100(6):756–760.

14 Knittle K, De Gucht V, Meas S. 2012. Lifestyle- and behaviour-change interventions in musculoskeletal conditions. *Clin Rheumatol.* 26(3):293–304.

15 Fleig L, Pomp S, Schwarzer R, Lippke S. 2013. Promoting exercise maintenance: how interventions with booster sessions improve long-term rehabilitation outcomes. *Rehabil Psychol.* 58(4):323–333.

16 Pears SM, Morton K, Bijker M, et al. 2015. Development and feasibility study of very brief interventions for physical activity in primary care. *BMC Public Health.* 15:333.

17 Killingback C, Tsofliou F, Clark C. 2017. Older people's adherence to community-based group exercise programmes: a multiple-case study. *BMC Public Health.* 17:115.

18 Bauman A, Reis R, Sallis J, et al. 2012. Correlates of physical activity: why are some people physically active and others not? *Lancet.* 380(9838):258–271.

19 Smith G, Banting L, Eime R, et al. 2017. The association between social support and physical activity in older adults: systematic review. *Int J Behav Nutr Phys Act.* 14:56.

20 Jack K, McLean SM, Moffett JK, Gardiner E. 2012. Barriers to treatment adherence in physiotherapy outpatient clinics: a systematic review. *Man Ther.* 15(3):220–228.

21 George ES, Kolt GS, Duncan MJ, et al. 2012. A review of the effectiveness of physical activity interventions for adult males. *Sports Med.* 42(4):281–300.

22 van Achterberg T, Huisman-de Waal GGJ, Ketelaar NABM, et al. 2011. How to promote healthy behaviours in patients? An overview of evidence for behaviour change techniques. *Health Promot Int.* 26(2):148–162.

23 Greaves CJ, Sheppard KE, Abraham C, et al. 2011. Systematic review of reviews of intervention components associated with increased effectiveness in dietary and physical activity interventions. *BMC Public Health.* 11:119.

24 McMahon S, Lewis B, Oakes J, et al. 2017. Assessing the effects of interpersonal and intrapersonal behavior change strategies on physical activity in older adults: a factorial experiment. *Ann Behav Med.* 51(3):376–390.

25 De Bourdeaudhuij I, Sallis J. 2002. Relative contribution of psychosocial variables to the explanation of physical activity in three population based adult samples. *Prev Med.* 34(2):279–288.

26 Olander E, Fletcher H, Williams S, et al. 2013. What are the most effective techniques in changing obese individuals' physical activity self-efficacy and behaviour: a systematic review and meta-analysis. *Int J Behav Nutr Phys Act.* 10:29.

27 Parschau L, Barz M, Richert J, et al. 2014. Physical activity among adults with obesity: testing the Health Action Process Approach. *Rehabil Psychol.* 59(1):42–49.

28 Gross J, Vancampfort D, Stubbs B, et al. 2015. A narrative synthesis investigating the use and value of social support to promote physical activity among individuals with schizophrenia. *Disabil Rehabil.* 38(2):123–150.

29 Qiu S, Sun Z, Cai X, et al. 2012. Improving patients' adherence to physical activity in diabetes mellitus: a review. *Diabetes Metab J.* 36(1):1–5.

30 Abaraogu U, Ezenwankwo E, Dall P, et al. 2018. Barriers and enablers to walking in individuals with intermittent claudication: a systematic review to conceptualize a relevant and patient-centered program. *PLoS One,* 13(7):e0201095.

31 Sterdt E, Liersch S, Walter U. 2014. Correlates of physical activity of children and adolescents: a systematic review of reviews. *Health Educ J.* 73(1):72–89.

32 Gellert P, Ziegelmann JP, Warner LM, Schwarzer R. 2011. Physical activity intervention in older adults: does a participating partner make a difference? *Eur J Ageing.* 8(3):211–219.

33   Li K, Cardinal B, Acock A. 2013. Concordance of physical activity trajectories among middle-aged and older married couples: impact of diseases and functional difficulties. *J Gerontol B Psychol Sci Soc Sci.* 68(5):794–806.

34   Liljas A, Walters K, Jovicic A, et al. 2017. Strategies to improve engagement of 'hard to reach' older people in research on health promotion: a systematic review. *BMC Public Health.* 17:349.

35   Booth ML, Bauman A, Owen N, Gore CJ. 1997. Physical activity preferences, preferred sources of assistance, and perceived barriers to increased activity among physically inactive Australians. *Prev Med.* 26(1):131–137.

36   Moore GF, Moore L, Murphy S. 2011. Facilitating adherence to physical activity: exercise professionals' experiences of the National Exercise Referral Scheme in Wales. A qualitative study. *BMC Public Health.* 11:935.

37   Picorelli A, Pereira L, Pereira D, et al. 2014. Adherence to exercise programs for older people is influenced by program characteristics and personal factors: a systematic review. *J Physiother.* 60(3):151–156.

38   Rackow P, Scholz U, Hornung R. 2015. Received social support and exercising: an intervention study to test the enabling hypothesis. *Br J Health Psychol.* 20(4):763–776.

39   Cobb L, Godino J, Selvin E, et al. 2016. Spousal influence on physical activity in middle-aged and older adults. *Am J Epidemiol.* 183(5):444–451.

40   Jackson S, Steptoe A, Wardle J. 2015. The influence of partner's behavior on health behavior change: The English Longitudinal Study of Ageing. *JAMA Int Med.* 175(3):385–392.

41   Edmunds S, Clow A. 2016. The role of peer physical activity champions in the workplace: a qualitative study. *Perspect Public Health.* 136(3):161–170.

42   Kwan B, Stevens C, Bryan A. 2017. What to expect when you're exercising: an experimental test of the anticipated affect-exercise relationship. *Health Psychol Rev.* 36(4):309–319.

43   Wang X. 2011. The role of anticipated negative emotions and past behavior in individuals' physical activity intentions and behaviors. *Psychol Sport Exerc.* 12(3):300–305.

44   Sudeck G, Schmid J, Conzelmann A. 2016. Exercise experiences and changes in affective attitude: direct and indirect effects of in situ measurements of experiences. *Front Psychol.* 7:900.

45   Nam S, Dobrosielski D, Stewart K. 2012. Predictors of exercise intervention dropout in sedentary individuals with type 2 diabetes. *J Cardiopulm Rehabil Prev.* 32(6):370–378.

46   King A, Hoppe R. 2013. 'Best practice' for patient-centered communication: a narrative review. *J Grad Med Educ.* 5(3):385–393.

47   Smith B, Thomas M, Batras D. 2016. Overcoming disparities in organized physical activity: findings from Australian community strategies. *Health Promot Int.* 31(3):572–581.

48   King D, Allen P, Jones D, et al. 2016. Safe, affordable, convenient: environmental features of malls and other public spaces used by older adults for walking. *J Phys Act Health.* 13(3):289–295.

49   Loprinzi P, Joyner C. 2016. Source and size of emotional and financial-related social support network on physical activity behavior among older adults. *J Phys Act Health.* 13(7).

50   Prince S, Reed J, Martinello N, et al. 2016. Why are adult women physically active? A systematic review of prospective cohort studies to identify intrapersonal, social environmental and physical environmental determinants. *Obes Rev.* 17(10):919–944.

51   Rhodes R, Quinlan A. 2015. Predictors of physical activity change among adults using observational designs. *Sports Med.* 45(3):423–441.

52   Engberg E, Alen M, Kukkonen-Harjula K, et al. 2012. Life events and change in leisure time physical activity: a systematic review. *Sports Med.* 42:433–447.

53   Abbasi I. 2014. Socio-cultural barriers to attaining recommended levels of physical activity among females: a review of literature. *Quest.* 66(4):448–467.

54   Oliveira A, Lopes C, Rostila M, et al. 2013. Gender differences in social support and leisure-time physical activity. *Rev Saude Publica.* 48(4):602–612.

55   Beck F, Gillison F, Koseva M, et al. 2016. The systematic identification of content and delivery style of an exercise intervention. *Psychol Health.* 31(5):605–621.

56   Enwald H, Kangas M, Keranen N, et al. 2017. Health information behaviour, attitudes towards health information and motivating factors for encouraging physical activity among older people: differences by sex and age. *Informat Res.* 22(1):810–829.

57   Rhodes R, Martin A, Taunton J, et al. 1999. Factors associated with exercise adherence among older adults. An individual perspective. *Sports Med.* 28(6):397–411.

58   Parry S, Knight L, Connolly B, et al. 2017. Factors influencing physical activity and rehabilitation in survivors of critical illness: a systematic review of quantitative and qualitative studies. *Intensive Care Med.* 43(4):531–542.

59   Cavallo D, Brown J, Tate D, et al. 2014. The role of companionship, esteem, and informational support in explaining physical activity among young women in an online social network intervention. *J Behav Med.* 37(5):955–966.

60   Wang Q, Egelandsdal B, Amdam G, et al. 2016. Diet and physical activity apps: perceived effectiveness by app users. *JMIR mhealth uhealth.* 2:e33.

61   McGowan E, Speed-Andrews A, Blanchard C, et al. 2013. Physical activity preferences among a population-based sample of colorectal cancer survivors. *Oncol Nurs Forum.* 40(1):44–52.

62   Trinh L, Plotnikoff R, Rhodes R, et al. 2012. Physical activity preferences in a population-based sample of kidney cancer survivors. *Support Care Cancer.* 20(8):1709–1717.

63   Belanger LJ, Plotnikoff RC, Clark A, Courneya KS. 2012. A survey of physical activity programming and counseling preferences in young-adult cancer survivors. *Cancer Nurs.* 35(1):48–54.

64   Ross A, Melzer T. 2016. Beliefs as barriers to healthy eating and physical activity. *Australian Journal of Psychology.* 68(4):251–260.

65   Farrance C, Tsofliou F, Clark C. 2016. Adherence to community based group exercise interventions for older people: a mixed-methods systematic review. *Prev Med.* 87:155–166.

66   Wurz A, St-Aubin A, Brunet J. 2015. Breast cancer survivors' barriers and motives for participating in a group-based physical activity program offered in the community. *Support Care Cancer*. 23(8):2407–2416.

67   Molanorouzi K, Khoo S, Morris T. 2015. Motives for adult participation in physical activity: type of activity, age, and gender. *BMC Public Health*. 15:66.

68   Devereux-Fitzgerald A, Powell R, Dewhurst A, French D. 2016. The acceptability of physical activity interventions to older adults: a systematic review and meta-synthesis. *Soc Sci Med*. 158:14–23.

69   Franco M, Tong A, Howard K, et al. 2015. Older people's perspectives on participation in physical activity: a systematic review and thematic synthesis of qualitative literature. *Br J Sports Med*. 49(19):70–78.

70   Withall J, Jago R, Fox KR. Why some do but most don't. 2011. Barriers and enablers to engaging low-income groups in physical activity programmes: a mixed methods study. *BMC Public Health*. 11:507.

71   Child S, Kaczynski A, Moore S. 2017. Meeting physical activity guidelines: the role of personal networks among residents of low-income communities. *Am J Prev Med*. 53(3):385–391.

72   Firestone M, Yi S, Bartley K, Eisenhower D. 2015. Perceptions and the role of group exercise among New York City adults,, 2010–2011: an examination of interpersonal factors and leisure-time physical activity. *Prev Med*. 72:50–55.

73   Ball K, Jeffery RW, Abbott G, et al. 2010. Is healthy behavior contagious: associations of social norms with physical activity and healthy eating. *Int J Behav Nutr Phys Act*. 7:86.

74   Rongen A, Robroek S, van Ginkel W, et al. 2014. Barriers and facilitators for participation in health promotion programs among employees: a six-month follow-up study. *BMC Public Health*. 14:573.

75   Van Dyck D, De Greef K, Deforche B, et al. 2011. Mediators of physical activity change in a behavioral modification program for type 2 diabetes patients. *Int J Behav Nutr Phys Act*. 8:105.

76   Best K, Miller W, Eng J, Routhier F. 2016. Systematic review and meta-analysis of peer-led self-management programs for increasing physical activity. *Int J Behav Med*. 23(5):527.

77   Webel A, Okonsky J, Trompeta J, Holzemer W. 2010. A systematic review of the effectiveness of peer-based interventions on health-related behaviors in adults. *Am J Public Health*. 100(2):247–253.

78   Burton E, Farrier K, Hill K, et al. 2018. Effectiveness of peers in delivering programs or motivating older people to increase their participation in physical activity: systematic review and meta-analysis. *J Sports Sci*. 36(6):666–678.

79   McArthur DD, Dumas A, Woodend K, et al. 2014. Factors influencing adherence to regular exercise in middle-aged women: a qualitative study to inform clinical practice. *BMC Women's Health*. 14:49.

80   Chapman G, Colby H, Convery K, Coups E. 2016. Goals and social comparisons promote walking behavior. *Med Decis Making*. 36(4):472–478.

81   Nakhasi A, Shen A, Passarella R, et al. 2014. Online social networks that connect users to physical activity partners: a review and descriptive analysis. *J Med Internet Res*. 16:e153.

82   Prochaska JO, Marcus BH. 1994. The transtheoretical model: applications to exercise. In: Dishman RK, editor. *Advances in Exercise Adherence*. Campaign, IL: Human Kinetics, pp. 161–180.

83   Husebø AD, Drystad SM, Søreide JA, Bru, E. 2012. Predicting exercise adherence in cancer patients and survivors: a systematic review and meta-analysis of motivational and behavioural factors. *J Clin Nurs*. 22(1–2):4–21.

84   Platt A, Green HJ, Jayasinghe R, Morrissey S. 2014. Understanding adherence in patients with coronary heart disease: illness representations and readiness to engage in healthy behaviours. *Austr Psychol*. 49(2).

85   Nigg CR, Geller MS, Motl RW, et al. 2011. A research agenda to examine the efficacy and relevance of the Transtheoretical Model for physical activity behavior. *Psychol Sport Exerc*. 12(1):7–12

86   Rhodes R, Janssen I, Bredin S, et al. 2017. Physical activity: health impact, prevalence, correlates and interventions. *Psychol Health*. 32(8):942–975.

87   Hardcastle S, Hancox J, Hattar A, et al. 2015. Motivating the unmotivated: how can health behavior be changed in those unwilling to change? *Front Psychol*. 6:835.

88   Miller W, Rollnick S. 2013. *Motivational Interviewing: Preparing People for Change*. 3rd ed. New York, NY: Guilford Press.

89   Khan A, Brown WJ, Burton NW. 2013. What physical activity contexts do adults with psychological distress prefer? *J Sci Med Sport*. 16(417–421).

90   Fraser S, Chapman J, Brown W, et al. 2016. Physical activity attitudes and preferences among inpatient adults with mental illness. *Int J Ment Health Nurs*. 24:413–420.

91   Burton NW, Khan A, Brown WJ. 2012. How, where and with whom? Physical activity context preferences of three adult groups at risk of inactivity. *Br J Sports Med*. 46:1125–1131.

92   Dunlop WL, Beauchamp MR. 2011. En-gendering choice: preferences for exercising in gender-segregated and gender-integrated groups and consideration of overweight status. *Int J Behav Med*. 18(3):216–220.

93   Peeters G, Brown W, Burton NW. 2014. Physical activity context preferences in people with arthritis and osteoporosis. *J Phys Act Health*. 11:536–542.

94   Burton NW, Walsh A, Brown WJ. 2008. It just doesn't speak to me: middle-aged men's reactions to 10,000 steps a day. *Health Promot J Austr*. 19(1):52–59.

95   Gavarkovs A, Burke S, Petrella R. 2016. Engaging men in chronic disease prevention and management programs: a scoping review. *Am J Men's Health*. 10(6):N145–N154.

96   Beauchamp MR, Carron AV, McCutcheon S, Harper O. 2007. Older adults' preferences for exercising alone versus in groups: considering contextual congruence. *Ann Behav Med*. 33(2):200–206.

97   Hogg L, Grant A, Garrod R, Fiddler H. 2012. People with COPD perceive ongoing, structured and socially supportive exercise opportunities to be important for maintaining an active lifestyle following pulmonary rehabilitation: a qualitative study. *J Physiother*. 58(3):189–195.

98   Morgan F, Battersby A, Weightman A, et al. 2016. Adherence to exercise referral schemes by participants - what do providers and commissioners need to know? A systematic review of barriers and facilitators. *BMC Public Health.* 16:227.

99   Hisler G, Phillips A, Krizan Z. 2017. Individual differences in diurnal preference and time-of-exercise interact to predict exercise frequency. *Ann Behav Med.* 51(3):391–401.

100 Abrantes AM, Battle CL, Strong DR, et al. 2011. Exercise preferences of patients in substance abuse treatment. *Ment Health Phys Act.* 4(2):79–87.

101 Desveaux L, Goldstein R, Mathur S, Brooks D. 2016. Barriers to physical activity following rehabilitation: perspectives of older adults with chronic disease. *J Aging Phys Act.* 24(2):223–233.

102 Dunlop WL, Schmader T. 2014. For the overweight, is proximity to in-shape, normal-weight exercisers a deterrent or an attractor? An examination of contextual preferences. *Int J Behav Med.* 21(1).

103 Forbes C, Blanchard C, Mummery W, Courneya K. 2015. A comparison of physical activity preferences among breast, prostate, and colorectal cancer survivors in Nova Scotia, Canada. *J Phys Act Health.* 12(6):823–833.

104 Chapman J, Fraser S, Brown W, Burton NW. 2016. Physical activity preferences, motivators, barries and attitudes of adults with mental illness. *J Ment Health.* 25(5):448–454.

105 Lowe SS, Watanabe SM, Baracos VE, Courneya KS. 2010. Physical activity interests and preferences in palliative cancer patients. *Support Care Cancer.* 18(11):1469–1475.

106 Rogers L, Malone J, Rao K, et al. 2009. Exercise preferences among patients with head and neck cancer: prevalence and associations with quality of life, symptom severity, depression, and rural residence. *Head Neck.* 31(8):994–1005.

107 Choi J, Lee M, Lee J-K, et al. 2017. Correlates associated with participation in physical activity among adults: a systematic review of reviews and update. *BMC Public Health.* 17:356.

108 Sugiyama T, Cerin E, Owen N, et al. 2014. Perceived neighbourhood environmental attributes associated with adults' recreational walking: IPEN Adult study in 12 countries. *Health Place.* 28:22–30.

109 Annear M, Keeling S, Wilkinson T, et al. 2014. Environmental influences on healthy and active ageing: a systematic review. *Ageing Soc.* 34(4):590–622.

110 Lee J, Kim Y. 2017. Application of the social ecological constructs to explain physical activity in middle aged adults. *Int J Sport Psychol.* 48(2):99–110.

111 Franco M, Howard K, Sherrington C, et al. 2015. Eliciting older people's preferences for exercise programs: a best-worst scaling choice experiment. *J Physiother.* 61(1):34–41.

112 Persson R, Cleal B, Jakobsen M, et al. 2014. Help preferences among employees who wish to change health behaviors. *Health Educ Behav,* 41(4):376–386.

113 Moran M, Van Cauwenberg J, Hercky-Linnewiel R, et al. 2014. Understanding the relationships between the physical environment and physical activity in older adults: a systematic review of qualitative studies. *Int J Behav Nutr Phys Act.* 11:79.

114 Farren L, Belza B, Allen P, et al. 2015. Mall walking program environments, features, and participants: a scoping review. *Prev Chronic Dis.* 12:E129.

115 Sugiyama T, Neuhaus M, Cole R, et al. 2012. Destination and route attributes associated with adults' walking: a review. *Med Sci Sports Exerc.* 44:1275–1286.

116 Rodrigues I, Armstrong J, Adachi J, MacDermid J. 2017. Facilitators and barriers to exercise adherence in patients with osteopenia and osteoporosis: a systematic review. *Osteoporos Int.* 28(3):735–745.

117 Borodulin K, Sipila N, Rahkonen O, et al. 2016. Socio-demographic and behavioral variation in barriers to leisure-time physical activity. *Scand J Public Health.* 44(1):62–69.

118 Sequeira S, Cruz C, Pinto D. 2012. Prevalence of barriers for physical activity in adults according to gender and socioeconomic status. *Br J Sports Med.* 45:A18–A19.

119 Leijon ME, Faskunger J, Bendtsen P, et al. 2011. Who is not adhering to physical activity referrals, and why? *Scand J Prim Health Care.* 29(4):234–240.

120 Strazdins L, Welsh J, Korda R, et al. 2016. Not all hours are equal: could time be a social determinant of health? *Sociol Health Illn.* 38(1):21–42.

121 Justine M, Azizan A, Hassan V, et al. 2013. Barriers to participation in physical activity and exercise among middle-aged and elderly individuals. *Singapore Med J.* 54(10):581–586.

122 Yang D, Hausien O, Aqeel M, et al. 2017. Physical activity levels and barriers to exercise referral among patients with cancer. *Patient Educ Couns.* 100(7):1402–1407.

123 Caudroit J, Boiche J, Stephan Y. 2014. The role of action and coping planning in the relationship between intention and physical activity: a moderated mediation analysis. *Psychol Health.* 29(7):768–780.

124 Koring M, Richert J, Parschau L, et al. 2012. A combined planning and self-efficacy intervention to promote physical activity: a multiple mediation analysis. *Psychol Health Med.* 17(4):488–498.

125 Bandura A. 1997. *Self Eefficacy: The Exercise of Control.* New York: Freeman.

126 Young M, Plotnikoff R, Collins C, et al. 2014. Social cognitive theory and physical activity: a systematic review and metaanalysis. *Obes Rev.* 15(12):983–995.

127 Szymlek-Gay E, Richards R, Egan R. 2011. Physical activity among cancer survivors: a literature review. *N Z Med J.* 124(1337):77–89.

128 Bui L, Mullan B, McCaffery K. 2013. Protection motivation theory and physical activity in the general population: a systematic literature review. *Psychol Health Med.* 18(5):522–542.

129 Amireault S, Godin G, Vezina-Im L. 2013. Determinants of physical activity maintenance: a systematic review and meta-analyses. *Health Psychol Rev.* 7(1):55–91.

130   Rhodes RE, Fiala B. 2009. Building motivation and sustainability into the prescription and recommendations for physical activity and exercise therapy. *Physiother Theory Pract.* 25:424–441.

131   Janssen I, Dugan S, Karavolos K, et al. 2014. Correlates of 15-Year maintenance of physical activity in middle-aged women. *Int J Behav Med.* 21(3):511–518.

132   McAlister A, Perry C, Parcel G. 2008. How individuals, environments, and health behavior interact. Social cognitive theory. In: Glanz K, Rimer BK, Viswanath K, Orleans C, editors. *Health Behavior and Health Education Theory, Research, and Practice.* 3rd ed. Hoboken NJ, USA: Wiley.

133   Ashford S, Edmunds J, French DP. 2010. What is the best way to change self-efficacy to promote lifestyle and recreational physical activity? A systematic review with meta-analysis. *Br J Health Psychol.* 15(2):265–288.

134   French D, Olander E, Chisholm A, Mc Sharry J. 2014. Which behaviour change techniques are most effective at increasing older adults' self-efficacy and physical activity behaviour? A systematic review. *Ann Behav Med.* 48(2):225–234.

135   Teixeira PC, Carraça EV, Marques MM, et al. 2015. Successful behavior change in obesity interventions in adults: a systematic review of self-regulation mediators. *BMC Med.* 13:84.

136   Rhodes R, Pfaeffli L. 2010. Mediators of physical activity behaviour change among adult non-clinical populations: a review update. *Int J Behav Nutr Phys Act.* 7:37.

137   Kwasnicka D, Dombrowski S, White M, Sniehotta F. 2016. Theoretical explanations for maintenance of behaviour change: a systematic review of behaviour theories. *Health Psychol Rev.* 10(3):277–296.

138   Sharpe P, Wilcox S, Schoffman D, Baruth M. 2016. Participation, satisfaction, perceived benefits, and maintenance of behavioral selfmanagement strategies in a self-directed exercise program for adults with arthritis. *Eval Program Plann.* 60:143–150.

139   Freene NW, Waddington G, Chesworth W, et al. 2014. Community group exercise versus physiotherapist-led home-based physical activity program: barriers, enablers and preferences in middle-aged adults. *Physiother Theory Pract.* 30(2):85–93.

140   Schuz B, Li A, Hardinge A, et al. 2017. Socioeconomic status as a moderator between social cognitions and physical activity: systematic review and meta-analysis based on the Theory of Planned Behavior. *Psychol Sport Exerc.* 30:186–195.

141   Rhodes R, Kaushal N, Quinlan A. 2016. Is physical activity a part of who I am? A review and meta-analysis of identity, schema and physical activity. *Health Psychol Rev.* 10(2):204–225.

142   Li K, Liu D, Haynie D, et al. 2016. Individual, social, and environmental influences on the transitions in physical activity among emerging adults. *BMC Public Health.* 16:682.

143   Pomp SF, Fleig L, Schwarzer R, Lippke S. 2013. Effects of a self-regulation intervention on exercise are moderated by depressive symptoms: a quasi-experimental study. *Int J Clin Health Psychol.* 13(1):1–8.

144   Michie S, Abraham C, Whittington C, et al. 2009. Effective techniques in healthy eating and physical activity interventions: a meta-regression. *Health Psychol.* 28(6):690–701.

145   Harkin B, Webb T, Chang B, et al. 2016. Does monitoring goal progress promote goal attainment? A metaanalysis of the experimental evidence. *Psychol Bull.* 142(2):198–229.

146   Al-Abri R, Al-Balushi A. 2014. Patient satisfaction survey as a tool towards quality improvement. *Oman Med J.* 29(1):3–7.

147   Rothman A, Baldwin A, Hertel A, Fuglestad P. 2011. Self regulation and behavior change: disentangling behavioral intention and behavioral maintenance. In: Vohs KD, Baumeister R, editors. *Handbook of Self-regulation Research, Theory and Applications.* Second ed. New York: Guilford Press.

148   Williams D, Lewis B, Dunsiger S, et al. 2008. Comparing psychosocial predictors of physical activity adoption and maintenance. *Ann Behav Med.* 36(2):186–194.

149   Fleig L, Lippke S, Pomp S, Schwarzer R. 2011. Exercise maintenance after rehabilitation: how experience can make a difference. *Psychol Sport Exerc.* 12:293–299.

150   Tak E, van Uffelen J, Paw M, et al. 2012. Adherence to exercise programs and determinants of maintenance in older adults with mild cognitive impairment. *J Aging Phys Act.* 20(1):32–46.

151   Krogh J, Lorentzen A, Subhi Y, Nordentoft M. 2014. Predictors of adherence to exercise interventions in patients with clinical depression – A pooled analysis from two clinical trials. *Ment Health Phys Act.* 7:50–54.

152   Wienke BJ, Jekauc D. 2016. A qualitative analysis of emotional facilitators in exercise. *Front Psychol.* 7:1296.

153   Maher J, Gottschall J, Conroy D. 2015. Perceptions of the activity, the social climate, and the self during group exercise classes regulate intrinsic satisfaction. *Front Psychol.* 6:1236.

154   Fox L, Rejeski W, Gauvin L. 2000. Effects of leadership style and group dynamics on enjoyment of physical activity. *Am J Health Promot.* 14(5).

155   Teixeira PJ, Carraça EV, Markland D, et al. 2012. Exercise, physical activity, and self-determination theory: a systematic review. *Int J Behav Nutr Phys Act.* 9:78.

PRACTICAL 17
BEHAVIOURAL COUNSELLING FOR EXERCISE

Nicola W. Burton

Introduction

Behavioural counselling is a conversation-based approach to assist clients to adopt, change and/or maintain behaviour. Counselling may be individual or group based, and use a range of modalities such as face to face, telephone or videoconferencing. The frequency and duration of counselling can vary from a single short consultation (e.g. 5 minutes) to multiple sessions over years. Some content of behaviour counselling will vary by practitioner personal style, and whether a specific theoretical approach to understanding and changing behaviour is used.

To date, much of the research evidence regarding behavioural counselling for exercise has focused on promoting physical activity via the primary care context. Empirical reviews of studies in this area indicate that physical activity counselling can provide positive effects[1-3] including among people with chronic conditions such as obesity, heart disease, diabetes and arthritis.[4] Physical activity counselling in clinical settings can be cost-effective and cost-competitive.[5-7]

Behavioural counselling can be used to promote motivation and resolve ambivalence regarding exercise, identify and problem-solve barriers to exercise and activate resources to support exercise adoption, adherence and maintenance. This practical will present a framework for behavioural counselling for exercise. This framework will provide a pragmatic means by which to integrate and apply information from previous practicals on understanding exercise non-adherence and promoting exercise adherence.

Client-centred Communication and Counselling

The quality of interpersonal communication between practitioners and clients is consistently recognised as a core aspect of the helping relationship. Good practitioner communication skills are associated with more client adherence, fewer complaints, client and practitioner satisfaction and improved client health outcomes.[8] The inherent health communication challenge is to incorporate the agendas of both the practitioner and the client: the practitioner's agenda to explain the issue and associated management, and the client's agenda to obtain understanding/assistance and personalise generic information.

Client-centred communication and counselling *prioritises* responsiveness to the client's needs and values, and *actively* includes the client in decision-making. The practitioner seeks to understand the client within her/his current (psychological, social and environmental) context, and works collaboratively with the client to develop a management plan that is in accordance with the client's values. In this approach, the client's perception of the practitioner's respect, empathy, positive regard and genuineness is a primary facilitator of behaviour change. Accordingly, key components for the practitioner include:

- eliciting the client's perspectives (e.g. priorities, concerns, expectations) and actively respecting these
- understanding the client's wider context beyond the immediate issue (i.e. social influences, physical setting)
- establishing and maintaining a partnership with the client to develop goals and associated strategies (i.e. shared decision-making)
- tailoring information and activities to the client's perspective.

Specific communication skills consistent with a client-centred approach include open-ended questioning, active listening (reflecting, paraphrasing, clarifying), expressing empathy, acknowledging and accepting ambivalence, a non-judgmental approach avoiding argument, collaborative agreement and discussions, providing support and encouragement and promoting flexibility and a sense of control.

Activity 17.1 Reflective listening

In pairs, identify who will be speaker 1 and listener 1.

Speaker 1: For 2 minutes describe what you want from your perfect holiday, without mentioning a specific destination.

Listener 1: Respond to this communication without any reference to yourself or others. Reflect and paraphrase what you hear, offer two suggestions for a holiday destination consistent with what you heard and determine how attractive each of your suggestions are to the talker and why that is.

Swap roles and repeat the activity.

_____

_____

_____

_____

5a Behavioural Counselling Framework

The 5A behavioural counselling framework is a client-centred evidence-based clinical tool for health behaviour change. It been endorsed by the United States Preventive Services Task Force,[9] the Canadian Task Force on Preventive Care[10] and the Swedish National Institute of Public Health[11] as a framework for physical activity counselling. This approach is applicable to a range of settings and practitioners, and can be used to promote exercise. The framework identifies five key communication tasks.

1. *Assess*: understand the client's current level of behaviour, related knowledge and thoughts/feelings about behaviour change.
2. *Advise*: clear and specific recommendations for behaviour, the potential benefits and risks of which are linked to the client's specific interests and concerns.
3. *Agree*: mutual commitment to the behaviour change, and collaboration between the client and practitioner on goals which are consistent with the client's interests.
4. *Assist*: collaboration between the client and practitioner to identify and use practical behaviour change strategies, problem-solve barriers, and activate (personal, social, environmental, professional) resources to support behaviour change. This may include identifying and sourcing additional types of assistance and resources.
5. *Arrange*: follow-up and evaluation of behaviour change efforts (which may also include adjustment of change strategies), plus organisation of referrals and resources if required.

Some representations of this framework are slightly different (e.g. ask, advise, assess, assist, arrange, assess again), and some actions within each stage can vary (e.g. goal setting may be part of the agree or assist process, referrals may be part of assist or arrange). However, the philosophy of the approach is constant in terms of eliciting the client's perspective, tailoring information to the client and working with the client to identify goals and activate change strategies that are consistent with the client's values and interests.

The 5A counselling framework is based on several behaviour change theories and strategies including the theory of planned behaviour,[12] goal-setting theory,[13] self-determination theory[14] and motivational interviewing,[15,16] which are each effective for promoting physical activity.[17-20] This is a unifying framework that can incorporate a range of strategies. Assessment may include formal tests (e.g. objective and subjective assessment); as well as determining client knowledge (affective and instrumental), attitudes and motivational readiness. Advice may encompass feedback on objective tests and providing information from clinical practice guidelines and associated recommendations. Assistance can comprise behavioural and cognitive techniques (e.g. action planning, self-monitoring, competing demands plans), target social and environmental factors, use multi-modal resources, include adjunct treatments and involve a range of practitioners or significant others of the client. What strategies are used within each stage, and to what extent, will vary by client need and the parameters of the counselling contract.

The advantage of this framework is that it provides a coherent way to structure and organise behaviour change communication with the client. It incorporates principles that are known to facilitate behaviour change, in particular individual tailoring. The rest of this practical will demonstrate how the framework can be used in an exercise context.

5a Behavioural Counselling for Exercise: Assess

The counselling *begins* by eliciting the *client's* perspectives. The key component of this stage is *gathering* information, rather than providing it. Key assessment information relates to:

- what the client understands about the 'problem' or desired outcome, and the salience of exercise to that (i.e. knowledge, personal meaning)
- what exercise is currently being done
- how the client thinks and feels about exercise and exercise change (i.e. attitudes).

This assessment can be done with a few direct questions, such as:

- 'What do you know about [specific condition or outcome]? What do you know about exercise in relation to [specific condition or outcome]?'
- 'What exercise did you do during [nominate period]?' (This may be clarified using the FITT dimensions of frequency, intensity, time and type.)
- 'How do you feel about doing exercise? What do you think will happen if you do more exercise?'
- 'What reasons do you have not to exercise?'/'What reasons do you have to exercise?'
- 'What might get in the way of doing exercise?'/'What could help you to exercise?'

This questioning provides insight into the factors that may motivate, facilitate or constrain exercise for the client. The information obtained establishes where the client is in terms of exercise knowledge, attitudes, expectations, interest and capacity, and can complement other formalised assessments. Gathering information from the client *first* is useful to minimise misleading/incorrect assumptions about the client. The open-ended style of questioning actively demonstrates an interest in the client and builds rapport. Responses are then used to individually tailor exercise-related communication and planning with the client, and will also inform the assist stage of the counselling.

The breadth and depth of assessment will be determined in part by the time available, as well as the client's insight and willingness to share information. It is not necessary for the practitioner to obtain a high level of detail, as a general understanding may be sufficient. Assessment information need not be limited to a health-related context, and can also include information related to, for example, emotions, personal situations and significant others. Practitioners can tend to focus on instrumental attitudes towards exercise (i.e. benefits for health and physical functioning). However, *affective* judgments towards exercise (i.e. thoughts about the overall pleasure/displeasure and feeling states expected from exercising) may be more important for engagement.[21,22]

Worked Case Study: Exercise Behaviour Counselling—Assess

You work in a rehabilitation centre. Susan is a 40-year-old woman who presents saying she needs to do more exercise to help her neck and shoulder pain and headaches. Consistent with the 5A behavioural counselling framework, you ask the following questions to elicit information on her knowledge, exercise behaviour and attitudes/feelings about exercise.

- What can you tell me about your pain?
- What do you know about exercise and pain?
- What exercise did you do last week?
- How do you feel about doing more exercise? What do you think will happen if you do more exercise?
- What reasons do you have not to exercise? What reasons do you have to do more exercise?
- What might get in the way of doing more exercise? What could help you to do more exercise?

Susan provides the following information. She is an office worker and spends all of her working day in front of a computer. The neck and shoulder pain has been present on and off for most of her working life; it gets worse when she has a busy and stressful day at work, but is not an everyday thing. She says the pain comes from working at her computer and she often feels stiff and sore at the end of the day, and on a bad day will also get headaches. The pain typically gets better with some general movement and stretching and a good night's sleep. Last week she did not do much exercise. She tries to do a weekly yoga class or go for a walk around the neighbourhood on the weekend, but she does not exercise if she has a headache, so as not to make it worse. Susan is concerned about doing more exercise as she is not the gym type, and she is also worried about making her headaches worse if she does the wrong type of exercise. Years ago she went to an exercise trainer who had her lifting heavy weights and that made the pain worse and gave her more headaches so she stopped going. So she does not want to do any exercise with weights. She feels hesitant about starting an exercise program, but knows she has to do something to try and help herself. If she did more exercise she might feel better but she would also have less time to get things done after work. The main reason to exercise is to try and manage her pain and reduce the frequency of her headaches, which are making it hard to do things after work and getting her down. She does not have a lot of free time to exercise and after work she is tired and just wants to relax: even though it would probably be good for her, it is just easier not to exercise. The main thing that would get in the way of exercise is lack of motivation and feeling too tired and sore after work. She can't really think of anything specific that would help her to do more exercise, though she would need her husband to help out with their kids after school if she attended a class, and she would need to see that exercise was making a difference.

From these responses, the key assessment outcomes are as follows.

Knowledge and exercise salience
- Reasonable understanding of her pain (what exacerbates, what helps)
- Knows that stretching/exercise can help pain management
- Thinks weights should be avoided
- Thinks exercise should be avoided if she has a headache

Current behaviour
- Little regular exercise
- Walking or yoga perhaps once per week

Feelings about change, anticipated outcomes
- Hesitant, worried about pain exacerbation
- Anticipates exercise may reduce pain and headaches
- Wants to help self

Reasons against/for exercise
- Against: exercise takes time and effort, easier not to exercise
- For: manage pain and reduce headaches which are interfering with after-work life and getting her down

Barriers
- Fear of exacerbating pain
- Low motivation
- Competing time demands (family commitments)
- Feeling tired and sore after work

Enablers
- Help with managing children after school
- Support from husband
- Seeing positive outcomes from change

Activity 17.2 Exercise behaviour counselling—Assess

You work in a retirement community. John is a 67-year-old man who presents saying that he needs to do more exercise to 'grow old gracefully'. Following the 5A behavioural counselling framework, you ask the following questions to elicit information on his knowledge, exercise behaviour and feelings about exercise.

- What can you tell me about 'growing old gracefully'?
- What do you know about exercise and 'growing old gracefully'?
- What exercise did you do last week?
- How do you feel about doing more exercise? What do you think will happen if you do more exercise?
- What reasons do you have not to exercise? What reasons do you have to do more exercise?
- What might get in the way of doing exercise? What could help you to do more exercise?

John provides the following information. Over the past 10 years his weight has gradually been increasing, and now he just feels fat and unfit. He puffs when he walks up the stairs and has aches and pains, particularly in his knees. He knows that there is not much that can be done to lose weight as you get older, especially for someone of his age who can no longer do the type of hard exercise that is necessary to lose weight (like jogging). However, he also knows you've got to 'use it or lose it', so he had better start now before things get any worse. He knows about the general recommendations to do exercise for 20 minutes three times a week. Last week he did a lot of exercise with an hour in the garden on most days: mowing, sweeping up leaves, pruning, weeding and watering the plants. He is somewhat interested in doing more exercise as he used to play football and go to the gym when he was younger, but that just gradually dropped off over time. If he did more exercise, he might be able to get around a bit better and not puff so much going up stairs. Doing more exercise would be good to keep him moving so he does not become one of those fat old men who can't do anything, as he wants to be able to spend time and play with his grandchildren. The main reason not to exercise is that exercise takes a lot of effort; these days he does not have the strength that he once did and he is not sure he can do vigorous exercise anymore. It would be hard to have to face up to how much condition he has lost over the years. His sore knees will also make exercise tough, and his weight would be embarrassing in the gym around all those fit people. The main help he needs is working out what he can do safely and sensibly. His wife is very supportive of him starting some exercise, as she has been doing exercise classes at the local community hall.

From these responses, identify key assessment outcomes.

Knowledge and exercise salience

_____
_____
_____
_____
_____

Current behaviour

_____
_____

Feelings about change, anticipated outcomes

_____
_____
_____
_____
_____

Reasons against/for exercise

_____
_____
_____
_____
_____
_____
_____
_____

Barriers

_____
_____
_____
_____
_____

Enablers

_____

_____

_____

_____

_____

5a Behavioural Counselling Framework for Exercise: Advise

Providing advice *after* eliciting the client's perspective is consistent with the client-centred communication philosophy of *prioritising* responsiveness to the client. Advice is offered in a warm and empathic manner, and at a level that is consistent with the health literacy demonstrated by the client during the assessment. After gathering information on the client's perspective, the practitioner:

- summarises *the client's* understanding and perceptions of risks and benefits
- provides *salient* information to confirm and clarify the client's knowledge and understanding
- provides *clear and strong* advice regarding change, linked to the *client's* specific interests.

To actively demonstrate understanding, the practitioner can provide a summary statement acknowledging *both* the pros and cons of exercise *from the client's perspective*. This creates an opportunity for the client to hear what information they provided, correct any misinterpretation and confirm priorities. Acknowledging both the pros and the cons personalises the information giving and demonstrates respect for the client. If a client does not identify specific pros or cons, then that can also be part of the summary statement. For example:

- 'There is a range of reasons why you don't currently exercise, and it is hard for you to think of any specific reasons for you to start.'

This acknowledgment of pros and cons also provides a basis for the practitioner to *gently* provide information to improve knowledge and correct any misunderstandings. Information on the potential benefits and risks of exercise are linked back to the *client's* specific interests and concerns. Such information could pertain to:

- the nature of the presenting problem/desired outcome in terms of causes, consequences and management practices
- the relationship between exercise and the presenting problem/desired outcome
- perceived risks associated with exercise and contraindications
- exercise targets or parameters
- various management options and clinical recommendations for management
- results of any formalised assessments.

The practitioner then provides clear and strong advice regarding exercise—the potential benefits of which are again linked back to the *client's* specific interests. Linking advice to the client's context increases recall,[23] which can be compromised by practitioner- or client-related factors. For example, practitioners may provide non-specific information in an attempt to present a balanced review of evidence, or with a desire to avoid discouraging clients. Clients may have competing attention demands (e.g. thinking about events unrelated to the counselling) or react to information with emotions that are distracting. Linking exercise advice to the client's anticipated benefits is consistent with positive message framing which can enable recall, enhance motivation and promote positive behaviour change.[24,25]

Worked Example: Exercise Behavioural Counselling—Advise

In response to Susan's assessment information, the following *acknowledgment of her feelings and thoughts* about exercise could be offered.

> 'There are some pros and cons for you in doing more exercise. Exercise may help your neck and shoulder pain and headaches; but you're also concerned that some types of exercise—like lifting weights—may make things worse, and it will take too much time after work when you're tired or sore and want to relax.'

The following *confirmation of her understanding* of her pain and the potential value of exercise could be provided.

'You're right in that prolonged desk and computer work can cause neck and shoulder pain and headaches, particularly after a busy and stressful day. As you say, this then makes it harder to get things done and can lead to feeling down. You are also right in that stretching and sleeping well can help reduce this.'

The following information could be offered to *clarify misperceptions and improve knowledge*.

'You said that you avoid exercise if you have a headache, but sometimes exercise can relieve muscle tension and so reduce the severity and duration of a headache. Also, exercise does not need to be in a gym, take a lot of time or involve weights to be helpful. There are many different types of exercise we can consider to see what works best for you. In addition to helping manage pain, exercise can also help fatigue and mood.'

The practitioner can then provide clear and strong advice linked to her interests.

'Exercise is one of the best things you can do to manage your neck and shoulder pain and headaches. Exercise can help you feel less stiff, sore and tired after work, and give you more energy to do things and feel happier.'

Note: In this case study, Susan's statements about avoiding lifting weights could be interpreted as poor knowledge regarding the potential benefits of resistance exercise and building strength to manage her pain symptoms. However, as client-centred communication *prioritises* responsiveness to the client, and lifting weights is not an essential component for her exercise program, it will be more helpful to consider this as a client preference and prescribe other exercise. When sufficient trust is established, from both her experience of the practitioner–client relationship and her exercise experiences, Susan may be willing to attempt weights as part of her exercise program.

Activity 17.3 Exercise behaviour counselling—Advise

In response to John's assessment information, how would you advise him in a way that is consistent with the 5A behavioural framework?

- How would you acknowledge his perceived benefits and risks/concerns?

_____

_____

_____

_____

_____

_____

_____

_____

_____

- What understandings could be confirmed?

_____

_____

_____

_____

_____

_____

_____

_____

_____

- What information could you provide to clarify misperceptions and improve knowledge?

_____

_____

_____

_____

_____

_____

_____

_____

_____

_____

- What clear and strong advice would you provide, linked to his perception of benefits?

_____

_____

_____

_____

_____

_____

_____

_____

_____

_____

_____

5a Behavioural Counselling Framework: Agree

For the agree component, the practitioner and client mutually commit to the change and *collaborate* to identify behavioural goals. Agreement is reached after considering potential options, consequences and client preferences. The practitioner contributes 'expert' information on exercise options, considerations and recommendations; and the client contributes information on what is acceptable, feasible and consistent with their interests and preferences.

This shared decision-making promotes client knowledge, trust and satisfaction.[26] Erroneous beliefs about shared decision-making may make it an uncomfortable or questionable process for some practitioners. Common a unsupported myths about shared decision-making are that clients make the decisions, the practitioner has no role and clients are not interested in a collaborative role; it is difficult to do when clients ask the practitioner what to do, state it takes too much time and that it is not compatible with clinical practice guidelines.[27] In contrast, however, shared decision-making[27]:

- is an *interdependent* process in which the client and practitioner each provide information, and the practitioner's knowledge is an important part of the process
- is desired by the majority of clients, including passive and vulnerable people, but potentially constrained by the client's confidence and the practitioner's attitude to do so
- includes a series of skills that can be taught and learned by both practitioners and clients
- has a variable effect on consultation times, but can be done in a short timeframe
- does not exclude the adoption of clinical practice guidelines.

Activity 17.4 Exercise behaviour counselling—Agree

Identify five ways you could share decision-making about an exercise prescription with a client.

1. _____

_____

_____

2. _____

_____

_____

3. _____

_____

_____

4. _____

_____

_____

5. _____

_____

_____

Seeking agreement for attempting change is needed *before* discussing the details of what change will be done and how. Actively engaging a client's agreement before proceeding further can reduce the likelihood of resistance.[28] Agreement can be sought by asking a direct question; for example:

- 'Are you willing to work together to develop a program of exercise that suits you?'

If the client agrees, this is acknowledged, with reference to the client's interests, and support offered for the change process; for example:

- 'It's great that you are willing to try more exercise. Exercise is a great way for you to [refer to client interests/outcomes].'
- 'I can help you in terms of [e.g. suggesting different types of exercises and supervising your sessions].'

During the agreement process, the client may demonstrate ambivalence; that is, have mixed or contradictory thoughts/feelings such as identifying both the potential benefits of exercise and the disadvantages. In a client-centred approach,[15,16] ambivalence is considered a normal and understandable part of the behaviour change process, and is responded to by:

- expressing empathy about and acceptance of ambivalence
- developing awareness of the discrepancy between the client's goals/values and behaviour
- avoiding argument and direct confrontation
- adjusting to the client's resistance
- supporting the client's self-efficacy (confidence) and being (appropriately) optimistic.

In practical terms this involves the practitioner:

- doing reflective listening and summary statements. This is different from identifying with the problem (e.g. sharing common experiences) which can compromise the counselling process
- asking open-ended questions
- encouraging *the client* to provide reasons to engage with exercise
- restating the *client's* goals/values and how exercise is consistent with this
- *gently* correcting misperceptions about exercise
- recognising client resistance as a signal to use different strategies
- affirming knowledge, attitudes, behaviour, efforts and experiences that demonstrate the client's potential and ability to engage with exercise
- offering assistance and support for the client to engage with exercise.

Table 17.1 provides examples of how to ask open-ended questions about exercise. Closed-ended questions (i.e. answered with one word or a yes or no response) can be an integral part of communication, but in this context should be limited in use. Closed-ended questions can be used for clarification and checking understanding, but are not the basis of the communication process.

Table 17.2 provides examples of questions to elicit motivational statements about exercise. These open-ended and motivational questions elicit thoughts and feeling in a neutral manner and encourage the client to do the talking.

TABLE 17.1 Examples of Open-ended Questions About Exercise

Closed-ended Question	Open-ended Question/Statement
Do you want an exercise program?	Tell me why you are here today.
Are you worried about not exercising?	How do you feel about not exercising? What do you think could happen if you don't exercise?
Has your doctor told you to do more exercise?	What has your doctor said about exercise?
Do you like exercise?	How do you feel about exercising?
Do you think it would help your condition if you did more exercise?	What do you know about exercise and your condition?
Do you know about the benefits of exercise?	How might exercise benefit you?
Is this exercise program something you can do?	What do you think about this program for you?
Is that possible for you?	What do you think about doing that?
Does that stop you doing the things you want?	How does that affect what you want to do?
Does that concern you?	How does that make you feel?
Is that something you can do this week?	What do you think about doing that this week?
Does that work for you?	How is that for you?
Do you know what exercise you should be doing?	What exercise do you think you should be doing?
Do you know what the recommended exercise is?	What do you know about exercise recommendations?
Do you understand that?	Tell me what you understand about that.

TABLE 17.2 Sample Questions to Elicit Motivational Statements About Exercise

- Why do you think you need to do exercise?
- What reasons do you have to do more exercise?
- Why do you think that not exercising is an issue?
- Why do you think exercise is important?
- What difficulties do you have from not doing exercise?

TABLE 17.2 Sample Questions to Elicit Motivational Statements About Exercise (continued)
• How has not doing exercise created problems for you? • Why might other people see exercise as important for you? • What do you think will happen if you don't exercise? • What makes you think it is time to do more exercise? • Why are you thinking about doing more exercise now? • How would things be better if you did do more exercise?

Activity 17.5 Exercise behavioural counselling—responding to ambivalence

In pairs, identify who will be speaker 1 and listener 1.

Speaker 1: Identify something potentially advantageous that you are not doing and have mixed feelings about. Identify this for the listener.

Listener 1: Explore this ambivalence by:

- asking open-ended questions to elicit thoughts and feelings about the issue
- using reflective listening and summary statements
- eliciting possible reasons for change and self-motivational statements
- providing statements to build confidence
- offering support.

Avoid talking about your own experiences, arguing with or correcting the talker. Sample questions to elicit motivational statements are:

- Why do you think you need to do that?
- What reasons do you have to do that?
- Why do you think that is an issue?
- Why do you think that is important?
- What difficulties have you had from not doing that?
- How has not doing that created problems for you?
- Why might other people see that as important for you?
- What do you think will happen if you don't do it?
- What makes you think it is time to change?
- Why are you thinking about this now?
- How would things be better if you did change?

Swap roles and repeat the activity.

Reflect and comment on your reactions as both the talker and the listener.

- What worked? Why do you think that was?

_____

_____

_____

_____

_____

- What was difficult? Why was that?

_____

_____

_____

_____

5a Behavioural Counselling Framework: Assist

For this component, the focus is on activating internal and external resources to support behaviour adoption, adherence and maintenance. The central tenet is that behaviour change typically requires more than information and instruction (i.e. education); it is instead a multilevel process influenced by intrapersonal, interpersonal and physical and contextual environmental factors.

Specific assistance techniques will vary by client need and presentation, practitioner style and the constraints and resources of the counselling context. However, consistent with the client-centred approach, the key principles of assistance are again for the practitioner and client to work together with a focus on the client's preferences and experiences. For the practitioner, this means:

- eliciting the client's opinions and experiences
- providing suggestions and potential options from their knowledge and experience (e.g. what has worked for other clients, aligning actions with client interests)
- promoting flexibility and a sense of control for the client with the exercise program
- recognising client efforts and highlighting gains (matched to the client's interests).

Initially, the practitioner can elicit client information to inform exercise programming; for example:

- 'What time can you commit to a program?'
- 'What duration would fit in with the other things you do?'
- 'How often do you think you can attend sessions?'
- 'What types of exercise do you like?'
- 'What types of exercise are you less interested in?'
- 'What time suits you to exercise?'

The practitioner collaborates by providing expert knowledge on, for example, exercise recommendations, more effective and less effective types of exercise, and exercise options and variations.

Assist also involves the use of behavioural and cognitive strategies to promote change. There is a range of behaviour change techniques that can be used to promote exercise.[29] Some of these were presented in the previous practical on promoting exercise adherence. Common examples are action planning, instruction, modelling, graded tasks, self-monitoring, reviews, feedback and rewards.

- _Action planning:_ Detailed planning of what the client will do, including when (time of day, frequency, duration), where and how. Collaboration between the client and practitioner can reflect negotiation between recommendations and options from the practitioner and what the client thinks is feasible.
- _Feedback:_ Providing the client with data about the exercise performance.
- _Graded tasks:_ Breaking down the exercise into smaller, more achievable tasks and enabling the client to build on small successes.
- _Instruction:_ Telling the client how to exercise: this may be verbal, written or pictorial.
- _Modelling/demonstration:_ Showing the client how to perform the exercise. This may be in person, pictorially or remotely.
- _Practice/rehearsal:_ Repeated performance of the behaviour in order to increase habit and skill.
- _Problem-solving:_ Identifying/analysing factors influencing the behaviour and generating and selecting strategies that include overcoming barriers and/or increasing facilitators.
- _Review:_ A behavioural review is an analysis of the extent to which the exercise was achieved (e.g. sets and repetitions done). An outcome review is an analysis of the extent to which outcomes (e.g. weight loss, improved balance) were achieved.

- *Rewards:* Providing praise/recognition for attempts and efforts towards the prescribed exercise (i.e. partial completion) or successful performance (i.e. full completion).
- *Self-monitoring:* The client keeps a record of the exercise and/or related outcomes.
- *Social support:* Advising, arranging and/or providing encouragement, praise, advice and practical help for performance of the behaviour.

In a client-centred approach, the *client* is prompted to consider what factors impact exercise engagement/maintenance *and* how these can be addressed. Exercise barriers may relate to behavioural (e.g. exercise complexity, effort required), intrapersonal (e.g. attitude, lack of enjoyment), interpersonal (e.g. criticism, needing help with time competing tasks) or contextual factors (e.g. competing time demands, exercise setting). Some barriers may have been identified in the assessment phase, and the practitioner may ask for the client's perception about the potential impact of barriers. The client is engaged in the problem-solving process by the practitioner asking open-ended questions such as:

- 'What might you do to overcome that?'
- 'How could you do that differently?'
- 'What have you done before or in other situations about that?'

The practitioner can also contribute to problem-solving by offering suggestions and sharing knowledge/information on what other clients have done. With this, it is important to check the client's reaction to such suggestions.

Clients may benefit from assistance with exercise-related cognitions; for example, developing realistic expectations, how to adaptively interpret poor achievement or lapses, and accepting setbacks and interruptions. The gap between expectations of exercise and reality can promote discouragement,[30] and clients who do not achieve exercise targets, or who think they are not competent, may develop negative affective judgments about exercise, which can adversely affect participation.[21,31]

Practitioners can assist clients to identify and access social support for exercise. Importantly, the preferred nature, source and type of social support for exercise will vary across clients. Consistent with a client-centred approach, the practitioner can elicit the client's interests and preferences for social support with a series of questions; for example:

- 'Who would be involved with/impacted by your exercise program?'
- 'Who could help you with your exercise? What can you ask them to do or not do?'
- 'Do you prefer to exercise alone or with others?'
- 'How can I help you with your exercise?'

Assistance may also involve enabling access to resources; for example, information aids on how to exercise, equipment, online tools, self-monitoring materials, site access, demonstrations, contacts. Again, the provision of such resources is checked with the client, rather than automatically assumed.

- 'What resources could help you with your exercise?'
- 'There are a range of resources I could help you with—which of these interests you?'

Worked Example (continued): Exercise Behaviour Counselling—Assist

Susan is worried about making her headaches worse, and finding time to do an exercise program with work and looking after her family. She is not confident of her physical abilities and does not know if she will be able to do what you want her to. Last time she tried an exercise program, the weights made the pain worse and it was hard to know if it was making a meaningful difference. She was not very good at the exercises and the exercise supervisor was not very sympathetic and only seemed interested in what weight she was lifting for each exercise. Susan felt like she was wasting the exercise consultant's time so stopped going after a month.

Susan could be assisted in the following ways.

1. Acknowledging exercise concerns and offering support.

   'There have been some problems for you in the past with exercise in terms of making your headaches worse and finding time to exercise while also working and looking after your family. You are not confident about exercise and whether it is helpful for you. It's great that you are willing to do more exercise now, and exercise can help with neck and shoulder pain and give you more energy. I can work with you to develop an exercise plan that suits you, and help you feel more confident and keep track of whether it is helpful.'

2. Action planning: elicit her exercise interests and preferences; for example:
   - ask what frequency, duration and time she can commit to exercise each week
   - ask what time suits her to exercise given her family commitments

- check her interest in exercise location (e.g. facility versus home-based exercises)
- ask how she prefers to do exercise (e.g. initially she may not want to do weights) and what she is willing to try.

3. Identify and problem-solve barriers (encouraging flexibility and a sense of control):
   - ask her how she could manage her family commitments to enable exercise
   - ask what could help her confidence in her exercise
   - develop an adapted exercise program for when she has less time/energy after work
   - discuss how to respond to potential feelings of low confidence/progress.

4. Behaviour change strategies:
   - self-monitoring: assess her interests in keeping a diary of her chosen outcomes (e.g. pain, headaches, energy, mood) to monitor progress
   - realistic expectations: setting up expectations of reasonable gains in a specified timeframe and what she might not be capable of at first
   - increasing confidence: demonstrations, rehearsals, setting graded tasks to create a sense of mastery and providing specific feedback
   - acknowledging effort (not just achievement).

5. Exploring options for social support:
   - ask who could support her exercise and how
   - ask how you as the practitioner can best support her (as her last exercise supervisor was not very sympathetic).

6. Resources:
   - check interest in and availability of resources (e.g. exercise equipment).

Activity 17.6 Exercise behaviour counselling—assist

Using the information from your assessment of John (who wants to 'grow old gracefully') how might you assist him?

_____

_____

_____

_____

_____

_____

_____

_____

_____

_____

_____

_____

_____

_____

_____

_____

_____

_____

_____

_____

5a Behavioural Counselling Framework: Arrange

The final stage of the counselling is to arrange additional resources and clarify any follow-up.

Clients may benefit from connecting with other professionals in the wider care context, or expertise and opportunities in the general community. This could address coexisting concerns and complementary issues (e.g. footcare, nutrition, poor mental health, pain management, medical care) or enable opportunities for exercise (e.g. access to facilities, equipment). With the client's agreement, these connections can be arranged or facilitated by the exercise practitioner.

Arrangements regarding further contact with the practitioner or other professionals needs to be clarified. If the counselling is limited to a single session, then that needs to be stated, and options for other assistance or enquiries provided. This is particularly important for clients with risk concerns. If the counselling is continuing, follow-up is best scheduled in a short time period initially or linked to a specific milestone. Future contacts can be spaced at successively longer intervals to promote self-regulation, and may use a range of modalities; for example, face to face, videoconferencing, telephone or text messages. This schedule is again developed in collaboration with the client, negotiating between the practitioner's availability and the client's interests.

The counselling closes with a final (tailored) statement of support and encouragement.

- 'I'm so pleased you are going to start exercising. Exercise is one of the best ways to [reflect client interests]. I'm supporting you all the way—great work!'

Follow-up Counselling Sessions

Behavioural counselling can be done in a single session or multiple sessions. In a single session, the conversation will focus on past experiences and anticipatory effects; that is, responses to questions about exercise feelings, barriers and enablers will come from the client's history and conjecture (including observations and information from others).

With multiple counselling sessions, the 5A format is repeated, with reference to the client's actual experiences of exercise. The time spent in each task may change over successive sessions; for example, less time on assessment and advice, and more time on assistance.

Assess

Follow-up assessment focuses on the exercise done since the last contact, and the actual exercise experiences of the client. The practitioner is listening for gains (to reinforce efforts) and barriers (to be problem-solved).

- 'What exercise did you do during [nominate period]?'
- 'How did you feel doing more exercise?'
- 'What did you notice doing more exercise?'
- 'What got in the way of your exercise or made it difficult?'
- 'What helped your exercise?'

Advise

Follow-up advice commences with a summary of the client's exercise experiences, including both the positive and the negative aspects. This summary includes an acknowledgment of efforts (not just achievements) and recognition of any gains. The practitioner can confirm the client's understanding and provide information to clarify misperceptions regarding exercise experiences. Clear and strong advice is then provided to *continue* with the exercise.

- 'There have been some pros and cons for you in doing more exercise [reflect client information].'
- (in the case of suboptimal performance) 'It may be hard at times, but it is important for [reflect client interests] and [other relevant information].'
- (in the case of optimal performance) 'That's great what you've been able to do. It is important for [reflect client interests] and [other relevant information].'
- 'It is important that you continue to exercise to [reflect client interests and any gains].'

Agree

Follow-up agreement confirms the client's willingness to continue, with the practitioner offering ongoing support and responding to ambivalence.

- 'Are you willing to continue working together on your exercise program?'
- 'It's great that you're going to keep going. Exercise is one of the best things to do for [personalised interests].'

- 'I can help you with [reflect information]. Let's check the plan to see what works for you and what might be changed.'
- 'It's hard for you to think about continuing …'

Assist

The practitioner and the client collaborate to review the action plan, social support, problem-solving strategies and resources. Information obtained during the assessment (e.g. difficulties, enablers) can be reintroduced and addressed here.

- 'Last time we agreed you would [information]. How was that?'
- 'How did people help with your exercise plan? How did people make it difficult? How can I best help you?'
- 'What made it difficult for you to exercise [reflect assessment information]? How could that be done differently?'

Arrange

The final stage of the follow-up counselling is to arrange additional resources and clarify follow-up.

Summary

Behavioural counselling is a conversation-based approach to assist clients to adopt, change and maintain behaviour. It is based on client-centred communication, which *prioritises* responsiveness to the client's needs and values, and *actively* includes the client in decision-making. The 5A counselling framework has been endorsed by a range of international organisations, is applicable to a range of settings and health practitioners and can be used as a standalone or adjunct strategy to promote exercise. The framework provides a coherent way to structure and organise behaviour change communication with the client, and incorporates principles that are known to facilitate behaviour change, in particular individual tailoring. It involves five key communication tasks.

1. Assess: the client's understanding, current behaviour, attitudes, enablers and barriers.
2. Advise: salient information to confirm the client's understanding and correct any misunderstandings, and clear and strong advice to change (linked to the client's interests).
3. Agree: mutual commitment and collaboration on behaviour change goals, resolving ambivalence to change.
4. Assist: identifying factors impacting on exercise and activating internal and external resources to support adherence and maintenance.
5. Arrange: enabling additional resources and clarifying follow-up.

References

1   Gagliardi A, Faulkner G, Ciliska D, Hicks A. 2015. Factors contributing to the effectiveness of physical activity counselling in primary care: A realist systematic review. *Patient Educ Couns.* 98(4):412–419.

2   Bock C, Jarczok M, Litaker D. 2014. Community-based efforts to promote physical activity: A systematic review of interventions considering mode of delivery, study quality and population subgroups. *J Sci Med Sport.* 17(3):276-282.

3   Noordman JvdW, T; van Dulmen, S. 2012. Communication-related behavior change techniques used in face-to-face lifestyle interventions in primary care: A systematic review of the literature. *Patient Educ Couns.* 89(2):227–244.

4   Kivela K, Elo S, Kyngas H, Kaariainen M. 2014. The effects of health coaching on adult patients with chronic diseases: A systematic review. *Patient Educ Couns.* 97(2):147–157.

5   Lin J, Zhuo X, Bardenheier B, et al. 2017. Cost-effectiveness of the 2014 US Preventive Services Task Force (USPSTF) Recommendations for Intensive Behavioral Counseling Interventions for Adults With Cardiovascular Risk Factors. *Diabetes Care.* 40(5):640–646.

6   Cowper P, Peterson M, Pieper C, et al. 2017. Economic analysis of primary care-based physical activity counseling in older men: The VA-LIFE Trial. *J Am Geriatr Soc.* 65(3):533–539.

7   Hogg WE, Zhao X, Angus D, et al. 2012. The cost of integrating a physical activity counselor in the primary health care team. *J Am Board Fam Med.* 25(2):250–252.

8   King A, Hoppe R. 2013. 'Best practice' for patient-centered communication: A narrative review. *J Grad Med Edu.* 5(3):385–393.

9   Whitlock E, Orleans C, Pender N, Allan J. 2002. Evaluating primary care behavioral counseling interventions: an evidence-based approach. *Am J Prev Med.* 22(4):267–284.

10   Elford R, MacMillan H, Wathern C, Canadian Task Force on Preventive Health Care. 2001. *Counselling for Risky Health Habits: A Conceptual Framework for Primary Care Practitioners.* London ON: CTFPHC Technical Support, Canadian Task Force.

11   Swedish National Institute of Public Health. 2011. *Physical Activity in the Prevention and Treatment of Disease.* Sweden: Professional Associations for Physical Activity, Swedish National Institute of Public Health.

12 Ajzen I. 1991. The theory of planned behavior. *Organ Behav Hum Dec.* 50:179–211.

13 Locke E, Latham G. 2002. Building a practically useful theory of goal setting and task motivation. *Am Psychol.* 57(9):705–717.

14 Deci E, Ryan R. 2002. *Handbook of Self Determination Theory.* Rochester, N.Y.: University of Rochester Press.

15 Rollnick S, Miller W, Butler C. 2008. *Motivational Interviewing in Health Care.* New York: The Guilford Press.

16 Miller W, Rollnick S. 2002. *Motivational Interviewing: Preparing People for Change.* New York: Guilford Press.

17 Hagger MS, Chatzisarantis NLD, Biddle SJH. 2002. A meta-analytic review of the theories of reasoned action and planned behavior in physical activity: predictive validity and the contribution of additional variables. *J Sport Exerc Psychol.* 4(1):3–32.

18 Teixeira PJ, Carraça EV, Markland D, et al. 2012. Exercise, physical activity, and self-determination theory: A systematic review. *Int J Behav Nutr Phys Act.* 9:78.

19 McEwan D, Harden S, Zumbo B, et al. 2016. The effectiveness of multi-component goal setting interventions for changing physical activity behaviour: a systematic review and meta-analysis. *Health Psychol Rev.* 10(1):67–88.

20 O'Halloran P, Blackstock F, Shields N, et al. 2014. Motivational interviewing to increase physical activity in people with chronic health conditions: a systematic review and meta-analysis. *Clin Rehabil.* 28(12):1159–1171.

21 Rhodes RE, Fiala B, Conner M. 2010. A review and meta-analysis of affective judgments and physical activity in adult populations. *Ann Behav Med.* 38(3):180–204.

22 Conner M, Rhodes RE, Morris B, et al. 2011. Changing exercise through targeting affective or cognitive attitudes. *Psychol Health.* 26(2):133–149.

23 Flocke S, Stange K. 2004. Direct observation and patient recall of health behavior advice. *Prev Med.* 38(3):343–349.

24 Notthoff N, Carstensen L. 2104. Positive messaging promotes walking in older adults. *Psychol Aging.* 29(2):329–341.

25 Gallagher K, Updegraff J. 2012. Health message framing effects on attitudes, intentions, and behavior: A meta-analytic review. *Ann Behav Med.* 43(1):101–16.

26 Shay L, Lafata J. 2015. Where is the evidence? A systematic review of shared decision making and patient outcomes. *Med Decis Making.* 35(1):114–131.

27 Légaré F, Thompson-Leduc P. 2014. Twelve myths about shared decision making. *Patient Educ Couns.* 96(3):281–288.

28 Rollnick S, Mason P, Butler C. 1999. *Health Behavior Change: A Guide for Practitioners.* Edinburgh and New York: Churchill Livingstone.

29 Michie S, Ashford S, Sniehotta F, et al. 2011. A refined taxonomy of behaviour change techniques to help people change their physical activity and healthy eating behaviours: the CALO-RE taxonomy. *Psychol Health.* 26(11):1479–1498.

30 Thomas D, Kyle T, Stanford F. 2015. The gap between expectations and reality of exercise-induced weight loss is associated with discouragement. *Prev Med.* 81:357–360.

31 Nasuti G, Rhodes R. 2013. Affective judgment and physical activity in youth: review and meta-Analyses. *Ann Behav Med.* 45(3):357–376.

APPENDIX A
BORG 6–20 RATING OF PERCEIVED EXERTION (RPE) SCALE®

Instructions

- Have the scale in full view at all times.
- Make the participant aware of what RPE stands for and that this is an 'all over' integrated rating which incorporates both peripheral muscular and central cardiorespiratory sensations.
- Focus the participant's attention on the verbal descriptors of the scale as much as on the numerical values.
- Anchor the top and bottom ratings to previously experienced sensations of 'no exertion at all' and 'extremely hard/maximal exertion'.
- Allow the participant to understand that there is no right or wrong rating; it represents how hard the participant felt they were working at the time of providing the rating.

6	
7	VERY, VERY LIGHT
8	
9	VERY LIGHT
10	
11	FAIRLY LIGHT
12	
13	SOMEWHAT HARD
14	
15	HARD
16	
17	VERY HARD
18	
19	VERY, VERY HARD
20	

APPENDIX B
ADULT OMNI-RESISTANCE EXERCISE RPE SCALE[1]

Instructions

- Have the scale in full view at all times.
- Make the participant aware that they are being asked to rate the level of exertion of their active muscles only, not for their chest/breathing or their overall body.
- Tell the participant to use both the pictures and the words to help them select one rating number that represents the level of exertion their active muscles are experiencing.
- Instruct the participant to use their memory of the least and greatest effort that they had experienced while lifting weights to help in establishing the visual-cognitive link.
- Use the following script: 'You should respond with a 0 when you are lifting a very light weight that is extremely easy to lift. Respond with a 10 when you are lifting the heaviest weight you can lift and you may not be able to lift for one more repetition.'

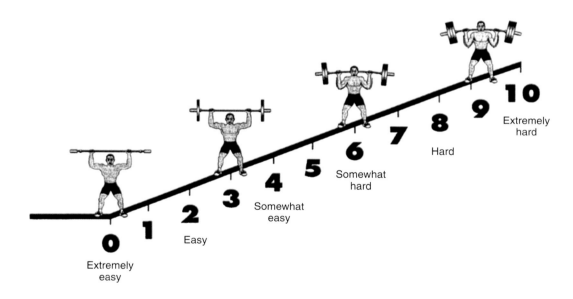

Reference

1.   Robertson RJ, Goss FL, Rutkowski J, et al. 2003. Concurrent validation of the OMNI perceived exertion scale for resistance exercise. Medicine and science in sports and exercise. 35:333–341.

APPENDIX C
PARmed-X FOR PREGNANCY

SCREENING TOOL
PHYSICAL ACTIVITY/EXERCISE DURING PREGNANCY

Name _____

Address _____

Phone _____ Birthdate   /   /

Current Health Professional _____ Contact _____

Current Gestational Age (weeks) _____ Due Date _____

STAGE 1 - GENERAL CONTRAINDICATIONS TO PHYSICAL ACTIVITY/EXERCISE
This section explores general health prior to pregnancy

1.	Has your medical practitioner ever told you that you have a heart condition or have you ever suffered a stroke?	YES	NO
2.	Do you ever experience unexplained pains or discomfort in your chest at rest or during physical activity/exercise?	YES	NO
3.	Do you ever feel faint, dizzy or lose balance during physical activity/exercise?	YES	NO
4.	Have you had an asthma attack requiring immediate medical attention at any time over the last 12 months?	YES	NO
5.	If you have diabetes (type I or type 2) have you had trouble controlling your blood sugar (glucose) in the last 3 months?	YES	NO
6.	Do you have any diagnosed muscle, bone or joint problems that you have been told could be made worse by participating in physical activity/exercise?	YES	NO
7.	Do you have any other conditions that may require special consideration for you to exercise?	YES	NO

IF YOU ANSWERED **YES** to any of the 7 questions above, you should seek guidance from a health professional before participating in any further physical activity/exercise.

IF YOU ANSWERED **NO** to all 7 questions above, please proceed to STAGE 2, which specifically considers your health during pregnancy.

This screening tool is to be used in conjunction with the Australian Physical Activity Guidelines for Pregnant Women https://www1.health.gov.au/

Pregnant women should discuss their physical activity / exercise behaviours with an appropriately qualified health professional as this tool does not constitute nor replace medical advice. No responsibility or liability whatsoever can be accepted by Exercise & Sport Science Australia, Fitness Australia, Sports Medicine Australia or Exercise is Medicine for any loss, damage, or injury that may arise from any person acting on any statement or information contained in this document. While care has been taken to ensure the information contained in the material is accurate at the date of publication, the organisations do not warrant its accuracy. If you intend to take any action or inaction based on this form, it is recommended that you obtain your own professional advice based on your specific circumstances.

SCREENING TOOL
PHYSICAL ACTIVITY/EXERCISE DURING PREGNANCY
VERSION 1 (MARCH 2021)

STAGE 2 - CONTRAINDICATIONS TO PHYSICAL ACTIVITY/EXERCISE DURING PREGNANCY
ABSOLUTE CONTRAINDICATIONS DURING PREGNANCY

Have you ever been told that you have any of the following contraindications to physical activity/exercise:

1.	Incompetent cervix	YES	NO
2.	Ruptured membranes, premature labour	YES	NO
3.	Persistant second or third trimester bleeding	YES	NO
4.	Placenta previa	YES	NO
5.	Pre-eclampsia	YES	NO
6.	Evidence of intrauterine growth restriction	YES	NO
7.	Multiple gestation (eg: triplets or higher number)	YES	NO
8.	Poorly controlled Type I diabetes, hypertension or thyroid disease	YES	NO
9.	Other serious cardiovascular, respiratory or systemic disorder	YES	NO

IF YOU ANSWERED **YES** to any of the 9 questions above, you should discuss opportunities to modify your physical activity/exercise with a health professional before participating in any further physical activity/exercise. It is still important that you avoid sitting for long periods of time.

IF YOU ANSWERED **NO** to all 9 questions above, please proceed to RELATIVE CONTRAINDICTIONS.

RELATIVE CONTRAINDICATIONS DURING PREGNANCY

Have you ever been told that you have any of the following contraindications to physical activity/exercise:

1.	History of spontaneous miscarriage, premature labour or fetal growth restriction	YES	NO
2.	Mild/moderate cardiovascular or chronic respiratory disease	YES	NO
3.	Pregnancy-induced hypertension	YES	NO
4.	Poorly controlled seizure disorder	YES	NO
5.	Type 1 diabetes	YES	NO
6.	Symptomatic anaemia	YES	NO
7.	Malnutrition, significantly underweight or eating disorder	YES	NO
8.	Twin pregnancy after the 28th week	YES	NO
9.	Other significant medical condition/s (Please detail below)	YES	NO

IF YOU ANSWERED **YES** to any of the 9 questions above, you should discuss opportunities to modify your physical activity/exercise with a health professional before participating in any further physical activity/exercise. It is still important that you move about frequently and avoid sitting for long periods of time.

IF YOU ANSWERED **NO** to all 9 questions above, please follow the physical activity/exercise guidelines on the next page.

IMPORTANT: Where physical activity/exercise is safe, health professionals should encourage physical activity/ exercise in accordance with the Australian Physical Activity Guidelines for Pregnant women, with the key messages being **Move more - Sit less - Be active during pregnancy!**

STAGE 3 - PHYSICAL ACTIVITY/EXERCISE GUIDELINES

DOSE: *HOW MUCH PHYSICAL ACTIVITY SHOULD I DO?*

IF YOU ARE:	SEDENTARY	ACTIVE BUT NOT MEETING GUIDELINES	MEETING GUIDELINES BETWEEN 150-300 MINS PER WEEK	EXCEEDING GUIDELINES
	Doing any physical activity is better than doing none If you currently do no physical activity, start slowly and progress towards meeting the guidelines	• Be active on most, preferably all, days every week • Accumulate 150 to 300 minutes (2 ½ to 5 hours) of moderate intensity physical activity or 75 to 150 minutes (1 ¼ to 2 ½ hours) of vigorous intensity physical activity, or an equivalent combination of both moderate and vigorous activities, each week • Do muscle strengthening activities on at least 2 days each week targeting large muscle groups • Minimise the amount of time spent in prolonged sitting • Break up long periods of sitting as often as possible		• Upper intensity limit for exercise during pregnancy is not known • To ensure safety and wellbeing, highly active women, including athletes, should have their physical/activity program overseen and managed by an informed health professional • May continue with current program, as long as necessary modifications are made as the pregnancy progresses

TYPE: *WHAT SORT OF ACTIVITY SHOULD I DO / NOT DO?*

Physical activities/exercises that are considered SAFE:

National guidelines concur that the following activities are considered to be generally safe for pregnant women with an uncomplicated pregnancy:

• Aerobic physical activity/exercise

• Muscle strengthening exercises using body weight, weights or resistance bands

• Pelvic floor muscle exercises

• Pregnancy specific classes

Physical activities/exercises that are considered UNSAFE:

Pregnant women are advised to avoid activities that involve:
• Significant changes in pressure (eg. sky diving, scuba diving etc.)
• Risk of contact / collision
• Risk of falling (ie. activities that require high levels of balance, coordination and agility)
• Heavy lifting
Women who are healthy and already active do not need to seek medical clearance for physical activity / exercise during pregnancy, but those who are considering high volumes of exercise training (high intensity, prolonged duration, heavy weights, etc) should seek advice and guidance from a health professional who is knowledgable about the effects of high level training on maternal and fetal outcomes.

INTENSITY: *HOW HARD SHOULD I EXERCISE?*

Rating of Perceived Exertion for Physical Activities

• Current PA guidelines recommend both moderate and vigorous intensity activities

• Use this RPE scale to judge the intensity of activities

• On this scale, where 1 is sedentary (not moving), and 10 is maximal effort, activities in the range 3-7 are considered safe and are recommended for health benefits in pregnant women

• Intensity may also be judged using the 'talk test'; in moderate intensity activities women should be able to carry on a conversation, while in vigorous activities they would find this difficult

1	Sedentary
2	Light
3	Moderate
4	
5	
6	Vigorous
7	
8	High Intensity
9	
10	

REASONS TO STOP EXERCISE AND CONSULT YOUR HEALTH CARE PROVIDER

• Chest pain
• Persistant excessive shortness of breath - that does not resolve with rest
• Severe headache
• Persistant dizziness/feeling faint - that does not resolve with rest
• Regular painful uterine contractions
• Vaginal bleeding
• Persistant loss of fluid from the vagina - indicating possible ruptured membrane

ADDITIONAL SAFETY PRECAUTIONS - WHAT TO AVOID?

• Avoid dehydration and inadequate nutrition. Stay well hydrated and try to ensure energy intake is in line with recommended gestational weight gain
• Avoid heat stress/hyperthermia in the first trimester. Adjust physical activity / exercise in excessively hot weather, especially when there is high humidity
• Avoid long periods of motionless posture (standing still, or lying in a supine position), especially if this causes light headedness or dizziness
• Avoid physical activity/exercise at high altitude (above 2000m) unless acclimatised and trained to do this prior to pregnancy
• Always wear appropriate shoes for the activity, non-restrictive clothing and a supportive bra

Developed by Hayman M, Brown WJ, Haakstad LAH, Mielke GI, Mena GP, Lamerton T, Green A, Keating SE, Gomes GAO, Coombes JS (2021)

SCREENING TOOL
PHYSICAL ACTIVITY/EXERCISE DURING PREGNANCY
VERSION 1 (MARCH 2021)

APPENDIX D
CONTRAINDICATIONS TO EXERCISING

Box D.1 provides absolute and relative contraindications to exercising based on the Contraindications to Exercise Testing from the American Heart Association.[1] Performing a pre-exercise screening and the careful review of a participant's medical history will help identify potential contraindications.

Box D.1   Contraindications to exercising (adapted from a Scientific Statement by the American Heart Association)[1]

Absolute contraindications

- Acute myocardial infarction (MI), within 2 days
- Ongoing unstable angina
- Uncontrolled cardiac arrhythmia with haemodynamic compromise
- Active endocarditis
- Symptomatic severe aortic stenosis
- Decompensated heart failure
- Acute pulmonary embolism, pulmonary infarction or deep vein thrombosis
- Acute myocarditis or pericarditis
- Acute aortic dissection
- Physical disability that precludes safe exercise

Relative contraindications

- Known obstructive left main coronary artery stenosis
- Moderate-to-severe aortic stenosis with uncertain relation to symptoms
- Tachyarrhythmias with uncontrolled ventricular rates
- Acquired advanced or complete heart block
- Hypertrophic obstructive cardiomyopathy with severe resting gradient
- Recent stroke or transient ischaemic attack
- Mental impairment with limited ability to cooperate
- Resting hypertension with systolic or diastolic blood pressures > 200/110 mmHg
- Uncorrected medical conditions, such as significant anaemia, important electrolyte imbalance and hyperthyroidism

Reprinted with permission Circulation. 2013;128:873–934 ©2013 American Heart Association, Inc.

Absolute Contraindications

An absolute contraindication is a reason or criterion that makes it inadvisable to exercise. Undertaking or continuing to exercise could place the participant at a higher risk of an untoward event (e.g. injury or medical condition) occurring as a result of exercising. Participants with absolute contraindications should not exercise until such conditions are stabilised or adequately treated.

Relative Contraindications

A relative contraindication is a reason or criterion that needs to be considered in deciding whether to exercise. Factors such as the risk versus benefit and access to medical support need to be considered. Participants with relative contraindications should not exercise until the risks and benefits are carefully assessed.

Reference

1.   Fletcher GF, Ades PA, Kligfield P, et al. 2013. On behalf of the American Heart Association Exercise, Cardiac Rehabilitation, and Prevention Committee of the Council on Clinical Cardiology, Council on Nutrition, Physical Activity and Metabolism, Council on Cardiovascular and Stroke Nursing, and Council on Epidemiology and Prevention. Exercise standards for testing and training: A scientific statement from the American Heart Association. Circulation. 128:873–934.

APPENDIX E
TREADMILL SAFETY

Treadmills are one of the most commonly used pieces of equipment for conducting aerobic exercise tests, and they are also one of the most dangerous. The following precautions will help to reduce the risk of injury when testing a participant on a treadmill.

Treadmill Location

The treadmill should be placed so that there is no possibility that a person who falls while on the treadmill could become trapped between the treadmill and something behind it (e.g. another piece of equipment). A minimum clearance of 0.5 m on each side of the treadmill and 2.0 m behind a treadmill is recommended.

Safety Features

It is important that the tester operating the treadmill is aware of the safety features of the treadmill (e.g. safety stop button, tether with a key/magnetic clip). Instruct the participant on the safety features of the treadmill prior to starting the test and establish a non-verbal sign that the participant can use to tell the tester to stop the treadmill (e.g. one hand in the air making a stop sign).

Treadmill Operation

Commonly used recreational treadmills now have multiple features. The tester should take the time to familiarise themselves with the different functions and understand the purpose of all the buttons. This includes if the treadmill can be programmed and how quickly/slowly the treadmill changes speed/grade can be changed within a program or when buttons (e.g. stop button) are pressed.

Starting the Treadmill

With the treadmill belt stationary, ask the participant to walk to the front of the treadmill, hold the handrail and straddle the belt. Ensure that no part of the participants' foot is in contact with the belt. Start the treadmill and increase until it reaches a speed that will allow the participant to start walking comfortably. Ask the participant to continue holding the handrail and carefully step on the belt and start walking when they are ready. Once the participant has achieved a normal walking pace, ask them to safely remove their hands from the handrail.

Handrails

For a person unaccustomed to walking on a treadmill, it is encouraged that the participant practise walking on the treadmill prior to running. Cues such as 'stand up tall', 'step out in front of you' and 'take longer strides' may help to correct unnatural walking techniques. Participants learning how to walk on a treadmill should hold on to the handrails until their walking technique has normalised.

Eyes

Instruct the participant to keep their eyes forwards, especially if the person is veering off to the side. It is common for people who are unaccustomed to a treadmill to look at their feet while exercising.

Positioning

Instruct the participant to stay in the centre of the belt—both left to right and front to back. If the participant is too close to the front of the belt, their foot can catch on the motor cover and trip. If too far down the belt, the participant may come off the back of the treadmill. As the participant becomes fatigued, they will usually shift towards the back of the treadmill. The supervisor should gently place their arm on the participant's back if they are getting too close to the end of the treadmill, and ask them to try and move forwards.

Stopping the Treadmill

The participant should stop/slow the treadmill themselves, and never step off a moving treadmill.

6	
7	VERY, VERY LIGHT
8	
9	VERY LIGHT
10	
11	FAIRLY LIGHT
12	
13	SOMEWHAT HARD
14	
15	HARD
16	
17	VERY HARD
18	
19	VERY, VERY HARD
20	

INDEX

Page numbers followed by "f" indicate figures, "t" indicate tables, and "b" indicate boxes.